I0034214

5G-Based Smart Hospitals and Healthcare Systems

With the increase in the development of the advanced cellular communication system, it is assumed that several sectors, such as the health industry, education, transport industry, business model, and so on, will rapidly grow. However, the requirements of the above-mentioned sectors are different and difficult to fulfill. Hence, 5G will be integral to several networks and will also need a unique management system for its successful rollout around the globe.

5G-Based Smart Hospitals and Healthcare Systems: Evaluation, Integration, and Deployment provides an overview of the role of advanced technologies in transforming the healthcare industry. It emphasizes the technical requirements of smart hospitals and the technologies associated with them along with explaining how technologies such as IoT, machine learning, and AI can be integrated with smart hospitals and 5G networks. The book evaluates several concerns such as privacy of data, infrastructure costs, and regular upgradability of technologies. Since the storage of information is a major concern with the implantation of 5G-based hospitals, this book will specifically address those issues, along with examining the potential pitfalls of 5G-based hospitals and the factors that cause their failures.

This book specifically targets professionals, academicians, engineers, researchers, management firms, technical institutes, R&D establishments, and individuals researching in the fields of 5G, healthcare, medical sensors, IoT, big data, and related fields. The main objectives of this book are to accumulate state-of-the-art IoT, 5G, AI, and machine learning–based approaches for resolving healthcare problems.

Advancements in Intelligent and Sustainable Technologies and Systems
Series Editor: Ajay Kumar

This book series aims to provide a platform for academicians, researchers, professionals, and individuals to participate and to provide novel systematic theoretical, experimental, computational work in the form of edited text or reference books and monographs in the area of intelligent and sustainable technologies and systems from engineering, management, applied science, healthcare, etc. domains. This book series will educate and inform the readers with a comprehensive overview of advancements in intelligent and sustainable techniques and systems with novel intelligent tools and algorithms to move industries from different domains from a data-centric community to a sustainable world. The book series covers ideas and innovations to help the research community and professionals to understand fundamentals, opportunities, challenges, future outlook, layout, life cycle, and framework of intelligent and sustainable technologies and systems for different sectors. It serves as a guide for computer science, mechanical, manufacturing, electrical, electronics, civil, automobile, industrial engineering, biomedical, healthcare, and management professionals.

If you are interested in writing or editing a book for the series or would like more information, please contact Cindy Carelli, cindy.carelli@taylorandfrancis.com

5G-Based Smart Hospitals and Healthcare Systems: Evaluation, Integration, and Deployment
Edited by Arun Kumar, Sumit Chakravarty, Aravinda K., and Mohit Kumar Sharma

5G-Based Smart Hospitals and Healthcare Systems

Evaluation, Integration, and Deployment

Edited by
Arun Kumar
Sumit Chakravarty
Aravinda K.
Mohit Kumar Sharma

CRC Press
Taylor & Francis Group
Boca Raton London New York

CRC Press is an imprint of the
Taylor & Francis Group, an **informa** business

Designed cover image: Shutterstock

MATLAB® is a trademark of The MathWorks, Inc. and is used with permission. The MathWorks does not warrant the accuracy of the text or exercises in this book. This book's use or discussion of MATLAB® software or related products does not constitute endorsement or sponsorship by The MathWorks of a particular pedagogical approach or particular use of the MATLAB® software.

First edition published 2024
by CRC Press
2385 NW Executive Center Drive, Suite 320, Boca Raton FL 33431

and by CRC Press
4 Park Square, Milton Park, Abingdon, Oxon, OX14 4RN

CRC Press is an imprint of Taylor & Francis Group, LLC

© 2024 selection and editorial matter, Arun Kumar, Sumit Chakravarty, Aravinda K., and Mohit Kumar Sharma; individual chapters, the contributors

Reasonable efforts have been made to publish reliable data and information, but the author and publisher cannot assume responsibility for the validity of all materials or the consequences of their use. The authors and publishers have attempted to trace the copyright holders of all material reproduced in this publication and apologize to copyright holders if permission to publish in this form has not been obtained. If any copyright material has not been acknowledged please write and let us know so we may rectify in any future reprint.

Except as permitted under U.S. Copyright Law, no part of this book may be reprinted, reproduced, transmitted, or utilized in any form by any electronic, mechanical, or other means, now known or hereafter invented, including photocopying, microfilming, and recording, or in any information storage or retrieval system, without written permission from the publishers.

For permission to photocopy or use material electronically from this work, access www.copyright.com or contact the Copyright Clearance Center, Inc. (CCC), 222 Rosewood Drive, Danvers, MA 01923, 978-750-8400. For works that are not available on CCC please contact mpkbookspermissions@tandf.co.uk

Trademark notice: Product or corporate names may be trademarks or registered trademarks and are used only for identification and explanation without intent to infringe.

Library of Congress Cataloging-in-Publication Data
Names: Kumar, Arun (Associate professor of electronics), editor. | Chakravarty, Sumit (Associate professor of electrical engineering), editor. | Aravinda, K., 1966- editor. | Sharma, Mohit Kumar (Assistant professor), editor.
Title: 5G-based smart hospitals and healthcare systems : evaluation, integration, and deployment / edited by Arun Kumar, Sumit Chakravarty, Aravinda K., and Mohit Kumar Sharma.
Description: First edition. | Boca Raton FL : CRC Press, 2024. | Includes bibliographical references and index.
Identifiers: LCCN 2023032745 (print) | LCCN 2023032746 (ebook) | ISBN 9781032515274 (hardback) | ISBN 9781032517278 (paperback) | ISBN 9781003403678 (ebook)
Subjects: MESH: Computer Communication Networks | Hospitals | Delivery of Health Care--methods | Artificial Intelligence | Wearable Electronic Devices
Classification: LCC RA971.6 (print) | LCC RA971.6 (ebook) | NLM WX 26.5 | DDC 362.110285--dc23/eng/20230828
LC record available at https://lccn.loc.gov/2023032745
LC ebook record available at https://lccn.loc.gov/2023032746

ISBN: 978-1-032-51527-4 (hbk)
ISBN: 978-1-032-51727-8 (pbk)
ISBN: 978-1-003-40367-8 (ebk)

DOI: 10.1201/9781003403678

Typeset in Times New Roman
by MPS Limited, Dehradun

Contents

            *Md. Asif Iqbal, Atul Kumar Dadhich, Javed Khan Bhutto,
            and Hina Shahnawaz*

            *R. Krishnamoorthy, Meenakshi Gupta, Gundala Swathi,
            Kazuaki Tanaka, Ch. Raja, and
            Janjhyam Venkata Naga Ramesh*

Preface

The field of smart healthcare has witnessed remarkable advancements in recent years, driven by the convergence of cutting-edge technologies and the increasing demand for personalized and efficient healthcare services. The integration of smartphones, computational power, and artificial intelligence has revolutionized wearable devices, enabling novel models and paradigms for athlete health monitoring, shoulder injury detection, patient movement tracking, and more. Moreover, policy frameworks and regulatory initiatives have shaped the healthcare landscape, paving the way for customized health services and patient-centric care.

In this book, we delve into the multifaceted world of smart healthcare, unveiling the potential of emerging technologies and innovative approaches to address various challenges faced by athletes, paraplegics, patients, and healthcare systems. Each chapter presents a unique perspective and offers insights into different aspects of smart healthcare, encompassing predictive analytics, image processing, wearable sensors, health policy, wireless communication, denoising techniques, and AI-based diagnosis. The journey begins with a focus on athlete health, where we introduce a groundbreaking method for forecasting the health of football players using recurrent neural networks and wearable technology. By leveraging real-time data and deep feature extraction, this approach provides reliable health predictions that can drive data-driven monitoring and instruction.

Moving forward, we explore the realm of paraplegics' health and the imperative need to prevent and detect shoulder damage. By integrating innovative technologies and data analytics, smart hospitals can monitor and analyze patient movement patterns, enabling timely interventions to mitigate the risk of shoulder injuries. We present a solution based on image processing techniques that detects improper wheelchair technique and posture, thus preventing potential shoulder discomfort or injury. The significance of wearable sensors in healthcare cannot be overstated, as they offer a wealth of applications in human movement detection, disease analysis, and patient monitoring. We delve into the use of wearable sensors to recognize precise movement patterns and sleep levels, presenting techniques and methodologies for gathering and analyzing long-term data. The chapter emphasizes the potential of wearables to revolutionize healthcare monitoring and self-assessment.

Shifting our focus to the Indian healthcare landscape, we delve into the comprehensive framework of health policies that aim to provide accessible and quality healthcare services to citizens. By exploring key policies and initiatives, such as Ayushman Bharat, Pradhan Mantri Jan Arogya Yojana, and the National Health Mission, we highlight the opportunities and challenges of designing new and customized health services for patients in India. A deep understanding of the policy landscape is crucial to aligning services with overarching goals and leveraging technology for enhanced accessibility and quality of care. As smart hospitals strive to optimize patient care and resource utilization through advanced technologies, they encounter various constraints related to data privacy, security, and interoperability. We examine the regulatory implications and challenges of integrating artificial intelligence, the Internet of Things, and fifth-generation wireless technology into smart hospitals. Additionally, we discuss the opportunities and complexities associated with the adoption of 5G networks worldwide.

The book then delves into the realm of brain tumor diagnosis, where computer-aided radiology methods and machine learning algorithms offer promising solutions. By effectively denoising phonocardiogram (PCG) signals and using adaptive filter models, we can enhance the accuracy of diagnosing different types of heart disorders. Furthermore, we explore the applications of wearable planar antennas, information aggregation mechanisms, and digital health data analysis, which contribute to the ongoing transformation of healthcare systems. The evolution of mobile communication architecture and the advent of 5G technology have revolutionized the healthcare industry. We discuss the complex transition requirements from fourth-generation to fifth-generation systems, emphasizing the need for reconfigurable and efficient communication solutions in smart hospitals. The low-latency capabilities and enhanced spectrum utilization of 5G networks empower real-time communication, telemedicine, and Internet of Medical Things connectivity, ultimately revolutionizing healthcare delivery and improving patient outcomes.

The energy efficiency of sensor nodes in wireless sensor networks (WSNs) is a critical concern. We compare Low Energy Adaptive Clustering Hierarchy (LEACH) and Energy Aware Multi-hop Multipath Hierarchy (EAMMH) routing algorithms to extend the network lifetime and reduce energy consumption. Through analytical results and insights, we shed light on the performance and efficiency of these protocols, paving the way for energy-efficient WSN designs.

The paradigm shift from specialist- and hospital-focused models to distributed and patient-centric approaches in smart healthcare sets the stage for a comprehensive exploration of IoT-based, 5G-supported wearable devices. By examining the challenges and opportunities in the deployment of smart healthcare systems, we navigate the path to seamless connectivity, improved performance, and enhanced coverage. Lastly, we introduce an intelligent healthcare monitoring system that combines the Internet of Things, optimization methods, and machine learning. Through the integration of these cutting-edge technologies, we aim to achieve early and accurate diagnosis of a wide range of diseases, thereby revolutionizing healthcare practices.

The chapters presented in this book provide a comprehensive overview of the advancements, challenges, and opportunities in the field of smart healthcare. From athlete health monitoring to brain tumor diagnosis, from wearable sensors to 5G-enabled smart hospitals, each chapter contributes to the collective knowledge and understanding of this rapidly evolving domain. We hope that this book inspires further research and innovation, leading to the development of intelligent healthcare systems that improve the lives of individuals and communities worldwide.

Arun Kumar
Sumit Chakravarty
Aravinda K.
Mohit Kumar Sharma

About the Editors

Dr. Arun Kumar, PhD, MTech, associate professor, Department of Electronics and Communication, New Horizon College of Engineering, Bengaluru, INDIA

Dr. Arun Kumar received his PhD in electronics and communication engineering from JECRC University, Jaipur, India. He is an associate professor in electronics and communication engineering at New Horizon College of Engineering in Bengaluru, India. Dr. Kumar has a total of 10 years of teaching experience and has published more than 95 research articles in SCI-E and Scopus Index journals, 2 books, and 3 International patents (granted). His research interests are advanced waveforms for 5G mobile communication systems and 5G-based smart hospitals, PAPR reduction techniques in the multicarrier waveform, and spectrum sensing techniques. Dr. Kumar has successfully implemented different reduction techniques for multi-carrier waveforms such as NOMA, FBMC, UFMC, and so on, and has also implemented and compared different waveform techniques for the 5G system. Currently, he is working on the requirements of a 5G-based smart hospital system. He is a member of the IEEE and a reviewer for many refereed, indexed journals. He was the lead guest editor of the special issue journal titled "Advanced 5G Communication System for Transforming Healthcare" in the *Journal CMC-Computers, Materials and Continua* (Q2, SCI, Scopus, Impact Factor: 3.7). He has served as co-convenor, Technical Programme Committee (TPC) Member, and reviewer at various international conferences such as ICPCCAI-2019, ICPCCAI-2020, IEEE ISMAC (2018), ESG2018, and so on.

Scopus Link: https://www.scopus.com/authid/detail.uri?authorId=56819583200

Dr. Sumit Chakravarty, Department of Electrical and Computer Engineering, Kennesaw State University, GA, USA

Dr. Sumit Chakravarty currently works as an assistant professor of electrical engineering at Kennesaw State University. He has completed his doctoral studies from the University of Maryland, Baltimore County, and his master of science from Texas A&M University, Kingsville, both in electrical engineering. His PhD dissertation is on analysis of hyperspectral signatures and data. He has multiple peer-reviewed journal publications, conference publications, a book chapter, and three granted patents (and one under review) besides the current work under progress. He has used his expertise in remote sensing by working as a scientist in industry where he also worked on other sensor modalities commonly used in remote sensing, like Multispectral, Lidar, and SAR. This includes working with a cross-disciplinary team comprised of specialists from industry, government bodies like NASA, Goddard, and academia like the University of Maryland. His other industrial experience in engineering and research includes working in various roles such as instrumentation engineer for Triune Projects, research intern at Siemens CAD and Apex Eclipse Communications, scientist for SGT Inc., and lead scientist for Honeywell Research (Automatic Control Solutions-Advanced Technology Labs). Some of his relevant experience includes instrumentation and plant logic design, noise reduction in communication systems, vibration analysis for equipment health monitoring, flare steam control loop design and modeling, image/video signal segmentation, and analysis and use of statistical techniques for remote sensing and medical CAD applications.

Prof. (Dr.) Aravinda K., PhD, MTech, BE, professor, Department of Electronics and Communication, New Horizon College of Engineering, Bengaluru, 560103, India

Dr. Aravinda K. currently works as professor and head of electronics and communication engineering at New Horizon College of Engineering, Bengaluru, India. He completed his doctoral studies at Amrita University and his master of science at Newport University. He has multiple peer-reviewed journal publications, conference publications, and a book chapter. He has received the Faculty Excellence Award, the Honor Award, the Certificate of Outstanding Contribution, and the Long Service Award at the national and international level.

Dr. Mohit Kumar Sharma, PhD, MTech, BE, assistant professor, Department of Electrical Engineering, Vivekananda Global University, Jaipur, Rajasthan, India

Dr. Sharma received his PhD in electronics and communication engineering from JECRC University, Jaipur (NAAC Accredited) in 2022. He completed his master's of technology from Malviya National Institute of Technology (MNIT), Jaipur in VLSI Design in the year 2014. He has published several articles in reputed international journals. His research areas are wireless communication, 5G waveform, and non-orthogonal multiple access (NOMA waveforms) with optimized PAPR algorithms. He is currently working as an assistant professor in the Department of Electrical Engineering, Vivekananda Global University (A+ Accredited, NAAC), Jaipur.

Acknowledgments

In the rapidly evolving area of 5G-based smart hospitals and healthcare systems, our work to develop the book culminated in the efforts of several academicians, scientists, and practitioners throughout the globe. The global fraternity has responded overwhelmingly to the invitation for contributions to this quickly expanding and dynamic topic. For this book, a total of 32 proposals have been received. Three independent reviewers who are acknowledged authorities in their respective fields have carefully examined and analyzed each of the submitted proposals. Sixteen outstanding submissions have been selected for final publication based on the results of peer review and the suitability of the revised manuscript for the book's topic. We would like to express our gratitude to all of our reviewers for giving up their time and expertise. We would also like to thank all of the authors for their excellent scholarly contributions to this book. We are also thankful to the New Horizon College of Engineering, Bengaluru (India); Kennesaw State University, USA; and VGU, Jaipur (India) for extending their support in every way possible for this book. Finally, we want to express our gratitude to the publisher, CRC Press, for their assistance and direction during the whole publishing process, which enabled us to complete this book on schedule. We believe that this book will be useful to both students and expert researchers working in this field.

1 A Hybrid Deep Learning–Based Remote Monitoring Healthcare System Using Wearable Devices

Diksha Srivastava
Department of Allied Medical Science and Technology,
NIMS University, Jaipur, Rajasthan, India

R. Krishnamoorthy
Centre for Advanced Wireless Integrated Technology,
Chennai Institute of Technology, Chennai,
Tamil Nadu, India

Doradla Bharadwaja
Department of Information Technology, Prasad V Potluri
Siddhartha Institute of Technology, Vijayawada,
Andhra Pradesh, India

Kavyashree Nagarajaiah
Department of MCA, Sri Siddhartha Institute of Technology,
Tumkur, Karnataka, India

Kazuaki Tanaka
Kyushu Institute of Technology, Japan

Janjhyam Venkata Naga Ramesh
Department of Computer Science and Engineering, Koneru
Lakshmaiah Education Foundation, Vaddeswaram, Guntur,
Andhra Pradesh, India

DOI: 10.1201/9781003403678-1

1.1 INTRODUCTION

The past few years have witnessed significant advancement in the areas of computer technology, communication, and AI trends and technologies. The ubiquitous accessibility of smart tools, computers for multimedia, and edge computing devices are trends that have been observed recently. The accessibility of data-gathering systems and information dispensation tools, such as cloud computing, are developments that have been observed recently [1]. The convergence of these developments has resulted in the development of innovative strategies and paradigms for intelligent wearables and innovations. This part will provide a quick overview of the development of AI in wearable devices (WDs), beginning with the necessity of wearables and continuing on to examine how AI may be utilized to the advantage of wearables as well as the primary hurdles. The subsequent sections of this paper will provide more in-depth discussions on the aforementioned topics and issues [2]. The market for the paybacks of stable scrutinization technology for medical, health, and well-being applications is expanding, as is the perception of those benefits. The number of people who are monitoring their health using wearable devices and using them to track their activities is steadily growing. The advancements in sensing and integrated electronic circuits have made it possible to construct sophisticated devices that are small and compact [3]. These devices can include a variety of sensors, including ones that measure temperature. Because these WDs and sensing devices are now readily available, new applications can be created for detecting a wide range of human actions in consumer and commercial settings. Some applications for wearable technology include the monitoring of sleep and circadian rhythms, the identification of weariness, the prevention of falls among the elderly, as well as the recognition of human emotions and stress. The observation of the behaviors and activities of animals and wild creatures is another potential application for the use of intelligent wearables. This method was described in [4], which provides an overview of the application of wearable technologies, with a particular emphasis on animal controlling.

Because the architecture of machine learning (ML) and AI tools is built in smart wearables, these technologies play an essential part in the development of these wearables. The majority of applications for artificial intelligence and connected wearables may be found in the medical healthcare industry, as well as in sports, therapy places, amusement, and shadowing in smart homes [5]. WDs like these enable medical professionals to keep an eye on patients' heart failure, diabetes, and overall cardiovascular activity. In addition to this, it is helpful in determining and categorizing human emotional states, as well as human posture and the stage of sleep. A grand deal of work has been put into the development of various AI and machine learning technologies. These artificial intelligence and ML strategies can be divided into two categories: traditional ML strategies [6] and more contemporary DL approaches.

For instance, the academics in [7] outlined a number of problems or difficulties that need to be solved before the introduction of intelligent wearables for activity identification. The necessity for an extensive quantity of training data in order to train the classifiers for movement acknowledgment is the first difficulty that must be overcome. When it comes to building deep learning classifiers, having access to a huge amount of training data is really important. Classifiers based on traditional approaches to ML can be passably taught with a smaller quantity of data. The selection of the necessary characteristics for recognition becomes the second challenge [8]. The practice of feature selection is traditionally carried out by hand, relying on the knowledge and experience of the machine learning designer. Classical approaches to machine learning. The procedure of feature selection can be carried out in a way similar to that of an end-to-end process, and it can also be incorporated as an element of the training procedure in deep learning systems [9]. The next obstacle is to differentiate amid activities that may have comparable inputs. For example, it can be difficult to tell the difference between an activity event that involves falling and an event that involves looking for something on the ground. In order for the smart wearables to be able to achieve the duties that are expected of them, it is necessary to have proficient techniques. This presents an additional obstacle for real-time deployments. These architectures for intelligent WDs would want to take into consideration exigent issues and hardware limits like space of the electronics chip and board, the amount of power that they would consume, and the costs associated with their production [10].

Figure 1.1 provides a high-level outline of the architecture of the smart wristband that incorporates iGenda. The bracelet is able to identify the exciting levels of people and then transmits those patterns to the iGenda. Then it shows those patterns to the caretakers. This presentation of information makes it possible to schedule new tasks taking into account the emotional states that people are now in [11]. This strategy deciphers biosignals into feelings by utilizing neural networks and the Pleasure, Arousal, and Dominance (PAD) approach.

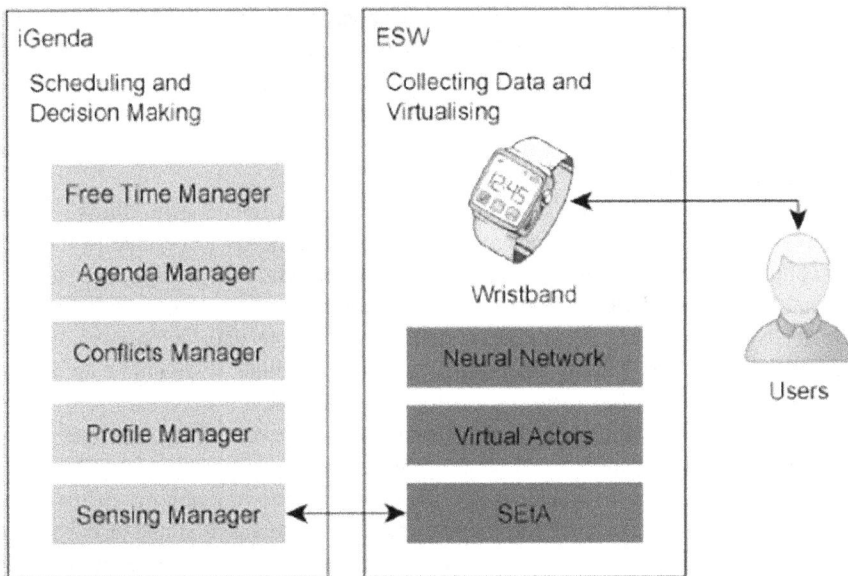

FIGURE 1.1 Concept diagram of smart wristband.

Assessing the dependability of wearable medical equipment is difficult. The paper describes the process of fine-tuning a wearable ambulatory monitoring device for use with COVID-19 patients in British isolation units. By using a chest patch and pulse oximeter, the system was able to continuously guess and convey critical sign data from patients to far-off nurse bays, protecting nurses from the spread of disease [12]. The system's ability to do remote patient monitoring was made possible by the use of a sheltered web-based structure and fault-tolerant smart methods. During the busiest time of year for hospital admissions, the plan was successfully implemented to monitor all patients in the ward. The technique has been improved and used in following pandemic waves in the United Kingdom. As the popularity of WDs continues to rise, scientists have created a wide variety of wearable devices that can track and record physical and mental health metrics like steps taken, hours slept, heart rate, skin temperature, etc. Symptoms of mental health issues like sadness, anxiety, and stress can be identified by patterns in the data acquired by these devices [13]. The raw sensor data can be linked to mental health issues, and behavioral markers can be identified with the use of machine learning. In this paper, we explore the current state of smartphone-based, wearable, and ambient sensors and their potential use in the detection, management, and treatment of mental health disorders [14].

As a result of advancements in machine learning (ML) and the Internet of Things (IoT), routine medical testing and healthcare services are increasingly being provided outside of hospitals, in the comfort of patients' own homes [15]. Employing an Android app in coincidence with IoT can improve the usability of medical devices, and portable sensors can deliver more accurate data. Because of its potential to enhance people's lives, the medical area stands to benefit greatly from the widespread adoption of many technologies, especially IoT [16]. With the proliferation of the Internet, access comes a shift away from traditional patient service methods and toward electronic healthcare systems, which in turn makes possible the widespread use of IoT-enabled, state-of-the-art medical equipment for both patients and doctors. There are several areas where ML and IoT devices can be useful, including healthcare, where they can facilitate remote monitoring, save costs, and boost patient satisfaction [17].

There are three distinguishing features that define a sensor as a "thing" in the context of the IoT healthcare system. At the outset, it needs to be able to identify and collect data on external factors like temperature, light, and precipitation, and on internal factors like ECG, blood sugar, and oxygen saturation. Second, it must be able to dynamically or via another system communicate data autonomously to a centralized controller. Finally, once the procedure is through, it should be able to go into standby mode, still alerting doctors to take swift action if necessary [18]. Two- and three-dimensional DNA origami designs have evolved as flexible nano-machines for transportation, sensing, and computation, respectively [19]. Electronic health records (EHRs) and medical photographs are just two examples of the types of data sources that have been the focus of pioneering research aimed at enhancing healthcare systems [20]. Even though the healthcare app and service development is customer-centric, it's evident that developers prioritize their own interests while crafting solutions. Recently, ML methods like CNN have been used in a wide range of applications, from proficiently ranking alcohol reliance to accurately anticipating the cruelty of brutal injuries in accidents to accurately estimating emotions in practical tools [21].

Significant improvements have been made in healthcare as a result of IoT and ML. By combining the Internet of Things, WDs, and ML, healthcare providers may monitor their patients' conditions in real time and intervene before they worsen. IoT devices have gained popularity in healthcare settings due to their efficiency, cost-effectiveness, and positive effect on patient satisfaction. Many different diseases and conditions can stem from mental and physical stress. The ability to continuously monitor physiological signals has been made possible by the convergence of WDs and IoT tools, allowing for the prior anticipation of stress-related issues and the implementation of preventative measures before the condition worsens. A wearable sensor system was presented in a study [22] to identify stress and monitor its development by combining physiological parameters like heart-rate inconsistency and skin conductance with relative data. Data from the user's wearable sensors was analyzed by ML algorithms in this system so that tailored recommendations and interventions could be made. Various sensors, including electroencephalography and electromyography sensors, have been investigated in other stress-monitoring research [23]. These sensors can monitor and potentially treat stress by gathering data on both mental and physical activity.

In this piece, we propose a tiny sensor patch that might be worn by a person and used for a range of remote health monitoring applications. This patch is easy to apply and can monitor several vital signs simultaneously. The concept of a health monitoring system for athletes that is powered by wearable sensors connected to the Internet of Things has been presented. This initiative seeks to construct sports clinics and team performance activities that craft more efficient utilize of expertise to hasten athletes' recoveries and facilitate their early return to a wider variety of sports. Wearable gadgets not only record an athlete's actions but also their health predictions made with an RNN [24]. The designed approach can examine an athlete's health in real time by gathering data from multiple physiological parameters, including heart rate. When used for sports medicine, wearable health monitoring technology has the potential to yield useful insights for trainers, doctors, and coaches. Athletes will have better health results in general thanks to this technology's ability to detect latent health risks and to deal with them. Furthermore, athletes may keep tabs on their development and get ready for future health problems with the use of wearable monitoring technologies [25]. WHM is a promising field of study in sports medicine. Data can be collected and analyzed in real time to aid in the prevention and treatment of accidents, the enhancement of training and performance, and the proliferation of the Internet of Things. Wearable gadgets will gradually play a more important role in the future of sports medicine and athlete health [26]. The following is an outline of how the remaining work will be organized: Recent studies on the Internet of Things (IoT) in healthcare systems are covered in Section 1.2, followed by the presentation of the suggested framework in Section 1.3, description of the experimental assessment in Section 1.4, and a wrap-up in Section 1.5.

1.2 RELATED WORKS

The essential physiological characteristics of the people can be evaluated with the help of numerous tiny sensors, including heart rate, blood pressure, and skin temperature. In wearable health monitoring systems (WHMSs), these sensors can be applied directly to the skin. Patients can get more in-depth and personalized health data via wearable health monitoring systems that include implanted devices [27]. The data is collected by the microsensor and, based on the clients opinions, is either wirelessly or cable transferred to a processing node for scrutiny. The motherboard of a microcontroller device acts as the system's brain, processing data and presenting it to the user. The healthcare provider shares what they've learned about the patient's present situation with the patient. Wearable technologies for stress monitoring, healthcare using the Internet of Things, and machine learning are all discussed in this section. Several studies have been conducted in the area of human behavior recognition applications. A unique Res-Bidir-LSTM network was proposed in [28] to address HAR issues. Although this method takes a lengthy period to deploy, early training results have shown remarkable accuracy. When sensor fusion is needed, the Res-Bidir-LSTM approach can be employed to difficult, complex HAR problems.

Time series should be part of the input to the HAR thanks to the LSTM's foundational architecture. The problem of the gradient disappearing into nothingness is circumvented thanks to this method. A system for automatic drug identification using deep learning methods was presented in [29] under the name ST-Med-Box. This method has the potential to improve the adherence of individuals with several prescriptions and chronic conditions. If a patient has an Android device, they can use a QR code scanner to record their prescription medicament information. Then we can ensure they are receiving timely medication reminders. Several RL strategies have been explored [30] to determine the best decision-making strategy for the IoT. Methods like Monte Carlo, Expected SARSA, and Q-learning are among them. Using RL methods, we can potentially reduce the fog node's idle time and maximize its utilization of available resources. Singh et al. [31] suggest an RL-based solution for reliable cloud administration. Several current investigations into the use of wearable-technology for stress recognition have served as inspiration for the proposed study. The Affective-Road data set monitored drivers' stress levels over the course of 10 drives. Ten drivers' stress levels were monitored as they drove different routes using a wearable glove equipped with a photoplethysmogram sensor developed [32].

The researchers behind this study are hoping their findings will help them create more accurate health and activity monitoring systems by shedding light on the impact self-tracking applications have on users' psyches. Patients with a higher disease load saw the greatest benefit, with a mean CAT score improvement of −0.9 points and a reduction in daily SABA use of −0.6 puffs. These results provide more evidence that EMMs can be utilized to passively observe COPD patients' illness saddle and cure outcomes [33]. Reddy et al. addressed the use of ML in contact tracking apps through the COVID-19 epidemic. Data collected by these apps can be used by ML to predict the spread of viruses and locate susceptible populations. However, in order to make trustworthy predictions, it is crucial to guarantee the data set's quality, reliability, and absence of biases. The article provides two guidelines for achieving high data quality for ML on a global scale. It pinpoints the regions where these needs can be satisfied, taking into account regional variations in contact tracking apps and smartphone penetration. Finally, the merits, drawbacks, and ethical implications of this method are examined.

There is a rising body of writing investigating the utility of wearable data in informing mental health therapy as more and more digital and wearable technologies are applied to the diagnosis, and observing of mental illnesses, especially in outpatient settings. When it comes to data analysis for smart wearable technology, DL is one of the significant methodologies [34]. The authors developed an innovative deep learning architecture based on sensors integrated into wearable technology to facilitate reliable human activity recognition systems. This novel deep architecture for model creation in data categorization combines a DNN with active learning. While the former makes use of a CNN with layered LSTM to learn a hierarchical representation of features and confine temporal dependencies in activity data, the latter chooses the optimal moment to retrain the deep network in a way that makes the system operational [35].

To predict the alleviation of anxiety and panic disorders during the whole day, the academicians of [36] developed a DL-paired system with WDs. In a similar vein, [37] presented a DL strategy using WDs to encourage physical activity among the visually impaired. The DL approach renders a 3D scene from the wearable camera, naming certain obstacles by name. The wearable tech alerts the user to potential hazards and provides details about how to avoid them. The depth estimator makes the obstructions appear closer than they actually are. To improve activity detection, [38] developed an unsupervised deep learning strategy to reconstructing the on-nodule WDs coder. To get rid of reconstruction error and boost precision, it combined the coder design with the Z-layer technique. In the Lab of Wireless Sensor Data Mining, researchers use wearable sensors to collect data for the DL approach. Six distinct movements are represented in the data, including standing, walking, sitting, and running, going upstairs, and going downstairs. In the sections that follow, we'll talk about the various deep learning network topologies and their potential uses in artificial intelligence and intelligent wearables [39].

According to the research conducted, there is some disagreement over the optimal method of measurement for physiological stress monitoring. Despite employing the identical physiological factors and classifiers, the classification accuracy attained by different studies was quite different. For instance, the accuracy of anticipating athletes' health utilizing WDs and RNNs was improved to 92% in the study "A Novel Deep Learning Method for Predicting Athletes' Health using Recurrent Neural Networks." Another work that used deep learning and wearable sensors to accurately identify physical activities was "Deep Learning–based Physical Activity Recognition using Wearable Sensors." This table summarizes the many ways in which wearable sensors and deep learning can be used to progress health monitoring and patient results. This area of study shows great promise for the future of healthcare management and monitoring.

1.3 PROPOSED METHODOLOGY

To begin, football players are outfitted with sensors that scrutinize their vital signs and accumulate data pertaining to their health. The sports person's medical record is then input into an RNN, which generates projections for the athlete's future fitness. When all of this information has been compiled, the training staff and the checkup staff can utilize it to develop individualized preparation plans and healing protocols, correspondingly [40]. It is essential to perform an in-depth investigation of the health of football players before coming up with a realistic and efficient training schedule to follow. Although these two premises are mutually exclusive, they both suggest that we proceed in the manner that has been described. The WHMS does not have a unified design as a result of the wide variety of methods that have been utilized by many systems during construction. Biological impulses are an example of the kind of patterns that can be transmitted via analog channels. If there isn't any communiqué going back and forth between the sensor and middle node, then there is no requirement for the middle node to perform any preprocessing [41].

The complexity and attention to detail required by the WHMS make its development a challenging endeavor. Designers often have to make concessions when there are many competing interests and not enough money to go around. The ideal method for building a system and its accompanying countermeasure settings will differ from one potential application to the next. The physiologic signal from the biosensor is transmitted to the central node in a WHMS system, and the measurement data from the wearable device is sent to the distant medical station or doctor [42]. The WHMS makes use of these two data sources for separate purposes. When it comes to managing data and other close-range broadcasts, some WHMSs offer both wired and wireless interconnection choices. However, the user's mobility and comfort are severely constrained by an HMS that needs wired data transmitted, not to mention the elevated danger of a system collapse. Sensor nodes are stitched into a selection of stretchy, smart textile clothing to form a body area network. Wearable health monitoring systems rely on conductive yarns developed by prestigious research institutions for data collection and transmission from sensor nodes. Data in the traditional star architecture is delivered to a single server, which can be thought of as any advanced microcontroller-based electrical device [43].

These include electronic tools like PDAs, mobile phones, and portable PCs. In Figure 1.2, we see a representation of an RNN, a form of NN optimized for processing time series data. Like a cyclic-dynamic-system, the outcome of each cycle is stored and utilized as an input in the subsequent cycle. The outcomes of previous cycles could be recalled and used as inputs for the present one. Compared to other types of neural networks, RNN is the superior option. No information is shared between neurons on the same layer in a conventional neural network. The RNN paradigm, in contrast, makes it possible for hidden layers to exchange information and for the outputs of individual brain units to be stored for later use. This data is easily accessible and can be put to many different uses [44].

Figure 1.4 is a simplified flowchart of the steps needed to analyze a motion capture of human actions. In order to classify human actions, video or image sequences are used in the analysis process. The image demonstrates that the first stage involves

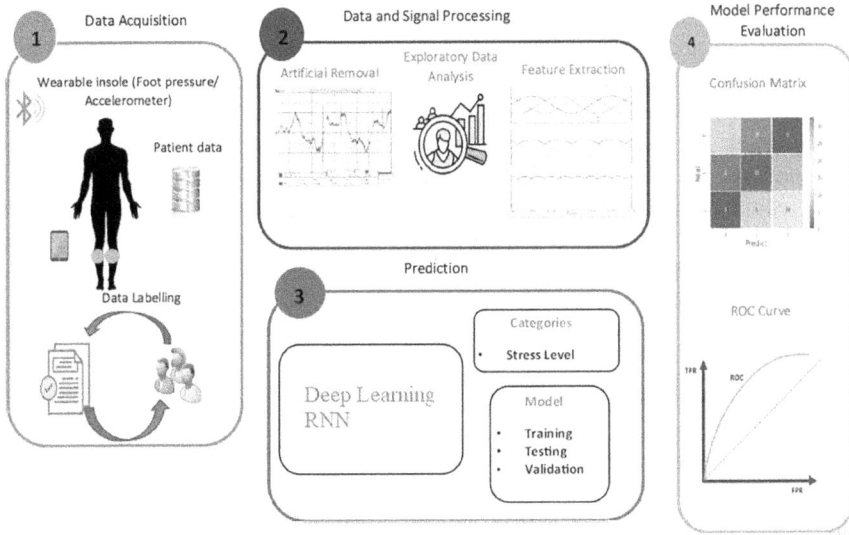

FIGURE 1.2   Architecture of the proposed model.

accessing information about human activities stored in a database. The next step is to perform some preliminary processing on the data, such as denoising or noise suppression. Features are extracted from the preprocessed data. After an activity has been recognized, a classifier is used to place it into a specific category. The efficacy of the technique is highly dependent on the quality of the feature appearance. The graphic demonstrates that the phase of extracting features is where the bulk of the work is required in calculating and evaluating the pattern discovery technique. Overall, the steps required to analyze motion representations of human motions are depicted graphically in Figure 1.2. Preprocessing, feature extraction, and pattern identification are all stressed for their significance in human action detection in sports [45].

1.3.1   SPORTS ACTION RECOGNITION AND BLOOD PRESSURE MONITORING

Because moving objects occupy such a tiny fraction of the screen compared to the background, in reality, this is a textbook case of sampling bias. Using DL to monitor player movement during games presents a number of challenges. Before we can analyze the training data, we need to normalize the samples to guarantee that they all have the same values. Context drawings are used to demonstrate the appearance of elements edges and to categorize them according to their distinguishing features, while most studies utilize outlines to indicate where individuals are. Data is commonly preprocessed and adjusted in DL prior to training; this includes values for the first layer's activation function, the weight-matrix spanning the first to the last layer. This measures how drastically the sum of all errors impacts the final product. To get the best possible results, we employ the DL method to categorize a picture of the athlete's current position. The model in this method is constructed by analyzing available data.

Both the time needed to train the model and the quality of the model it produces are affected by the initial parameters used to construct it. The recommended procedure is depicted in Figure 1.4 of an online flowchart. The strategy considers both the allusion BP and PPG signal when searching for inputs. In both the training and testing stages, the reference BP signal is used to calculate the systolic and diastolic blood pressure values. Each of the VGs that were given into the CNN can be turned into a feature vector with the help of forward propagation and certain pre-trained CNNs. That way, we can get a feature vector for each VGG. Using ridge regression, initial values for BP and weights and variances between the vectors are determined during training (Figure 1.3).

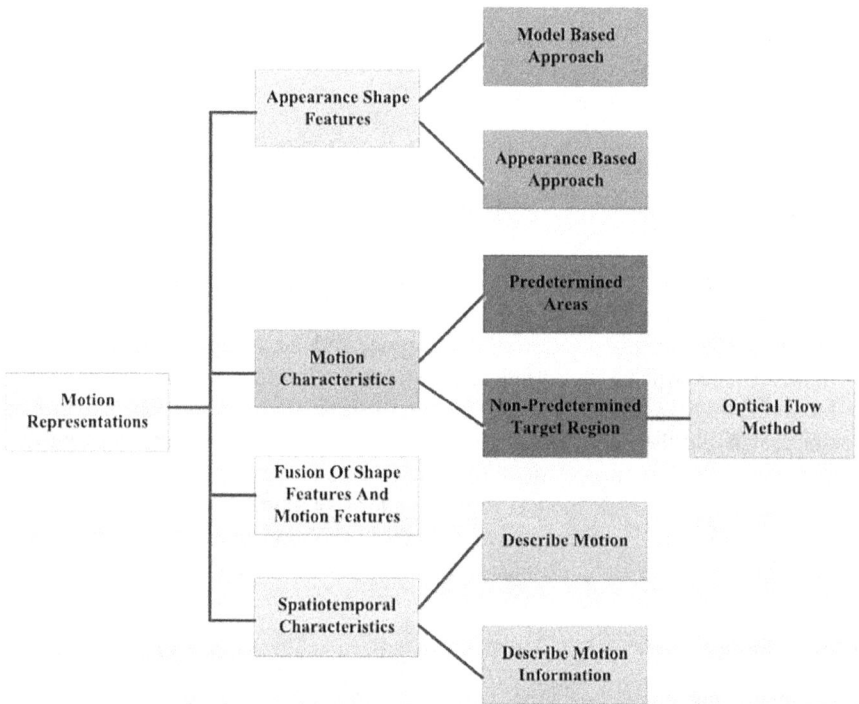

FIGURE 1.3   Investigation of motion representation in different stages.

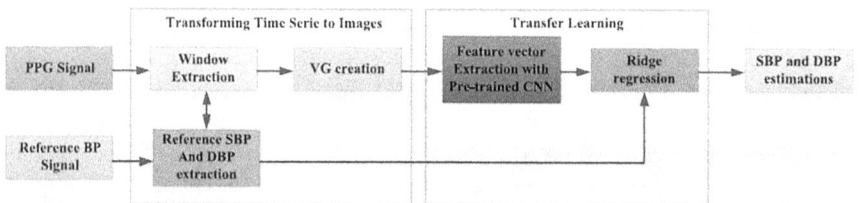

FIGURE 1.4   The framework proposed for anticipation of BP utilizing PPG.

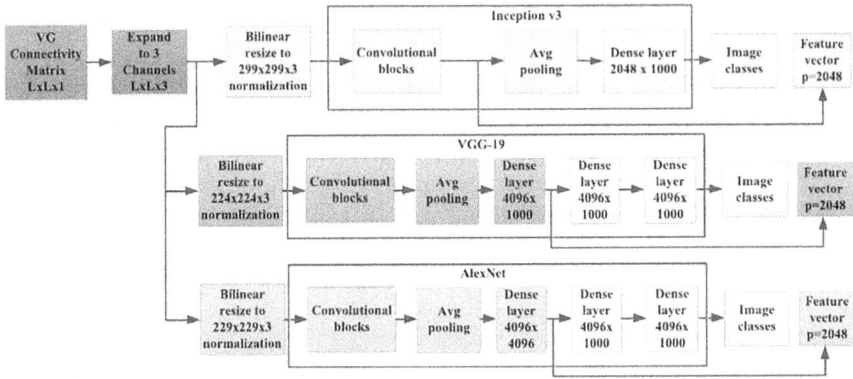

FIGURE 1.5 Flow diagram of the transfer learning.

In this investigation, we will discuss how to separate systolic peaks from a PPG signal by applying the methodology described in [46]. Specifically, we will use this method. Two separate measurements, known as the moving-average-peak (MApeak) and moving-average-beat (MAbeat), are utilized in order to pinpoint the precise location of the hypertension peak inside each beat. In actual use, there is no meaningful distinction to be made between these values. The first thing you need to do is remove all of the files that are currently saved there. Second, cut each record into ten-second chunks that do not overlap with one another. The windowing function calls for a time window that is ten seconds long. Third, eliminate the saturated portion of the PPG signal if there is a break in addition to saturation in the signal. In pace 4, eliminate the portions that have less than eight systolic peaks altogether. We utilized the methodology outlined in [47] in order to pinpoint the location of the systolic peak. The first thing that we did when putting this strategy into action was to calculate the square of every sample of PPG signals. Because we utilized different moving-average filters called MApeak and the other called MAbeat, we obtained two distinct curves.

The MApeak and MAbeat curves are depicted in Figure 1.5, with the previous being shown by a blue line and latter being represented by magenta line. Below, you can see examples of both curves. After that, we will be able to identify the provinces of concern by determining wherever the amplitude of the MApeak curve is greater than that of the MAbeat curve. The divisions are shown in the diagram as dashed lines. It is an effective method for drawing attention to the highest points of the systolic cycle of the heart. During the course of ten seconds, there should be in excess of ten peaks that represent the systolic phase. It should come as no surprise that this is the case given that the human heart beats at a rate of more than 60 times per minute on average.

1.4 RESULTS AND DISCUSSIONS

The positions of athletic motions are reflected in the joint points of the human skeleton, which are illustrated by three-dimensional skeleton matches. This provides insight not only into the large formation of the human body, but also into the specific architectural makeup of the human body. To perform athletic movements that are both more powerful and more fluid, it is essential to have a solid understanding of the interactions that take place between the various components of the skeleton [48]. On the other hand, learning about individual bones is not something that is useful in day-to-day living. After that, the generated pictures were scaled down via bilinear tuning so that they would match the input parameters for CNN, and the results of those CNNs were included in models that were already in existence. We employed the ridge regression method to estimate SBP and DBP, which needed us to first assess the linear weighting and then determine the bias [49]. Both of these steps were necessary for accurate results.

According to the findings, bringing the all temporal properties up to three contributes to an increase in the level of precision that can be achieved by classification and identification systems. The manner in which the pool will be utilized is the single most significant consideration to make regarding the dimensions of the center of the pool. The output of a research that investigated the capacity of CKs of varying sizes to discern amid unlike types of athletic actions is presented in Figure 1.6. Specifically, the work was motivated by the need to learn how to do both. The purpose of this study was to evaluate how well convolution kernels of varying sizes can differentiate between different athletic events.

In addition, removing joint points calls for more mathematical work to be done in order to establish the appropriate locations for the points. In the course of the inquiry, two separate data sets were utilized, and the results of several experiments were subsequently gathered and published. The training errors and test errors are

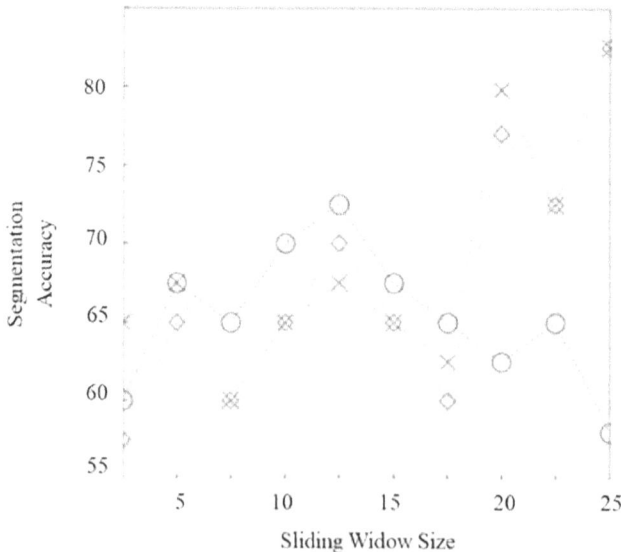

FIGURE 1.6 Various masses of convolution kernels (CKs) influence the efficiency of partition for identifying sports activities.

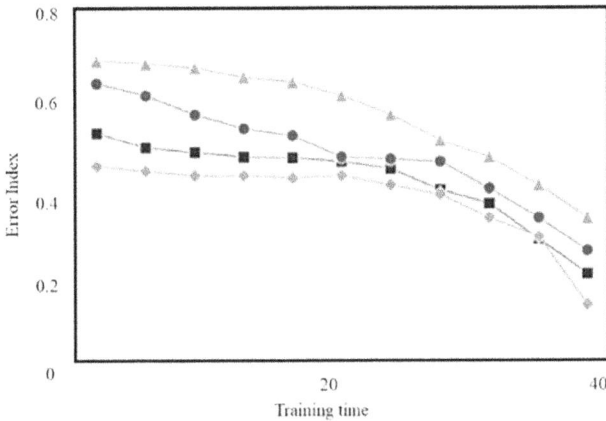

FIGURE 1.7   Error distribution of the design (before data set).

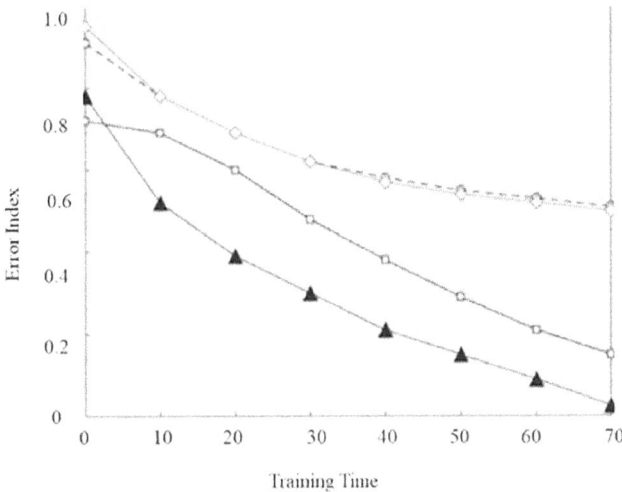

FIGURE 1.8   Error distribution of the approach (after data set).

depicted in Figures 1.7 and 1.8, respectively. These represent the findings of a study that required evaluating the effectiveness of a model using two separate data sets in order to come to a conclusion.

When compared to the correctness of DBP inference, the accuracy of SBP estimation is often similar to that of the B-level. The presentation must include all facets of the topic, right down to the very last fraction of a second. The model was trained and evaluated using the ABP labels. During the process of putting this into action, each of our comments was given careful consideration. On this page, you can find the findings of the experiment that we conducted. By contrasting the LSTM's authentic performance with our most optimistic projection, we were able to arrive at this conclusion [50]. This is what we found out when we contrasted the

TABLE 1.1
Investigation of BPM Based on LSTM

Parameters	BPM Value (mm Hg)		
	< 5	< 10	< 15
Systolic BP (SBP)	65.24	84.37	95.31
Diastolic BP (DBP)	89.27	97.28	98.59

LSTM outcome to the forecast that we considered to be perfect. The results of BP estimate methods that make use of randomly generated weights are outlined in Table 1.1, which may be found here. It gathers the findings of the numerous LSTM-based BPM estimating approaches that have been proposed and provides an outline of those contributions.

During the training stage of the study, we are going to look at the data in great detail. This is the first work that we are aware of that proposes utilizing VG for the purpose of synthesizing images from PPG data; therefore, we have every reason to believe that this assumption is accurate. In conclusion, the second research that was stated earlier showed that the LSTM had a satisfactory performance when it came to estimation. Nevertheless, in order to construct a useful LSTM design, permanent annotations of the allusion BP, which in this instance was ABP wave, were necessary. In the majority of instances, having unfettered entrée to the noting of the allusion BP plus is neither feasible nor practicable due to the nature of the situation. Blood pressure monitors that are designed in the form of cuffs are typically easy to use, which enables them to correctly construe the findings. As long as there is a need for more investigation into the matter, the proposed strategy cannot be implemented in WDs. There is also a risk of co-linearity and redundant data because the outcomes of the BP evaluation utilizing the feature vectors created by VGPOS and VGINV are comparable to one another. It is possible that this will assist in enhancing the efficiency of our methods and reducing the number of feature vectors that are available.

1.5 CONCLUSIONS AND FUTURE WORK

Earlier research has laid the groundwork for identifying motion samples through an understanding of general motion properties. In the context of this study, we present a synopsis of pertinent DL information. DL is a type of "deep model" that excels at generalization, processing speed for complex situations, and analysis. Our work here presents a novel approach to image transformation that makes use of the temporal information included in the PPG signal to achieve impressive speeds. All of the aims of our proposed method were attained, including the elimination of the require for entity alignment and physical feature engineering, the use of a tiny PPG signal range, and the application of DL models to data sets for BP anticipation on humble dispensation funds. All of these features are essential for achieving higher precision. Since our method is noninvasive, it represents a competitive alternative to traditional cuff-based blood pressure monitoring. After evaluating the kinetic properties of local segments, the approach identifies action examples. Both DL- and non-DL-based feature extraction methods are discussed in this research as two distinct categories of sports action identification systems. Due to its reliance on fictitious backdrop information, the non-DL method requires more photos featuring actual athletic events in motion. The use of DL is a straightforward strategy that can be applied to sports action video gatherings, permitting viewers to more efficiently comprehend data connected to action and build a more trustworthy portrait. In this chapter, we introduce a strategy for incorporating RNNs into WDs with the purpose of providing accurate health anticipations for sports players. The initial step of this project is to implement a system of sensors for monitoring the health of football players. Data about the athletes' recent levels of corporal fitness is crucial. Following this, an RNN is used to extract deep features from the data at every time step, and finally, the results of the health prediction are obtained. One hundred professional football players were chosen at random for our research. The experimental results showed an accuracy rate of 81%, which is a big boost above the effectiveness of other options. The results show that the approach recommended in this research is the best and most effective one. By contrasting the proposed algorithm with the methods used in established research, its efficacy may be gauged. Experiments show that the technique is both conventional and trustworthy. Incredibly accurate recognition can be achieved in a relatively short quantity of time.

REFERENCES

1. Islam, M.R., Kabir, M.M., Mridha, M.F., Alfarhood, S., Safran, M. and Che, D., 2023. Deep learning-based IoT system for remote monitoring and early detection of health issues in real-time. *Sensors*, *23*(11), p. 5204.
2. Balamurugan, D., Aravinth, S.S., Reddy, P.C.S., Rupani, A. and Manikandan, A., 2022. Multiview objects recognition using deep learning-based wrap-CNN with voting scheme. *Neural Processing Letters*, *54*(3), pp. 1495–1521.
3. Kumar, A., Dhana, G. R., Albreem, M. and Le, D., 2021. A comprehensive study on the role of advanced technologies in 5G based Smart hospital. *Alexandria Engineering Journal*, *2021*(60), pp. 5527–5536.
4. Ramakrishnan, B, Kumar, A, Chakravarty, S, Masud, M, and Baz, M., 2021. Analysis of FBMC Waveform for 5G Network Based Smart Hospitals. *Applied Sciences*, *11*(19), p. 8895. 10.3390/app11198895
5. Arikumar, K.S., Prathiba, S.B., Alazab, M., Gadekallu, T.R., Pandya, S., Khan, J.M. and Moorthy, R.S., 2022. FL-PMI: federated learning-based person movement identification through wearable devices in smart healthcare systems. *Sensors*, *22*(4), p. 1377.
6. Krishnamoorthy, R., Liya, B. S., Padmapriya, S., Gunasundari, B. and Thiagarajan, R., 2021. Categorizing the heart syndrome condition by predictive analysis using machine learning approach, *3rd International Conference on Advances in Computing, Communication Control and Networking (ICAC3N)*, pp. 104–108, 10.1109/ICAC3 N53548.2021.9725725.
7. Li, W., Chai, Y., Khan, F., Jan, S.R.U., Verma, S., Menon, V.G. and Li, X., 2021a. A comprehensive survey on machine learning-based big data analytics for IoT-enabled smart healthcare system. *Mobile Networks and Applications*, *26*, pp. 234–252.

8. Ashreetha, B., Devi, M.R., Kumar, U.P., Mani, M.K., Sahu, D.N. and Reddy, P.C.S., 2022. Soft optimization techniques for automatic liver cancer detection in abdominal liver images. *International Journal of Health Sciences*, *6*, pp. 32–41.

9. Souri, A., Ghafour, M.Y., Ahmed, A.M., Safara, F., Yamini, A. and Hoseyninezhad, M., 2020. A new machine learning-based healthcare monitoring model for student's condition diagnosis in Internet of Things environment. *Soft Computing*, *24*(22), pp. 17111–17121.

10. Chakravarty, S. and Kumar, A., 2023. PAPR reduction of GFDM signals using encoder-decoder neural network (Autoencoder). *National Academy of Science and Letters* 10.1007/s40009-023-01230-1.

11. Li, Y., Shan, B., Li, B., Liu, X. and Pu, Y., 2021b. Literature review on the applications of machine learning and blockchain technology in smart healthcare industry: A bibliometric analysis. *Journal of Healthcare Engineering*. 2023, pp. 1–12.

12. Kumar, K., Pande, S.V., Kumar, T., Saini, P., Chaturvedi, A., Reddy, P.C.S. and Shah, K.B., 2023. Intelligent controller design and fault prediction using machine learning model. *International Transactions on Electrical Energy Systems*. 2023, pp. 1–9.

13. Lokesh, S., Priya, A., Sakhare, D.T., Devi, R.M., Sahu, D.N. and Reddy, P.C.S., 2022. CNN based deep learning methods for precise analysis of cardiac arrhythmias. *International Journal of Health Sciences*, *6*, pp. 1–8.

14. Wang, Y., Nazir, S. and Shafiq, M., 2021. An overview on analyzing deep learning and transfer learning approaches for health monitoring. *Computational and Mathematical Methods in Medicine*, *2021*, pp. 1–10.

15. Lokesh, K., Srivastava, S., Kumar, M. P., Padmapriya, S. and Krishnamoorthy, R., 2021. Detection of stomach cancer using deep neural network in healthcare sector, *3rd International Conference on Advances in Computing, Communication Control and Networking (ICAC3N)*, pp. 521–526, 10.1109/ICAC3N53548.2021.9725656.

16. Bordoloi, D., Singh, V., Sanober, S., Buhari, S.M., Ujjan, J.A. and Boddu, R., 2022. Deep learning in healthcare system for quality of service. *Journal of Healthcare Engineering*. 2022, pp. 1–12.

17. Ashok, K., Boddu, R., Syed, S.A., Sonawane, V.R., Dabhade, R.G. and Reddy, P.C.S., 2022. GAN Base feedback analysis system for industrial IOT networks. *Automatika*, pp. 1–9.

18. Sabitha, R., Shukla, A.P., Mehbodniya, A., Shakkeera, L. and Reddy, P.C.S., 2022. A fuzzy trust evaluation of cloud collaboration outlier detection in wireless sensor networks. *Adhoc & Sensor Wireless Networks*, *53*, pp. 1–13.

19. Sundaravadivel, P., Kesavan, K., Kesavan, L., Mohanty, S.P. and Kougianos, E., 2018. Smart-log: A deep-learning based automated nutrition monitoring system in the IoT. *IEEE Transactions on Consumer Electronics*, *64*(3), pp. 390–398.

20. Muthappa, K.A., Nisha, A.S.A., Shastri, R., Avasthi, V. and Reddy, P.C.S., 2023. Design of high-speed, low-power non-volatile master slave flip flop (NVMSFF) for memory registers designs. *Applied Nanoscience*, *16*, pp. 1–10.

21. Prasath, A.S.S., Lokesh, S., Krishnakumar, N.J., Vandarkuzhali, T., Sahu, D.N. and Reddy, P.C.S., 2022. Classification of EEG signals using machine learning and deep learning techniques. *International Journal of Health Sciences*, *2022*, pp. 10794–10807.

22. Wang, Z. and Gao, Z., 2021. Analysis of real-time heartbeat monitoring using wearable device Internet of Things system in sports environment. *Computational Intelligence*, *37*(3), pp. 1080–1097.

23. Dhanalakshmi, R., Bhavani, N.P.G., Raju, S.S., Shaker Reddy, P.C., Marvaluru, D., Singh, D.P. and Batu, A., 2022. Onboard pointing error detection and estimation of observation satellite data using extended kalman filter. *Computational Intelligence and Neuroscience*, *22*, pp. 1–8.

24. Alnaim, A.K. and Alwakeel, A.M., 2023. Machine-learning-based IoT–edge computing healthcare solutions. *Electronics*, *12*(4), p. 1027.
25. Kadu, A., Singh, M. and Ogudo, K., 2022. A novel scheme for classification of epilepsy using machine learning and a fuzzy inference system based on wearable-sensor health parameters. *Sustainability*, *14*(22), p. 15079.
26. Sucharitha, Y., Reddy, P.C.S. and Suryanarayana, G., 2023. Network intrusion detection of drones using recurrent neural networks. *Drone Technology: Future Trends and Practical Applications*, pp. 375–392.
27. Sabry, F., Eltaras, T., Labda, W., Alzoubi, K. and Malluhi, Q., 2022. Machine learning for healthcare wearable devices: the big picture. *Journal of Healthcare Engineering*, *2022*, pp. 1–15.
28. Hayyolalam, V., Aloqaily, M., Özkasap, Ö. and Guizani, M., 2021. Edge intelligence for empowering IoT-based healthcare systems. *IEEE Wireless Communications*, *28*(3), pp. 6–14.
29. Shanmugaraja, P., Bhardwaj, M., Mehbodniya, A., Vali, S. and Reddy, P.C.S., 2023. An Efficient Clustered M-path Sinkhole Attack Detection (MSAD) Algorithm for Wireless Sensor Networks. *Adhoc & Sensor Wireless Networks*, *55*, pp. 1–27.
30. Jaber, M.M., Alameri, T., Ali, M.H., Alsyouf, A., Al-Bsheish, M., Aldhmadi, B.K., Ali, S.Y., Abd, S.K., Ali, S.M., Albaker, W. and Jarrar, M.T., 2022. Remotely monitoring COVID-19 patient health condition using metaheuristics convolute networks from IoT-based wearable device health data. *Sensors*, *22*(3), p. 1205.
31. Singh, B., Somasekhar, K., Anand, K., Gopikrishnan, M. and Krishnamoorthy, R., 2022. Machine learning based predictive modeling of plasma treatment in biomedical surfaces, *Second International Conference on Artificial Intelligence and Smart Energy (ICAIS)*, pp. 1043–1046, 10.1109/ICAIS53314.2022.9743031.
32. Ijaz, M., Li, G., Wang, H., El-Sherbeny, A.M., Moro Awelisah, Y., Lin, L., Koubaa, A. and Noor, A., 2020. Intelligent fog-enabled smart healthcare system for wearable physiological parameter detection. *Electronics*, *9*(12), p. 2015.
33. Hameed, K., Bajwa, I.S., Ramzan, S., Anwar, W. and Khan, A., 2020. An intelligent IoT based healthcare system using fuzzy neural networks. *Scientific Programming*, *2020*, pp. 1–15.
34. Qureshi, M.A., Qureshi, K.N., Jeon, G. and Piccialli, F., 2021. Deep learning-based ambient assisted living for self-management of cardiovascular conditions. *Neural Computing and Applications*, *34*, pp. 1–19.
35. Nancy, A.A., Ravindran, D., Raj Vincent, P.D., Srinivasan, K. and Gutierrez Reina, D., 2022. Iot-cloud-based smart healthcare monitoring system for heart disease prediction via deep learning. *Electronics*, *11*(15), p. 2292.
36. Aldabbas, H., Albashish, D., Khatatneh, K. and Amin, R., 2022. An architecture of IoT-aware healthcare smart system by leveraging machine learning. *International Arab Journal of Information Technology*, *19*(2), pp. 160–172.
37. Boursalie, O., Samavi, R. and Doyle, T.E., 2015. M4CVD: Mobile machine learning model for monitoring cardiovascular disease. *Procedia Computer Science*, *63*, pp. 384–391.
38. Nurmi, J. and Lohan, E.S., 2021. Systematic review on machine-learning algorithms used in wearable-based eHealth data analysis. *IEEE Access*, *9*, pp. 112221–112235.
39. Anand, A., Rani, S., Anand, D., Aljahdali, H.M. and Kerr, D., 2021. An efficient CNN-based deep learning model to detect malware attacks (CNN-DMA) in 5G-IoT healthcare applications. *Sensors*, *21*(19), p. 6346.
40. Begli, M., Derakhshan, F. and Karimipour, H., 2019. August. A layered intrusion detection system for critical infrastructure using machine learning. In *2019 IEEE 7th International Conference on Smart Energy Grid Engineering (SEGE)* (pp. 120–124). IEEE.

41. Hussain, A., Ali, S. and Kim, H.C., 2022. Activity detection for the wellbeing of dogs using wearable sensors based on deep learning. *IEEE Access*, *10*, pp. 53153–53163.

42. Kumar, A. and Gupta, M., 2017. A review on activities of fifth generation mobile communication system. *Alexandria Engineering Journal*, *57*(2), pp. 1125–1135. https://www.sciencedirect.com/science/article/pii/S1110016817300601.

43. Kumar, A., Albreem, M. A., Gupta, M., Alsharif, M. H. and Kim, S., 2020. Future 5G network based smart hospitals: Hybrid detection technique for latency improvement. *in IEEE Access*, 8, pp. 153240–153249, 10.1109/ACCESS.2020.3017625.

44. Shi, Q., Zhang, Z., He, T., Sun, Z., Wang, B., Feng, Y., Shan, X., Salam, B. and Lee, C., 2020. Deep learning enabled smart mats as a scalable floor monitoring system. *Nature Communications*, *11*(1), p. 4609.

45. Nahavandi, D., Alizadehsani, R., Khosravi, A. and Acharya, U.R., 2022. Application of artificial intelligence in wearable devices: Opportunities and challenges. *Computer Methods and Programs in Biomedicine*, *213*, p. 106541.

46. Reddy, P.C.S., Pradeepa, M., Venkatakiran, S., Walia, R. and Saravanan, M., 2021b. Image and signal processing in the underwater environment. *Journal of Nuclear Energy Science & Power Generation Technology*, *10*(9), p. 2.

47. Elbagoury, B.M., Vladareanu, L., Vlădăreanu, V., Salem, A.B., Travediu, A.M. and Roushdy, M.I., 2023. A hybrid stacked CNN and residual feedback GMDH-LSTM deep learning model for stroke prediction applied on mobile AI smart hospital platform. *Sensors*, *23*(7), p. 3500.

48. Vivekananda, G. N., Ali, A. R. H., Mishra, P., Sengar, R. and Krishnamoorthy, R., 2022. Cloud based effective health care management system with artificial intelligence, *IEEE 7th International Conference for Convergence in Technology (I2CT)*, pp. 1–6, 10.1109/I2CT54291.2022.9825457.

49. Reddy, P.C., Nachiyappan, S., Ramakrishna, V., Senthil, R. and Sajid Anwer, M.D., 2021a. Hybrid model using scrum methodology for software development system. *Journal of Nuclear Energy Science & Power Generation Technology*, *10*(9), p. 2.

50. Kumar, A., Gour, N., Yadav, S. K., Gaur, N., & Sharma, H. (2023). A comparative PAPR, BER, and PSD for optical NOMA communication framework. *Optical and Quantum Electronics*, *55*. 10.1007/s11082-023-05148-2

2 Advancements of Smart Hospital Integration with Health Services for Early Recognition of Shoulder Damage in Paraplegics

Improving Healthcare Standards Using Manual Assistive 5G Devices

Sumit Chakravarty
Department of Electrical and Computer Engineering, Kennesaw State University, GA, USA

Ying Xie
College of Computing and Software Engineering, Kennesaw State University, GA, USA

2.1 INTRODUCTION

To guarantee that a wheelchair handler does not damage themselves while operating their wheelchair, there is a correct way to propel themselves in their wheelchair. The Consortium for Spinal Cord Medicine created a guide called "Preservation of Upper Limb Function: What You Should Know," which lays out ways to prevent shoulder injuries [1]. Avoiding certain surfaces and using long, smooth strokes when propelling the wheelchair will reduce the stress put on the user's shoulders. The work aims to design and create a program that will be able to track the motion of users in wheelchairs, specifically paraplegics, and detect if they will develop shoulder issues or injuries from their motion in a wheelchair. Since many wheelchair users develop shoulder injuries due to the pressure they may or may not know they are applying to their shoulders, this chapter aims to create a working program that will present data that pertains to the movement and kinematics of the

DOI: 10.1201/9781003403678-2

19

wheelchair user for interpretation. The applied force of the user pressing down on the wheels can cause their arms to push up and away from their shoulders, which can put unneeded stress on that joint. This behavior is due to the many degrees of freedom that the shoulder possesses [2]. While there is no way to fully reduce the pressure on a manual wheelchair user's shoulder. With the utilization of MATLAB® and its different toolboxes, a program will be created to analyze a wheelchair user's motion to present data that is relevant to the kinematics data provided by the smart-wheel wheelchair. Using a video of the subject from their side profile, a chart will be output that tracks the motion of the subject. This chart will record the user's motion over time and can be correlated to the kinematics data. The main focus of this chapter is geared toward detecting tracking points on a subject while they propel themselves in a wheelchair. This will be accomplished through the use of image processing using the program MATLAB. A videotape will be composed of different subjects propelling themselves in a wheelchair, and the program will track the motion of their arms. Tracking their arms will determine if their wheelchair propulsion technique is correct and is not placing unwanted stress on their shoulders. A few motions that are detrimental to shoulder health include short, jerky motions; elbow distance from the body; and pressure applied to the rim of the wheelchair. One of the major ways to reduce shoulder muscle strain is the technique used to propel the wheelchair. A study found that the tangential forces applied to the wheel put an increased amount of stress on the shoulder muscles, specifically the anterior deltoid, which induces movement in the humeral head, causing shoulder pain. Another study focused on the difference between geared and non-geared manual wheelchairs, and they found a connection between muscle activity and the stroke cycle, which in turn decreases the forces applied to the shoulder joint [3]. The Consortium for Spinal Cord Medicine also mentions wheelchair users using long, smooth motions to reduce the strain on their shoulders [1]. With all of this in mind, the proper technique to reduce the strain put on shoulder joints is to reduce the amount of muscle activity in the user's shoulders. This is accomplished by the user using long strokes less often to propel themselves, which reduces the muscle activity that can lead to shoulder pain. Another study looked at the movement of different joints when a wheelchair user performed different maneuvers. They found that joint movement can be exaggerated by the swiftness of the maneuver, parquet substantial, flatness of the impulsion, and propulsion style [4]. The main takeaway from this study is that the actual motion and technique of the wheelchair maneuver can affect the strain applied to the shoulder joint.

2.1.1 MOTIVATION

Paraplegia, a condition resulting in the loss of motor and sensory function in the lower limbs, affects thousands of individuals worldwide. While advances in medical technology and rehabilitation have improved the quality of life for paraplegics, they continue to face unique challenges, particularly concerning upper extremity function. The shoulders, crucial for wheelchair mobility and activities of daily living, are highly susceptible to damage in paraplegics due to chronic overuse and increased stress [5]. This essay explores the motivation for early recognition of shoulder damage in paraplegics, emphasizing the importance of timely intervention, prevention of long-term complications, and the enhancement of overall quality of life [6].

- Implications of Shoulder Damage in Paraplegics:

  Shoulder damage in paraplegics can lead to significant functional impairment and reduce their independence and participation in daily activities. The repetitive stress placed on the shoulders during wheelchair propulsion, transfers, and overhead tasks can result in a range of injuries, including rotator cuff tears, tendonitis, impingement syndrome, and shoulder instability. These conditions can cause pain, weakness, restricted range of motion, and joint deformities, limiting the individual's ability to perform essential tasks and affecting their overall well-being [7].

- Importance of Early Recognition:

  Early recognition of shoulder damage plays a pivotal role in preventing the progression of injuries and minimizing long-term complications. Paraplegics often experience reduced pain perception below the level of injury, making it difficult to detect shoulder problems at an early stage. Ignoring or neglecting initial symptoms can lead to chronic pain, functional limitations, and the need for invasive interventions like surgeries. Timely recognition enables healthcare professionals to implement appropriate interventions, such as physical therapy, assistive devices, and lifestyle modifications, to address the issues before they worsen. Additionally, early detection allows for the inclusion of preventive strategies, such as education on proper wheelchair propulsion techniques and exercises to strengthen shoulder muscles, ultimately reducing the risk of shoulder damage [8].

- Preservation of Independence and Quality of Life:

  The ability to maintain independence is paramount for individuals with paraplegia. Healthy shoulders are vital for wheelchair mobility, transfers, self-care activities, and participating in recreational and social pursuits. Early recognition and intervention for shoulder damage can help preserve and enhance independence, allowing paraplegics to continue engaging in activities they enjoy. By addressing shoulder issues promptly, individuals can maintain their functional abilities and reduce the reliance on caregivers or assistive devices, promoting a sense of autonomy and self-esteem [2].

  Furthermore, early recognition and treatment of shoulder damage contribute to an improved quality of life. Pain and functional limitations resulting from untreated shoulder injuries can have a profound impact on an individual's emotional well-being and overall satisfaction. By proactively managing shoulder problems, paraplegics can minimize discomfort, maximize physical function, and experience an enhanced quality of life. This, in turn, positively affects their mental health, social interactions, and overall participation in the community. Early recognition of shoulder damage in paraplegics is crucial for mitigating the consequences of chronic overuse, preventing long-term complications, and preserving independence and quality of life. By promptly identifying and addressing shoulder issues, healthcare professionals can implement appropriate interventions and preventive measures, improving functional outcomes and reducing the burden on individuals with paraplegia. Efforts should be made to raise awareness among both healthcare providers and paraplegics themselves about the importance of regular shoulder assessments, the significance of early intervention, and the potential benefits of maintaining healthy shoulders.

2.1.2 USE OF SMART HEALTHCARE FOR SHOULDER DAMAGE IN PARAPLEGICS

Early recognition of shoulder damage in paraplegics is a critical aspect of their healthcare management, as it can significantly impact their quality of life and independence. Smart hospital technologies offer innovative solutions to enhance the identification and management of shoulder injuries in this population. By integrating remote monitoring, wearable devices, telemedicine, data analytics, and integrated health monitoring systems, smart hospitals can revolutionize the early recognition of shoulder damage in paraplegics, providing timely interventions and personalized care [9]. Remote monitoring and wearable devices play a crucial role in tracking and analyzing the shoulder movements and patterns of paraplegics. Sensors and accelerometers embedded in wheelchairs or wearable devices can capture data on the frequency, intensity, and duration of wheelchair propulsion and transfers. Machine learning algorithms can then analyze this data in real time to identify abnormal movement patterns and detect early signs of shoulder damage, such as excessive stress or repetitive movements. Healthcare professionals can intervene proactively by providing personalized recommendations for proper techniques, exercise regimens, and assistive devices to mitigate the risk of further injury [10]. Telemedicine and virtual consultations offer a convenient and accessible avenue for early recognition of shoulder damage in paraplegics, particularly for those facing geographical or logistical barriers in accessing specialized healthcare services [11]. Through videoconferencing and telecommunication technologies, healthcare providers can remotely assess the individual's shoulder function, range of motion, and pain levels. Patients can demonstrate their movements, guided by healthcare professionals, who can provide real-time feedback and instructions for exercises or modifications to prevent or address shoulder injuries. Telemedicine also allows for regular follow-ups and monitoring of progress, ensuring early detection of any changes in shoulder health and enabling timely interventions [12]. Data analytics and predictive models can aid in identifying risk factors and developing personalized approaches for paraplegics at higher risk of shoulder damage. By analyzing historical patient data, including demographics, medical history, lifestyle factors, and patterns of wheelchair use, machine learning algorithms can identify patterns and correlations between specific parameters and the likelihood of developing shoulder injuries. This information assists healthcare providers in identifying high-risk individuals and implementing preventive measures tailored to their needs [13]. Predictive models can also forecast the progression of shoulder damage based on individual characteristics, enabling early recognition and intervention before severe complications arise. Integrated health monitoring systems, encompassing electronic health records (EHRs), wearable sensors, and mobile applications, are instrumental in creating a comprehensive shoulder health monitoring platform. By integrating these systems, healthcare providers can access and share relevant information about the individual's shoulder health seamlessly. This holistic view allows for tracking changes over time and identifying potential red flags [14]. Moreover, individuals themselves can actively engage in self-monitoring through user-friendly applications, reporting symptoms, documenting daily activities, and receiving timely reminders for exercises and proper shoulder care. The integration of health monitoring systems empowers paraplegics to take an active role in their shoulder health, reduces the burden of physical assessments, and improves access to specialized care. In conclusion, smart hospital technologies hold immense potential in solving the challenge of early recognition of shoulder damage in paraplegics. By leveraging remote monitoring, wearable devices, telemedicine, data analytics, and integrated health monitoring systems, healthcare providers can identify shoulder injuries at an early stage, deliver timely interventions, and personalize preventive measures. Smart hospitals empower paraplegics to actively participate in their healthcare, improve their quality of life, and maintain their independence. As technology continues to advance, the integration of smart hospital solutions in the early recognition of shoulder damage in paraplegics will revolutionize their care, optimizing outcomes and enhancing their overall well-being [15].

2.1.3 SMART HEALTHCARE VS. CONVENTION HOSPITAL IN EARLY RECOGNITION OF INJURIES

A smart healthcare hospital offers several advantages over conventional hospitals when it comes to the early recognition of shoulder damage in paraplegics. The integration of advanced technologies and data-driven approaches in a smart hospital environment significantly enhances the ability to identify, monitor, and manage shoulder injuries in paraplegic patients [16]. With remote monitoring capabilities, smart hospitals can promptly identify any deviations from normal shoulder movements and provide immediate interventions. Healthcare professionals can remotely assess the data, analyze trends, and offer personalized recommendations for proper techniques, exercises, or modifications to prevent further damage and promote recovery. This real-time feedback enables timely adjustments to the individual's wheelchair use, daily activities, and exercise routines. In contrast, conventional hospitals may rely on periodic assessments, leading to delayed interventions and potential worsening of shoulder injuries. Smart hospitals harness the power of data analytics and predictive models to identify risk factors and develop personalized approaches for paraplegics at higher risk of shoulder damage. By analyzing historical patient data, including demographics, medical history, lifestyle factors, and patterns of wheelchair use, machine learning algorithms can identify patterns and correlations between specific parameters and the likelihood of developing shoulder injuries. This information assists healthcare providers in identifying high-risk individuals and implementing preventive measures tailored to their needs. Predictive models can also forecast the progression of shoulder damage based on individual characteristics, enabling early recognition and intervention before severe complications arise. Conventional hospitals often rely on manual record-keeping and limited data analysis capabilities, making it challenging to identify and address shoulder injuries at an early stage [17]. Integrated Health Monitoring Systems: Smart hospitals integrate various health monitoring systems, such as electronic health records (EHRs), wearable sensors, and mobile applications, to create a comprehensive shoulder health monitoring platform. This integration allows for seamless data sharing among healthcare providers, ensuring that all relevant information about the individual's shoulder health is readily available. By consolidating data from different sources, healthcare professionals can gain a holistic view of the individual's shoulder status, track changes over time, and identify potential red flags. Moreover, individuals themselves can actively engage in self-monitoring through user-friendly applications, reporting symptoms, documenting daily activities, and receiving timely reminders for exercises and proper shoulder care. This level of integration and patient engagement is challenging to achieve in conventional hospitals. Smart healthcare hospitals offer significant advantages over conventional hospitals in the early recognition of shoulder damage in paraplegics. Through remote monitoring, wearable devices, telemedicine, data analytics, and integrated health monitoring systems, smart hospitals provide continuous monitoring, timely intervention, and personalized care. These advancements empower paraplegics to actively participate in their shoulder health management, reduce the risk of further damage, and enhance their overall quality of life. As smart hospital technologies continue to evolve, their application in the early recognition of shoulder damage holds great promise for improving outcomes and optimizing the healthcare experience for paraplegic individuals [18].

2.2   PROBLEM REVIEW

Initially, the main issue with the chapter was associated with the data collected. The first round of videos had issues that were related to the cameras themselves and the environment in which the videos were taken. The videos were taken outside in a partially shady area, and the sunspots became an issue for the infrared videos. The reflected sunlight off of light-colored objects such as the concrete sidewalk has become a problem (Figure 2.1).

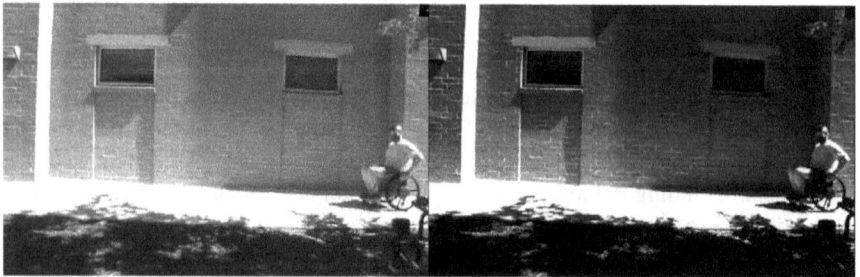

FIGURE 2.1   Gamma correction comparison for infrared video.

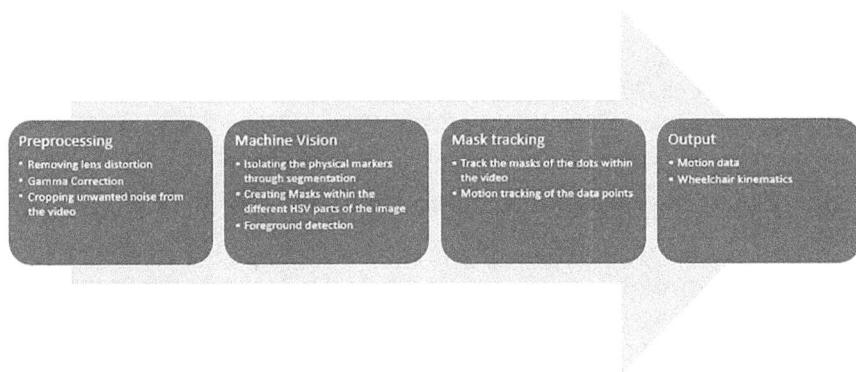

FIGURE 2.2 Algorithm flowchart.

Attempts at gamma correcting the videos were made, but the sunlight turned out to be much brighter than the reflective markers on the subject's arm. As indicated in Figure 2.2, with the maximum amount of gamma correction shown on the right, the reflected sunlight was too bright and whitewashed the whole image. Then the GoPro footage that was taken and was initially ignored. With the practice of Premiere Pro, the wide-angle electron lens distortion was removed from the footage and it was able to be used, but the markers were still very small and difficult to pick up with the initial image processing algorithm. The second round of videos that were taken were only GoPro videos, and they were also sent through Premiere Pro to remove the fisheye lens distortion. The second algorithm design includes the Open-Pose to detect the subject's arms. This became problematic trouble with using the library in conjunction with MATLAB. The MATLAB example code has errors due to a missing file that MATLAB did not supply with the example. They have resolute this matter, nevertheless the example code continues to produce unknown errors. With these errors, a new algorithm had to be created because Open-Pose was no longer a viable option. The current algorithm focuses on the detection of the dots along the subjects' arms. The dots that were intended to be used as the tracking points are too small to be picked up accurately, but the white stickers that the markers were placed on along the subject's arm remained immense enough that it was separated from the subject's arm and tracked. This led to better results but left room for increased noise due to the environment in which the footage was shot. Through morphology techniques and cropping of the footage, most of the noise was removed. Through entire of the data points filtered out, it was noted that the shoulder marker was only detected 70% of the time, the elbow marker was detected 55% of the time, and the wrist marker was only detected 34% of the time. These errors were caused by a few different factors that remained associated to the subject on the test. The markers changed shape due to the circumstance that they were placed on the subject's sleeve and as the subject moved, their sleeve would wrinkle and in turn change the shape of the markers. This caused the algorithm to filter out the marker due to its decreased size. The wrist marker would also change because the HSV color segmentation would detect both the color of the marker and the color of the subject's pants. Their pants fit within the saturation and value threshold of the marker, and this would cause the algorithm to combine the marker and the subject's pants into one large blob. This increased the side of the blob for the wrist marker, and the algorithm then filtered it out.

2.2.1 Present Technologies for Early Recognition of Shoulder Injury

Present technologies for early recognition of shoulder injury include [19–21]:

- Wearable Sensors:

    Wearable sensors, such as accelerometers and gyroscopes, can be attached to the upper body or worn on the affected shoulder to monitor movement patterns and detect abnormal motions or excessive stress. These sensors capture data on range of motion, acceleration, and orientation, providing valuable insights into the biomechanics of shoulder movements. By analyzing this data, healthcare professionals can identify deviations from normal patterns and detect early signs of shoulder injury.
- Motion Capture Systems:

    Motion capture systems utilize cameras and markers placed on the body to track movement in real-time. This technology enables precise measurement of joint angles and kinematics during shoulder movements. By comparing the captured data to established norms or predetermined thresholds, healthcare providers can identify abnormal movement patterns or asymmetries that may indicate a shoulder injury. Motion capture systems are often used in research or specialized clinics to assess shoulder function and detect subtle abnormalities.
- Electromyography (EMG):

    EMG is a technique that measures the electrical activity of muscles. It involves placing electrodes on the skin or using implantable sensors to detect muscle activation patterns. EMG can be used to assess muscle activity during shoulder movements and identify any imbalances or abnormal muscle recruitment patterns. Changes in muscle activation patterns may indicate muscle weakness, fatigue, or compensatory movements, which can be early signs of shoulder injury.
- Pressure Mapping:

    Pressure mapping systems use pressure sensors embedded in seating surfaces or wheelchair cushions to measure the distribution of pressure on the shoulder and surrounding areas. By monitoring pressure distribution during activities such as wheelchair propulsion or transfers, healthcare professionals can identify areas of high pressure or prolonged pressure that may contribute to shoulder injury. This information can guide recommendations for proper seating posture, cushion selection, and pressure relief techniques to minimize the risk of shoulder damage.
- Machine Learning and Artificial Intelligence:

    Machine learning and artificial intelligence algorithms can analyze large data sets of patient information, including demographics, medical

history, and movement data, to identify patterns and correlations associated with shoulder injuries. By training these algorithms on known cases
of shoulder injury and healthy individuals, predictive models can be
developed to assess the risk of developing shoulder injury in specific
populations. These models can help healthcare providers prioritize interventions and allocate resources effectively.

• Imaging Techniques:

    Imaging techniques such as magnetic resonance imaging (MRI) or
ultrasound can be used to visualize the structures of the shoulder joint,
including tendons, ligaments, and cartilage. These imaging modalities can
identify structural abnormalities or signs of inflammation that may be
indicative of a shoulder injury. While imaging techniques are not neces-
sarily considered early recognition tools, they can provide valuable diagnostic information when other symptoms or clinical findings suggest the
presence of a shoulder injury.

    It's important to note that while these technologies offer valuable in-
sights and aid in the early recognition of shoulder injuries, they should be
used in conjunction with clinical evaluation and expertise. Healthcare
professionals play a crucial role in interpreting the data provided by these
technologies and making informed decisions regarding the diagnosis and
management of shoulder injuries.

2.3   ALGORITHM DESIGN

The algorithm for this chapter follows the same algorithm that is used to detect
white blood cells with a few variations [22, 23]. The preprocessing required
for this chapter is to remove the fish-eye lens distortion and slightly increase
the gamma to decrease the contrast created by the lights caught in the frame.
From there, the code will take in the video and perform several image processing
operations on the individual video frames. Initially, the processing is to apply a
Gabor filter and perform a k-means clustering segmentation to isolate the white
markers in the frames. This method divides the frames into four parts, and each
pixel is given a mean value that is used to place them within the area of the
centroid of one of the four cluster parts. That process is repeated until convergence is reached and a final segmented image is produced, which reduces the
amount of processing required per frame. From there, the segmented image is
transformed from RGB to HSV. Then, using the saturation and value layers,
masks are created from the layers using color detection. Morphology is implemented in the form of removing objects that have a higher area of pixels than
the desired object. Morphology is then used again by bit-anding the two HSV
layers to isolate the parts of the image that were detected in each layer. The
combined layered image undergoes the process to remove larger and smaller
blobs than the white markers. The blobs that are left undergo one more process
with the foreground detection blob. The blobs from the initial detection are
applied to the foreground detection filter, and any blobs within this area will
be counted and their centroid locations recorded. From those recorded values, a

marker is placed over the blob, which marks the location of the detected blobs in the video. Different values will be recorded from the locations of the tracking points and will be output to the graph. The flowchart for the algorithm can be seen in the figure below.

The data collected for the initial tests includes two different types of cameras and the data collected from the wheelchair. The camera managed to record a side and front view of the subject while the assessments were being conducted. At the start of each trial, the subject started at the very far right of the side view cameras' field of view. Before any of the devices can be turned on, the subject must ensure that they are not touching the push rims of the wheelchair to prevent miscalibration of the wheelchair when it begins collecting data. The cameras and the wheelchair had remote starts, so each of them was started individually and then the subject was given the signal to start moving. Multiple videos were taken to give a wide range of motion, from slow and smooth to fast and jerky. Once the first set of data was collected, the preprocessing steps had to be implemented. The infrared videos had to undergo gamma correction, and the GoPro footage had to undergo fish-eye lens distortion removal. With all this completed, the first round of data collection was concluded. The footage for the second session of data collection was captured exclusively with GoPro cameras. This set of data was recorded in a similar manner; the first round of data was collected, with the exclusion of the infrared cameras. This provides a wider range of variation in motion because of the different subjects used and how they go about propelling themselves in the wheelchair. To increase the accuracy of the tracking data, the videos must be filmed with a featureless background and nothing the individual is wearing should match the tracking points. This will guarantee that the tracking data is accurate and noise free to ensure the best results.

2.4 SIMULATION RESULTS

The first round of recording ended with a few different issues. Initially, the GoPro footage could not be used due to the fish-eye lens distortion, which would have thrown off the position tracking of the markers on the subject as they moved across the camera's field of view. A solution to remove this distortion had not been found, so the GoPro footage remained unused. The infrared footage was used as a substitute of the GoPro video because the tracking markers were infrared reflectors and would show up very well in that type of footage. The issue with the infrared footage was the amount of reflected light from the sun off of the concrete and wall around the subject that can be seen in Figure 2.2. Gamma correction was implemented but was unable to remove enough of the reflected light while also leaving the detection markers still visible. The second round of recording was much better but presented a number of new issues. The fish-eye lens distortion was present, but with the use of Premiere Pro, the distortion was removed from the footage. The new problems were the amount of noise from the background around the subject and the subject itself. The background noise was from the extra people moving in the background, which prevented the foreground detection code from working properly. There is also noise from the surroundings, including white labels and the pants the subject is wearing,

Clustered Image

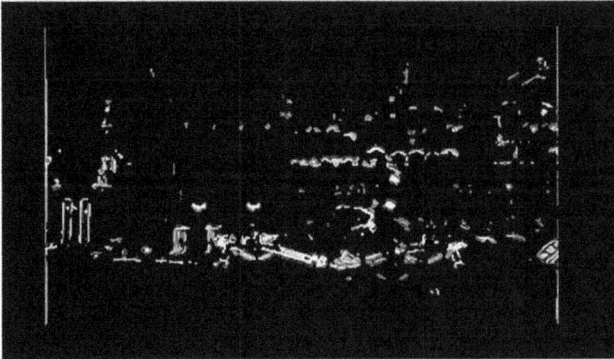

FIGURE 2.3 A frame after undergoing segmentation.

which appear in the mask of the video. Although most of the noise from the unwanted detected objects was able to be removed, some of the noise still remains and it has become challenging to remove. The first detection method used was clustering segmentation, which removed an abundance of the noise from the video. The segmentation scheme used was K-means. When integrated with a Gabor filter, this improves segmentation by adding texture and spatial aspects. Thirty Gabor filters were used with ten different wavelengths ranging from 0 to 2 and 3 orientations from 0 to 120 degrees. When segmented into four regions, most of the background was removed.

The segmentation in Figure 2.3 made it much easier to process all of the frames of the video because the segmentation removed most of the framework around the markers on the subject. The HSV color detection helped to detect the markers in the segmented image. This worked in amalgamation with morphology to remove detected objects larger than the markers themselves from the mask.

This method of detection, seen in Figure 2.4, also included the other blobs in the video that were considered noise. This method left a lot of blobs that were not about the video and, in the end, ended up throwing off the detection since the high number of detected objects. The final addition to the algorithm was the foreground detection mask given in Figure 2.5.

Saturation Mask   Value Mask

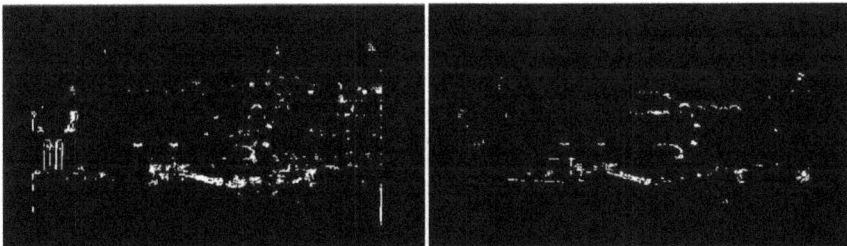

FIGURE 2.4 The color detection saturation and value masks.

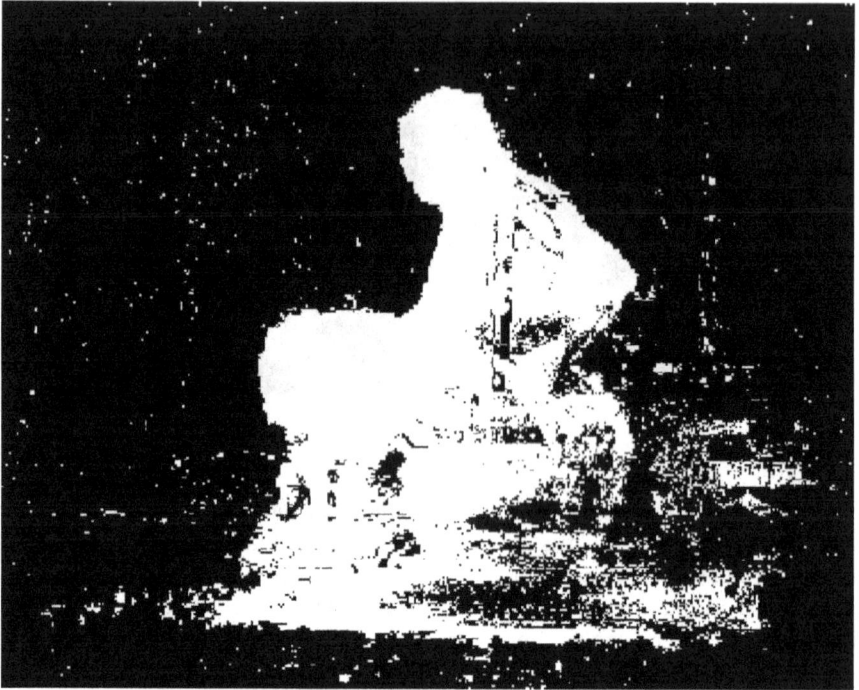

FIGURE 2.5   Foreground detection mask.

This was bit ANDed with the mask created from the segmentation and HSV color detection masks. This led to an increased reduction of noise from the background in the frames throughout the whole video. Unfortunately, this led to an increase in noise from the subject. The foreground detection ended up including more noise on the subject in the first 20 frames of the video due to the low variance of the foreground detection and the training slides required at the beginning of the video. This was overcome by visual detection of the markers from the blobs and their locations, which were exported to an Excel file. The error for the detection of the markers in each frame can be seen in Figure 2.6. The error is high for most of the video, but the detection rate for the shoulder and elbow is high enough that it is suitable to prove the data needs for this chapter.

Another issue is the amount of time required to process a video. Isolating the markers through segmentation and the HSV color isolation only takes a few seconds, but processing a whole video requires more time depending on the quantity of frames per video. Isolating only 15 frames' code changes were tested, and that takes around five minutes. Processing a whole video with roughly 300 frames can take up to an hour or more, depending on the dimensions of the images and their resolution. The tracking data that was collected from the program was exported to an Excel file. From there, the data markers had to be manually filtered to distinguish between noise and the data points.

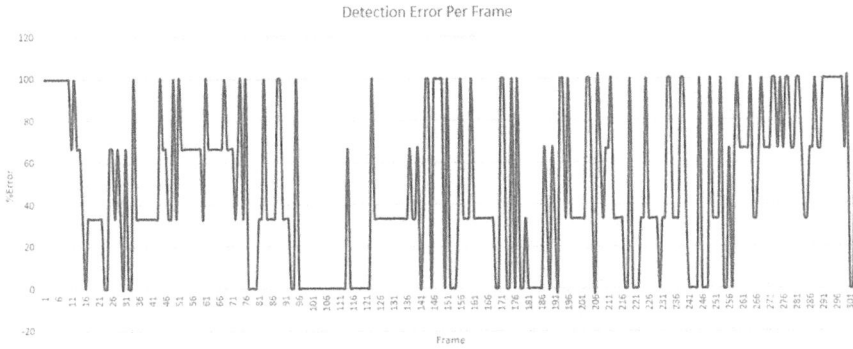

FIGURE 2.6   Error per frame of the detected markers.

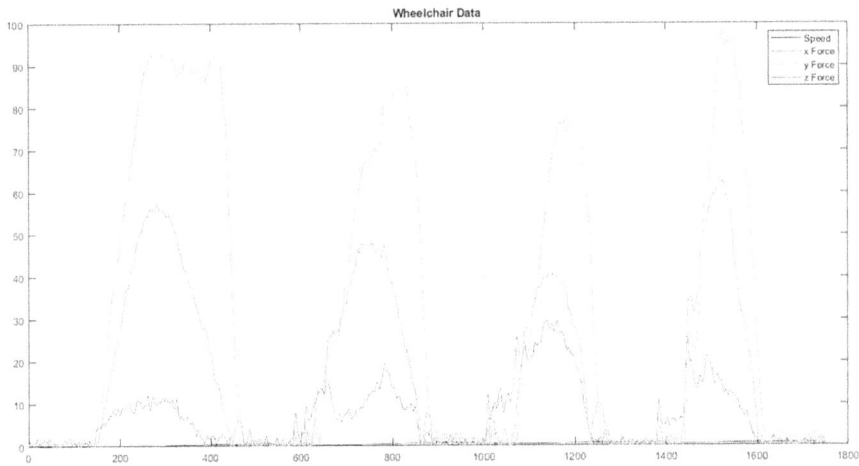

FIGURE 2.7   The smartwheel data collected for this trial.

Since the very low detection rate of the wrist and elbow markers, only the shoulder had enough data to print out a complete tracking data graph in Figure 2.8. The data in Figure 2.8 tracks the change in position on the y-axis for the shoulder tracking marker. When the data is at its peak, this means an individual has positioned their hand on the push rim and is in the process of propelling the wheelchair forward, which correlates to the graph in Figure 2.7 by displaying the force that is applied at the y-axis motion's peak. This shows that there is a connection between the amount of movement in the subject's shoulders and body and the amount of force that is being applied to the wheelchair. Most of the power that is applied to push a wheelchair forward comes from the movement of the person's body and not only their arms. This y-axis data shows there is a connection between the amount of motion a subject's body undergoes in the y-direction and the amount of force they apply in the y-direction. The more drastic the change in the motion of the shoulder tracking marker and the

Top Marker Y-Axis Movement

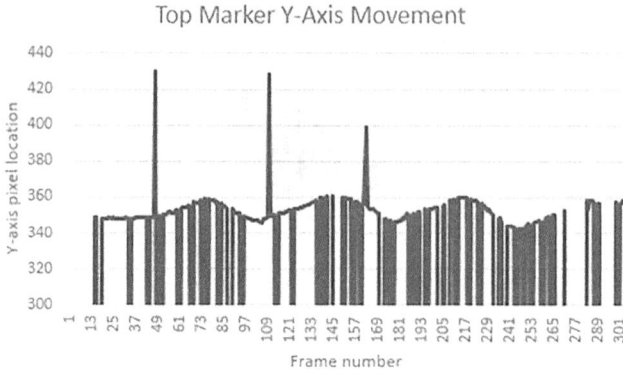

FIGURE 2.8   Shoulder marker y-axis tracking data.

Shoulder to Elbow Distance

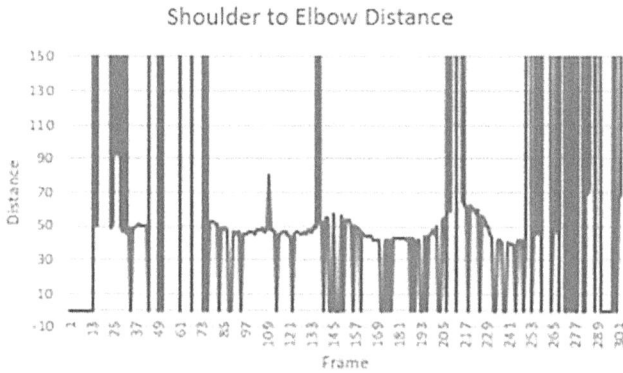

FIGURE 2.9   Distance between the shoulder and elbow of the subject as they move over time.

higher the pressure applied to the push rim, the more likely it is that the subject will develop shoulder-related complications.

Another connection between the tracking data and the wheelchair data that can be made is the change in distance between each of the tracking points, given in Figure 2.9. Since the shoulder and elbow detection rates were higher, only the remoteness between these two points can be used. As the subject places their hands on the push rim, their elbow is bent, and from the side view angle, the distance between the shoulder and elbow is smaller. When the subject finishes one push, their arm is extended and the distance between the points from the viewpoint of the camera is increased. The connection between the tracking data and the wheelchair kinematic data is that the faster the distance increases in the tracking data, the faster the wheelchair moves and more pressure is applied. The smaller the distance and the higher the pressure applied to the push rim, the more likely it could lead to shoulder injuries because of the pressure applied to the shoulders.

2.5 CHALLENGES IN IMPLEMENTATION OF SMART HEALTHCARE FOR INJURY DETECTION

While smart healthcare technologies offer numerous advantages for the early recognition of shoulder injuries, there are also some potential disadvantages to consider [24, 25, 26]:

- Cost: Implementing smart healthcare solutions can be costly, requiring investments in technology infrastructure, software development, training, and maintenance. The expenses associated with acquiring and maintaining the necessary devices, sensors, and data analytics systems may pose a financial burden for healthcare providers and limit widespread adoption.
- Technical Complexity: Smart healthcare technologies involve complex systems, including wearable devices, remote monitoring platforms, data analytics algorithms, and integration with existing healthcare systems. Managing and maintaining these systems may require specialized technical expertise and resources. Healthcare providers may face challenges in training staff and ensuring the seamless integration and interoperability of different components.
- Privacy and Security Concerns: With the use of smart healthcare technologies, there is a need to collect, store, and transmit sensitive patient data. This raises concerns regarding privacy and security. Safeguarding patient information from unauthorized access, data breaches, or cyber-attacks is of utmost importance. Stricter regulations and robust security measures need to be in place to protect patient confidentiality and maintain data integrity.
- Patient Acceptance and Compliance: The successful implementation of smart healthcare technologies relies on patient acceptance and compliance. Some individuals may be hesitant to embrace new technologies or find it challenging to incorporate wearable devices into their daily routines. Moreover, continuous monitoring may require patients to adhere to specific protocols, perform regular self-assessments, and actively engage in reporting symptoms or following recommended exercises. Lack of patient compliance can limit the effectiveness of early recognition efforts.
- Limitations in Accuracy and Interpretation: Although smart healthcare technologies provide valuable data, they may have limitations in accuracy and interpretation. Wearable sensors and motion tracking systems may have inherent errors or require calibration for accurate measurements. Data analytics algorithms may not always capture the full complexity of shoulder movements or account for individual variations. Healthcare providers need to carefully interpret the data provided by these technologies and consider it in conjunction with clinical evaluation to avoid false positives or false negatives.
- Access and Equity: The availability and accessibility of smart healthcare technologies may not be evenly distributed across all populations, potentially exacerbating existing healthcare disparities. Limited access to technology or internet connectivity, especially in rural or underserved areas, may hinder the implementation of smart healthcare solutions. Ensuring

equitable access to these technologies and addressing disparities in healthcare delivery should be a priority to maximize their benefits.

In conclusion, while smart healthcare technologies offer significant advantages for the early recognition of shoulder injuries, there are challenges and potential drawbacks that need to be addressed. Healthcare providers and technology developers should carefully consider the cost-effectiveness, technical complexity, privacy and security concerns, patient acceptance, accuracy limitations, and equitable access to ensure the successful integration and utilization of smart healthcare solutions in the early recognition of shoulder injuries.

2.6 DISCUSSIONS AND CONCLUSIONS

With the completion of this chapter, the prototype created output graphs of the position data from the tracking markers on the subject's arm and presents a graph of the kinematics data collected from the wheelchair side by side. This code allows for the autonomous tracking of the motion of a wheelchair user and provides pertinent information relating to the subject's motion while operating their wheelchair. This chapter, if continued, would be able to detect whether a paraplegic wheelchair user is doing something harmful while operating their wheelchair with greater accuracy and from multiple angles. While the prototype is able to isolate the tracking markers placed on a subject's arm and output the results from one camera perspective, this chapter could be manipulated to correlate the information gathered from multiple views and provide an accurate display of the angle and position data in a three-dimensional space. From there, the data collected could accurately describe and pinpoint which wheelchair arm motions are harmful to the user's shoulders.

FUNDING

There is no funding support in this work.

Compliance with ethical standards.

ETHICAL APPROVAL

This article does not contain any studies with human participants or animals performed by any of the authors.

All authors do not have any conflict of interest.

REFERENCES

1. Consortium for Spinal Cord Medicine and Paralyzed Veterans of America, *Preservation of upper limb function: what you should know*. Washington, DC: Consortium for Spinal Cord Medicine, 2008.

2. C. Kertesz, "Physiotherapy exercises recognition based on RGB-D human skeleton models," in Proceedings of European Modelling Symposium, Nov. 2013, pp. 21–29.
3. A. Kumar, H. Sharma, N. Gour, and R. Pareek, "A hybrid technique for the PAPR reduction of NOMA waveform", *International Journal of Communication Systems*, 10.1002/dac.5412.O.
4. W. N. Lam, A. F. T. Mak, W. C. Tam and R. A. Cooper, "Kinematics of the wrist, elbow and shoulder during manual wheelchair maneuvers," Proceedings of the Second Joint 24th Annual Conference and the Annual Fall Meeting of the Biomedical Engineering Society] [Engineering in Medicine and Biology, Houston, TX, USA, 2002, pp. 2573–2576 vol. 3, doi: 10.1109/IEMBS.2002.1053433.
5. A. Bevilacqua, L. Brennan, R. Argent, B. Caulfield, and T. Kechadi, "Rehabilitation exercise segmentation for autonomous biofeedback systems with ConvFSM," in Proceedings of 41st Annual International Conference IEEE Engineering Medical Biological Society (EMBC), July 2019, pp. 574–579.
6. K. Chapron, V. Plantevin, F. Thullier, K. Bouchard, E. Duchesne, and S. Gaboury, "A more efficient transportable and scalable system for real-time activities and exercises recognition," *Sensors*, vol. 18, no. 1, p. 268, 2018.
7. F. Escalona, E. Martinez-Martin, E. Cruz, M. Cazorla, and F. Gomez-Donoso, "EVA: EVAluating at-home rehabilitation exercises using augmented reality and low-cost sensors," *Virtual Reality*, vol. 2019, pp. 1–15, Dec. 2019.
8. M. W. van Ooijen, M. Roerdink, M. Trekop, J. Visschedijk, T. W. Janssen, and P. J. Beek, "Functional gait rehabilitation in elderly people following a fall-related hip fracture using a treadmill with visual context: Design of a randomized controlled trial," *BMC Geriatrics*, vol. 13, no. 1, p. 34, Dec. 2013.
9. B. Bonnecháre, V. Sholukha, L. Omelina, S. Van Sint Jan, and B. Jansen, "3D analysis of upper limbs motion during rehabilitation exercises using the KinectTM sensor: Development, laboratory validation and clinical application," *Sensors*, vol. 18, no. 7, p. 2216, 2018.
10. F. Gu, K. Khoshhelham, S. Valaee, J. Shang, and R. Zhang, "Locomotion activity recognition using stacked denoising autoencoders," *IEEE Internet Things Journal*, vol. 5, no. 3, pp. 2085–2093, Jun. 2018.
11. T. T. Um, V. Babakeshizadeh, and D. Kulic, "Exercise motion classification from large-scale wearable sensor data using convolutional neural networks," in Proceedings of IEEE/RSJ International Conference on Intelligent Robots System (IROS), Sep. 2017, pp. 2385–239.
12. V. V. Quiñones, M. J. Macawile, A. Ballado, J. D. Cruz and M. V. Caya, "Leukocyte segmentation and counting based on microscopic blood images using HSV saturation component with blob analysis," *2018 3rd International Conference on Control and Robotics Engineering (ICCRE)*, Nagoya, 2018, pp. 254–258, 10.1109/ICCRE. 2018.8376475.
13. S. M. Sundara and R. Aarthi, "Segmentation and Evaluation of White Blood Cells using Segmentation Algorithms," *2019 3rd International Conference on Trends in Electronics and Informatics (ICOEI)*, Tirunelveli, India, 2019, pp. 1143–1146, 10.1109/ICOEI.2019.8862724.
14. S. Kobashi, N. Shibanuma, K. Kondo, M. Kurosaka and Y. Hata, "Robust estimation of knee kinematics after total knee arthroplasty with evolutional computing approach," *2007 IEEE International Conference on Image Processing*, San Antonio, TX, 2007, pp. VI-9–VI-12, 10.1109/ICIP.2007.4379508.
15. A. Kumar and H. Sharma, "Intelligent cognitive radio spectrum sensing based on energy detection for advanced waveforms," *Radio Electronics and Communication Systems*, vol. 65, no.3, pp. 175–181, 2022, Scopus Indexed.

16. M. K. Sharma and A. Kumar, "NOMA waveform technique using orthogonal supplementary signal for advanced 5g networks security", *Journal of Discrete Mathematical Sciences and Cryptography*, 2022. 10.1080/09720529.2022.2075088.

17. S. Hwang, S. Kim and Y. Kim, "Torque and power outputs on skilled and unskilled users during manual wheelchair propulsion," *2012 Annual International Conference of the IEEE Engineering in Medicine and Biology Society*, San Diego, CA, 2012, pp. 4820–4822, 10.1109/EMBC.2012.6347072.

18. A. Kumar and M. Gupta "A review on activities of fifth generation mobile communication system," *Alexandria Engineering Journal*, vol. 57, no. 2, pp. 1125–1135, 2017. https://www.sciencedirect.com/science/article/pii/S1110016817300601

19. A. Kumar, M. A. Albreem, M. Gupta, M. H. Alsharif and S. Kim, "Future 5G network based smart hospitals: Hybrid detection technique for latency improvement," in *IEEE Access*, vol. 8, pp. 153240–153249, 2020, 10.1109/ACCESS.2020.3017625. UI-PRMD-Analysis. [Online]. Available: https://github.com/niemasd/UIPRMD-Analysis

20. R. Lun and W. Zhao, "A survey of applications and human motion recognition with microsoftkinect," *International Journal of Pattern Recognition and Artificial Intelligence*, vol. 29, no. 5, 2015, Art. no. 1555008, pp. 32–41.

21. M. Capecci, M. G. Ceravolo, F. Ferracuti, S. Iarlori, V. Kyrki, A. Monteriá, and F. Verdini, "A hidden semi-Markov model-based approach for rehabilitation exercise assessment," *Journal of Biomedical Information*, vol. 78, pp. 1–11, May 2018.

22. A. Kumar, G. R. Dhana, M. Albreem and D. Le, "A comprehensive study on the role of advanced technologies in 5G based smart hospital," *Alexandria Engineering Journal*, vol. 2021, no. 60, pp. 5527–5536, 2021.

23. B. Ramakrishnan, A. Kumar, S. Chakravarty, M. Masud, and M. Baz, "Analysis of FBMC Waveform for 5G Network Based Smart Hospitals," *Applied Sciences*, vol. 11, no. 19, p. 8895, 2021. 10.3390/app11198895J.

24. Wang, Y. Chen, S. Hao, X. Peng, and L. Hu, "Deep learning for sensor-based activity recognition: A survey," *Pattern Recognition Letters*, vol. 119, pp. 3–11, Mar. 2019.

25. J. Qi, P. Yang, A. Waraich, Z. Deng, Y. Zhao, and Y. Yang, "Examining sensor-based physical activity recognition and monitoring for healthcare using Internet of Things: A systematic review," *Journal of Biomedical Informatics*, vol. 87, pp. 138–153, Nov. 2018.

26. S. Chakravarty and A. Kumar, "PAPR Reduction of GFDM Signals Using Encoder-Decoder Neural Network (Autoencoder)". *National Academy of Science Letters* (2023). 10.1007/s40009-023-01230-1.

3 Fulfilling the Vision of Worldwide Communication in Healthcare

A Study of Implant Wearable Devices for Healthcare

Deekshitha S Nayak
Mangalore Institute of Technology & Engineering,
Moodabidri, Karnataka, India

Korhan Cengiz
Department of Computer Engineering, Istinye University,
Istanbul, Turkey

3.1 INTRODUCTION

The development of new technologies like smart sensing, the emergence of mobile medicine, and the acceptance of customised health concepts have all contributed to substantial advancements in the field of smart wearable devices in recent years. One of them has come to light as being the most promising: medical wearable technology. These intelligent devices actively gather physiological indicators and track metabolic state, which not only inspire people to live healthier but also give a stable supply of healthcare data for illness finding and treatment [1]. Thus, the development of the mobile medical sector may be led by wearable medical technology. Wearable sensor technologies are gradually being used in more recognized customer and medical products. Wearable technology can offer real-time information concerning an individual's health issues in circumstances including the elderly, people in rehabilitation, and people with various disabilities. The five main characteristics of wearable technology as a standard healthcare intervention are (1) sustainability and durability, (2) interactivity and intelligence, (3) wireless mobility, (4) wearability and portability, and (5) easy operation and downsizing. As a result, they can provide an impartial option for managing and tracking the development of chronic diseases [2].

DOI: 10.1201/9781003403678-3

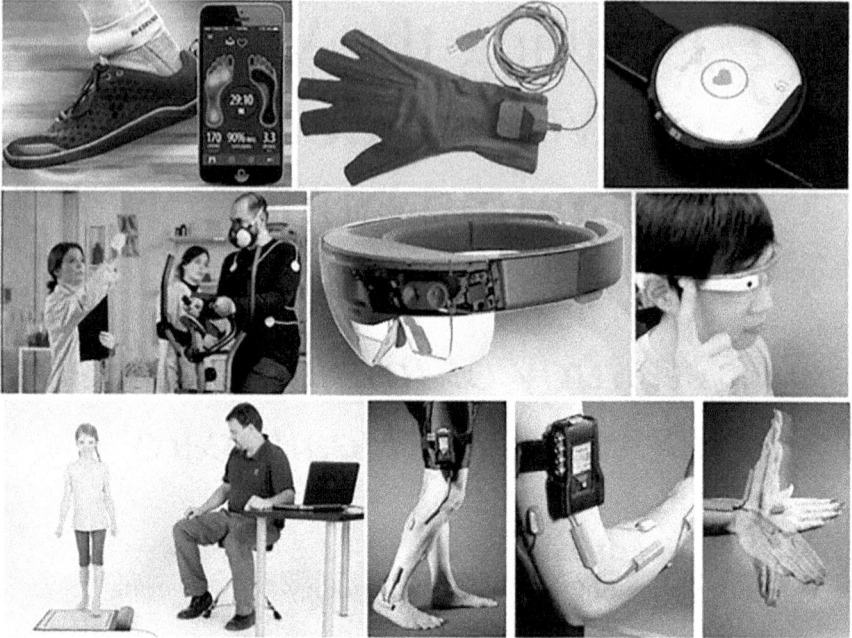

FIGURE 3.1 Various sensors in the wearable devices of healthcare [1].

Wearable technology could provide innovative solutions to healthcare problems. Applications for wearable technology like activity tracking and weight management were developed with disease prevention and health maintenance in mind [3]. Another application for wearable technology is the treatment of patients and disorders. Wearable apps may have a direct impact on clinical decision making. In order to create applications for fitness and healthcare, automatic human movement identification is important [4]. Step counts, altitudes climbed, distance travelled, and rate of running/walking are fitness tracking metrics that are incorporated into cell phones. Position sensing is especially suitable since time spent inactively is a reliable predictor of upcoming health problems. Sleep detection can also be done with movement sensors. Professional sports are using Inertial Measurement Unit (IMU) sensors more frequently, and athletes are using a variety of dedicated sensor-based applications [5]. These programmes typically cost too much to be used on a regular basis in the healthcare industry. Figure 3.1 shows the typical sensors for sensing human activity.

A smart watch's accelerometer can monitor activity and sleeping patterns. Sensors placed on the lower back and neck can be used to collect information regarding the motion range (ROM) of the upper body and head. In athletics, sensors are widely employed to monitor metrics like velocity, speed, and long-term fitness improvement. They may be placed on the leg following clinical management to aid with rehabilitation. Data on head and neck mobility is collected using headbands. The ability of data gloves to record information on finger movements, tremors, and restrictions of the finger joint is being studied at the research level. These devices are readily available on the market and are often used for health and fitness tracking.

3.2   LITERATURE REVIEW

IMU-based research investigations are becoming increasingly prevalent, however, the majority of these studies are conducted in a regulated clinical setting under close supervision. To achieve unrestricted patient monitoring and to extract the psychological and physical conditions of patients, they concentrate on processing multivariate sensor data. Earlier a wearable device may be used for research or clinical reasons, it is essential to recognize the many types of data that may be essential over time from data collection. In a therapeutic setting, IMU sensors are most frequently employed to monitor and record patient's movement. IMUs are affixed to particular parts of the patient's body, like the back, neck, wrist, or waist [6], and under the supervision of a doctor or an expert technical specialist, the wearer's gestures are accurately detected and recorded. Patients may be evaluated during a clinical assessment on particular functional tests that are pertinent to the ailment being examined. The information gathered from each sensor which is used as supplementary material to help a clinician determine whether a patient's health status has improved or declined [7]. IMU sensor data is typically stored in a monitoring device, like a microcontroller unit, which also controls data collection from the sensor and can enhance signal quality. Participants in clinical trial sensors and execute a series of preset movements as specified by the study protocol. For instance, axial spondyloarthritis progression can be detected by changes in spinal motion, but until recently, clinicians lacked an accurate way to monitor this. The different kinds and data sources that can be used in a medical trial are depicted in Figure 3.2.

3.3   WEARABLE TECHNOLOGY IN THE HEALTHCARE SECTOR

IMU sensors are the common type of sensor found in home monitoring systems and are widely used to track patient activity and healing at home. A patient may be asked to wear IMU sensors for a duration lengthier than 24 hours for each evaluation session in an ambulatory observing state. While data is being continuously

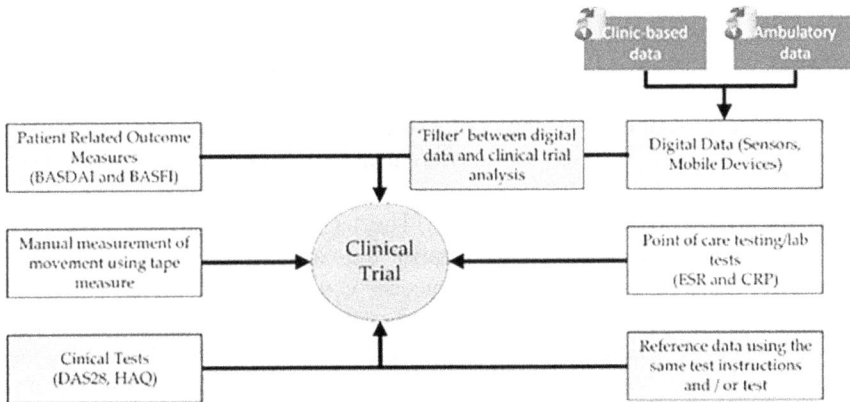

FIGURE 3.2   Data sources that could be applied in clinical research [1].

logged from each wearable sensor during this time, the wearer is typically expected to perform standard well-designed assessments as regular day activities. According to clinical studies, wearable technology is increasingly frequently used to track activity at home and examine patients' worries about their lifestyle, obesity, and symptoms of diseases like pulmonary problems, hypertension, diabetes, and cardiac disease. These are seen in a wearable device that is appropriately pertinent, typically equipped with the IMU sensor and managed by a smartphone application [8]. Musculoskeletal fitness may be tracked successfully with wearable sensors. These sensors are capable of precisely measuring head rotation, neck movement, flexion and extension motion, and joint angle [9]. Standardized functional tests can be used to evaluate a person's independence in performing tasks like washing, clothing, feeding, grooming, moving around, climbing stairs, using the restroom, and transitioning. They are widely used to compare human functionality to pre-determined functional standards. The results of both assessments are used to measure the patient's level of mobility.

3.4 QUANTIFIED SELF-WEARABLE TECHNOLOGY

The procedure of collecting personalised data on life and welfare via wearable equipment and other cutting-edge apparatus is called the "quantified self." Data gathering and analysis approaches are more prevalent as a result of the use of smartphones and wearables with plenty of sensors. As a result, the field of life cataloging and QS is growing quickly. Wearable tech gadgets can help the user increase productivity, reduce stress, and improve sleep habits [10]. These devices can deliver adequately thorough data to track wearers' disease development if they have chronic disease conditions. Numerous wearable gadgets are displayed in Figure 3.3 along with where on the body they are placed. Numerous typical wearable devices include headbands, smartwatches, cameras, sociometric badges, and textile sensors. Multiple sensors that gather information from the human body are integrated into these gadgets.

3.5 ACCURACY MEASUREMENT

Accuracy is the ability of a sensor to generate an evaluation that is equivalent to "gold-standard" computing tools. Repetition ability is the definition of dependability for a computation. The ability of a sensor to consistently detect and produce the same result, even when the measurement is inaccurate, is referred to as repeatability [11]. Validating a wearable device requires proving its relevance, reliability, consistency, and adaptability. The technological needs for wearable equipment in medical applications comprise the capacity to record data in real-world circumstances, as well as being precise, consistent, and having undergone testing in the healthcare community where they would be employed. Additionally, the kind of data essential for handling as part of medical applications or the significance of sensors within a precise research project governs the right selection of appropriate wearable sensors. For tracking activity in a controlled environment, several wearable sensors, such as textile and headbands sensors, are reliable in the

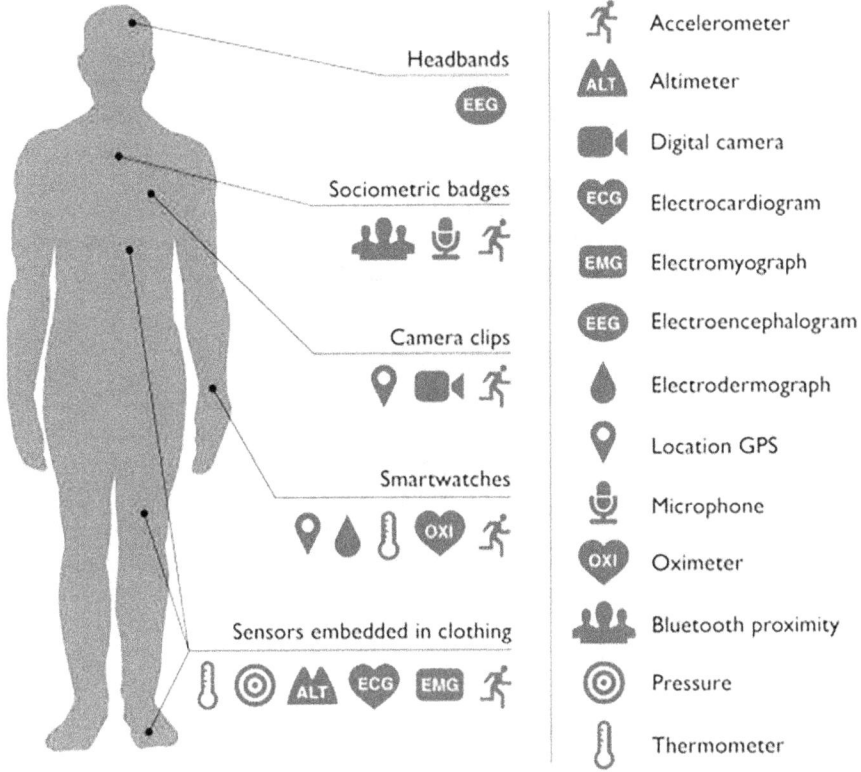

FIGURE 3.3 Wearable technology and the body parts to which they are attached [1].

short term but inaccurate over time [12]. Studies have demonstrated that a variety of wearable optical heart rate sensors are astonishingly accurate and stable both at rest and through prolonged high heart rate. But there are noticeable differences in how certain gadgets react to alterations in behaviour. Particularly when long-term heart rate observation is being done, gesture artefact is a doubted issue with wrist-worn sensors [13]. Nearly all smartphones and smart watches can now calculate step count, and several systems claim an accuracy rate of >95%. Wearable technology has an accuracy and precision of 92% to 99%. Due to the limitations on movement, some tools are more suitable to interior activities than others. While some gadgets may be better at tracking heart rate, others may be better at correctly counting steps. As a result, depending on the application and device, wearable technology's accuracy varies.

3.6 DETECTING HUMAN ACTIVITY USING DEEP LEARNING METHODS

Deep learning (DL) methods for human activity detection are a recent area of wearable technology innovation. With the aid of DL approaches, a taught system may recognise patterns in a variety of activities with the same intuition as a human. Specific movement patterns have been extracted from long-term data sets gathered by wearable devices, particularly those outfitted with IMUs and accelerometers, using pattern recognition and pattern matching approaches [14]. A data set is often classified using pattern recognition techniques based on training data and knowledge gleaned from previously observed patterns. The pattern matching module searches a big data set for particular patterns, and the results show whether the patterns were found or not. A wide range of data science applications, including spam filtering, web search engines, natural language processing, and digital libraries, have also used pattern matching.

Machine learning algorithms come in three types: semi-supervised, supervised, and unsupervised. Fully labelled data sets are used to train supervised learning algorithms, which can subsequently make calculations on fresh data. Predictive mapping of inputs to outputs can be assessed using a clear system. The categorization of a discrete-class issue is the main application of supervised learning [15]. Bayesian networks, support vector machines (SVMs), decision trees, and instance-based learning (IBL) are the most significant classifiers for supervised learning methods. Systems for offline human activity recognition (HAR) generate output utilising supervised learning strategies. For instance, supervised learning techniques are used to train the computer in HAR applications that monitor dietary habits and physical activity in people with obesity, disease of heart as well as in programmes that calculate the quantity of calories burned through a workout [16].

3.6.1 CONTRIBUTIONS

This chapter contributes a study on the various approaches in the wearable technology in the field of healthcare. The wearable device embedded with many sensors to monitor the health of human beings can prevent from health diseases.

3.6.1.1 Case Study

3.6.1.1.1 Case Study 1

Smartphones are used in fall detection systems owing to recent advancements in technology. These systems frequently combine drop detection with locating the person who fell using a GPS-based technique. A fall detection system made use of the accelerometers included in smartphones and included various algorithms for reliable fall detection. The features of the Android 2 functioning system were utilised in their implementation. To achieve great accuracy in the detection of falls, the sophisticated signal processing techniques are used. The system additionally delivered the subject's position using Google Maps. With this method, an alert regarding the fall and the position of the theme being watched is sent to a caregiver or member of the family by email, SMS, and Twitter messages. The objective of ongoing study is to reduce damages brought on by falls. The use of airbag technology has led to the development of numerous systems. When a fall is sensed by these systems, wearable accelerometers and gyroscopes cause the airbag to inflate. The airbag system that shields the subject before an influence is made needs to be miniaturised, even if these systems may be able to reduce injuries caused by falls.

3.6.1.1.2   *Case Study 2*

The detection of epileptic seizures is a further use of wearable sensors and system that has drawn significant interest from researchers and doctors. An abrupt loss of consciousness results from primary and subsequent compulsive epileptic crises. Stereotypical movements can be seen in conjunction with these episodes, as well as distinctive changes in the electroencephalogram. Systems and procedures using wearable sensors have been assessed to detect an electroencephalogram. Methods to identify electroencephalogram from regular motor actions have been developed using electroencephalographic sensors, 3D accelerometer on a wrist, a grouping of electromyography and accelerometer, and electrodermal activity. To find seizures, use the SHIMMER of wearable sensors and the Nokia N810 are used.

3.6.1.1.3   *Case Study 3*

It has been deemed of utmost importance to monitor the actions taken by older persons and those with chronic diseases who are taking part in "ageing in place" programmes. As a result, significant research has been done to evaluate the efficacy of wearable sensors in categorising daily life activities (ADL). Accelerometers can be used to track the ADL performed by older people being observed in their homes, as demonstrated. An in-shoe pressure and acceleration system was created to identify activities comprising standing, sitting, and walking while also being able to determine whether participants were simultaneously engaging in arm-reaching actions. An accelerometer-based gadget for step counting in Parkinson's disease patients was discovered. Wearable sensors were utilised to track patient's recovery from abdominal surgery. Activity tracking for wellness applications has been shown in numerous research studies to significantly improve workout compliance in population at risk. For instance, wearable equipment has been used to track physical activity in obese people and to make treatment interventions centred on promoting an active and healthy lifestyle more easily implemented.

3.7   RESULTS

The outcomes of clinical trial or self-care evaluations can be predicted by measuring wearable data. Apps for wearable technology therefore deal with a lot of physiological data supplied by the user. As a result, wearable technology's psychological aspects as well as data security and privacy should be carefully studied. The comfort and mental health of the wearer are included in the psychological element of a wearable technology. Additionally, the data that a wearable device collects, stores, and transmits must be suitably isolated and secure, and it must be kept and sent with both features. Wearable technology must be seen in the perspective of data security and privacy. A lot of wearable technology stores information locally without encryption or data security. NFC, Bluetooth, or Wi-Fi are the connections approaches for wearable devices to smartphones. Data protection against a brute-force attack is insufficient with

TABLE 3.1

Summary of the Existing Methods of Wearable Sensor Technology [1]

Model Type	Test for Analysis	Results
Hierarchical Dirichlet Process Model	Accuracy (79.20%)	The input data is used to automatically determine the levels of physical activity.
1D Convolutional Neural Network and Recurrent Neutral Network Model with Long Short Term Memory	Accuracy (90.15%)	For lower sample rates, the model performs well. But with regards to big data set accuracy is decreasing.
Convolutional Neural Network and Long Short-Term Memory – Recurrent Neutral Network	Accuracy (83.7%)	CNNs accomplish improved than LSTM-RNN for real-time data sets.
CNN with the Deep Q Neural Network	Accuracy (98.4%)	The CNN model outperforms the LSTM model.

insecure wireless connection channels. For data transfer, wearable sensors are continually coordinated with smartphones, and having third-party apps loaded on cell phones makes data hacking more likely. Wearable technology poses both passive and active attacks as data protection threats. Malicious nodes aim to gain access to the user's password and individual data stored on the smart device. This method has no negative effects or interference with the target device. Active attacks try to harm or change the device. A potential attacker can easily obtain data during a passive attack on a wearable device due to absence of protection on the communication line (Table 3.1).

3.8   CONCLUSION

Human motion analysis is an exciting area of study that is gaining more and more attention as wearable technology is used more frequently in ambulatory and home care settings. Wearable technology users might be able to measure their own health. This can be attained by using a variation of methods to monitor a range of sensor parameters. Therefore, wearable sensors can gather material about a patient's regular actions invisibly. Clinicians can gain more insight into a patient's health with sensor data due to its increased accessibility than with more constrained, subjective techniques. Producing precise, accurate, and clear results is one of the core aims of wearable technology. Completing explicitly quantified task packages, such as hardware validation assessment, clinical protocol formulation and testing, and feasibility study implementation and assessment, are requirements for this field of research. Future developments in this field will give therapists more in-depth knowledge of the numerous movements contained in home recording data. Due to this data, users will obtain a better understanding of their health, and experts will be able to analyse patients' fitness in greater detail and gain particular insights into their physical mobility.

REFERENCES

1. Vijayan, V., Connolly, J. P., Condell, J., McKelvey, N., and Gardiner, P. "Review of Wearable Devices and Data Collection Considerations for Connected Health" *Sensors*, vol. 21, no. 16, pp. 55–89, 2021, 10.3390/s21165589.
2. Kumar, A., Rajagopal, K., Gugapriya, G., Sharma, H., Gour, N., Masud, M., AlZain, M.A., and Alajmani, S.H. "Reducing PAPR with Low Complexity Filtered NOMA Using Novel Algorithm". *Sustainability*, vol. 14, p. 9631, 2022. 10.3390/su14159631.
3. Song, M. S., Kang, S. G., Lee, K.-T., and Kim, J. "Wireless, Skin-Mountable EMG Sensor for Human–Machine Interface Appl". *Micromachines*, vol. 10, pp. 879–892, 2019, 10.3390/mi10120879.
4. Kumar, A., and Chakravarty, S. "Dynamic Power Allocation to Improve an Existing SWIPT Cooperative NOMA Network". *Natl. Acad. Sci. Lett.* vol. 45, pp. 507–510, 2022. 10.1007/s40009-022-01141-7.
5. Jouffroy, R., Jost, D., and Prunet, B. "Prehospital Pulse Oximetry: A Red Flag for Early Detection of Silent Hypoxemia in COVID-19 Patients". *Crit. Care*, vol 24, pp. 1–12, 2020, 10.1186/s13054-020-03036-9.
6. Lee, J., Kim, D., Ryoo, H.-Y., Shin, B.-S. "Sustainable Wearables: Wearable Technology for Enhancing the Quality of Human Life". *Sustainability*, vol. 8, pp. 466–475, 2016, 10.3390/su8050466.
7. Kumar, A. and Gupta, M. "A Review on Activities of Fifth Generation Mobile Communication System". *Alexandria Engineering Journal*, vol. 57, no. 2, pp. 1125–1135, 2018, 10.1016/j.aej.2017.01.043.
8. Guner, U., Canbolat, H., and Unluturk A. "Design and Implementation of Adaptive Vibration Filter for MEMS Based Low Cost IMU". In Proceedings International Conference on Electrical and Electronics Engineering (ELECO), Bursa, Turkey, pp. 130–134, 2015, 10.1109/ELECO.2015.7394499.
9. De Arriba-Perez, F., Caeiro-Rodríguez, M., and Santos-Gago J.M. "Collection and Processing of Data from Wrist Wearable Devices in Heterogeneous and Multiple-User Scenarios". *Sensors*, vol. 16, pp. 1538–1549, 2016, 10.3390/s16091538.
10. Ramakrishnan, B., Kumar, A., Chakravarty, S., Masud, M., and Baz, M. "Analysis of FBMC Waveform for 5G Network Based Smart Hospitals". *Appl. Sci.*, vol. 11, p. 8895, 2021, 10.3390/app11198895.
11. Shen, Z., Yi, J., Li, X., Lo, M.H.P., Chen, M.Z.Q., Hu, Y., and Wang, Z. "A Soft Stretchable Bending Sensor and Data Glove Applications". *Robot. Biomimetics*, vol. 3, pp. 1–8, 2016, 10.1186/s40638-016-0051-1.
12. Henderson, J., Condell, J., Connolly, J., Kelly, D., and Curran, K. "Review of Wearable Sensor-Based Health Monitoring Glove Devices for Rheumatoid Arthritis". *Sensors*, vol. 21, pp. 1576–1592, 2021, 10.3390/s21051576.
13. De Pasquale, G. "Glove-Based Systems for Medical Applications: Review of Recent Advancements". *J. Text. Eng. Fash. Technol.*, vol. 4, pp. 10–22, 2018, 10.15406/jteft.2018.04.00153.
14. Djurić-Jovičić, M., Jovičić, N.S., Roby-Brami, A., Popović, M.B., Kostić, V.S., and Djordjević, A.R. "Quantification of Finger-Tapping Angle Based on Wearable Sensors". *Sensors*, vol. 17, pp. 203–215, 2017, 10.3390/s17020203.
15. Shyr, T.-W., Shie, J.-W., Jiang, C.-H., and Li, J.-J. "A Textile-Based Wearable Sensing Device Designed for Monitoring the Flexion Angle of Elbow and Knee Movements". *Sensors*, vol. 14, pp. 4050–4059, 2014, 10.3390/s140304050
16. Totaro, M., Poliero, T., Mondini, A., Lucarotti, C., Cairoli, G., Ortiz, J., and Beccai, L. "Soft Smart Garments for Lower Limb Joint Position Analysis". *Sensors*, vol. 17, pp. 2314–2325, 2017, 10.3390/s17102314.

4 An Overview of Healthcare Policy in India for Designing New Customised Health Services for the Patient

Akshaya Nidhi Bhati
Department of Electrical Engineering, School of Engineering
and Applied Science, University of Pennsylvania

Arun Kumar
Department of Electronics and Communication,
New Horizon College of Engineering, Bengaluru, India

Mehedi Masud
Department of Computer Science, College of Computers
and Information Technology, Taif University, Taif,
Saudi Arabia

Dac-Nhuong Le
Haiphong University, Haiphong, Vietnam

4.1 INTRODUCTION

Government policies have a significant impact on healthcare systems, influencing access, affordability, quality of care, health information systems, public health initiatives, and research and innovation. In this essay, we will delve deeper into each of these areas to understand the effects of government policy in healthcare. Access to healthcare is a fundamental aspect of any healthcare system, and government policies play a pivotal role in ensuring equitable access for all individuals. In many countries, governments have implemented universal healthcare systems or health insurance programs to provide coverage to a larger portion of the population. These policies aim to reduce disparities in healthcare access based on income or social status [1]. By guaranteeing access to healthcare services, governments strive to improve overall health outcomes and enhance social well-being.

DOI: 10.1201/9781003403678-4

Affordability and cost control are critical factors in healthcare, as high healthcare costs can be a barrier to access for many individuals. Governments employ various policies to address this issue. They may regulate the prices of medical services, prescription drugs, and health insurance premiums to ensure affordability. Additionally, governments may establish subsidies or assistance programs to help low-income individuals afford necessary medical care. These policies not only make healthcare more accessible but also aim to alleviate the financial burden on individuals and families. Quality of care is another key aspect influenced by government policies. Governments have the authority to set standards and regulations that healthcare providers must adhere to. These standards cover areas such as patient safety, infection control, and clinical guidelines [2]. By implementing and enforcing these policies, governments strive to ensure that healthcare services are of high quality and meet established benchmarks. Governments may also incentivize healthcare providers to adopt evidence-based practices and participate in quality improvement initiatives. These efforts contribute to improved patient outcomes and a higher level of healthcare quality. Health information systems have become increasingly important in healthcare delivery, and government policies can shape their development and adoption [3]. Governments may implement policies that encourage the use of electronic medical records (EMRs) and set inter-operability standards to facilitate the exchange of patient data among healthcare providers. These policies promote efficient and coordinated care delivery, reduce medical errors, and enable better management of patient information. Moreover, governments can invest in health information technology infrastructure and support the implementation of telehealth services, which have become crucial during the COVID-19 pandemic. These policies enhance the overall efficiency and effectiveness of healthcare systems. Public health initiatives are a vital component of government policies in healthcare. Governments have a responsibility to protect public health and prevent the spread of diseases [4]. Policies may focus on promoting vaccination programs, establishing disease surveillance systems, and developing public health campaigns to raise awareness about health risks and encourage healthy behaviours. These initiatives contribute to disease prevention, early detection, and effective management of public health crises. By implementing such policies, governments aim to improve population health outcomes and reduce the burden of preventable diseases. Research and innovation are essential for advancing healthcare and improving patient care [5]. Governments often play a significant role in funding and supporting medical research and development. Through policies and grants, governments provide resources to universities, research institutions, and healthcare organizations to conduct studies and develop innovative healthcare solutions. These policies encourage scientific advancements, the discovery of new treatments and therapies, and the translation of research findings into clinical practice. By fostering research and innovation, governments contribute to the growth and improvement of the healthcare sector, benefiting both individuals and society as a whole. In conclusion, government policies have a profound impact on healthcare systems. They influence access to healthcare services, affordability, quality of care, health information systems, public health initiatives, and research and innovation.

By implementing policies that prioritize equitable access, affordability, and high-quality care, governments can enhance population health outcomes, reduce healthcare disparities, and promote overall well-being. It is crucial for governments to continually assess and adapt their policies to meet the evolving needs of their populations and address emerging healthcare challenges [6].

4.1.1 MOTIVATION

Research on Indian government policies in healthcare is motivated by several factors that recognize the importance of understanding, evaluating, and improving the impact of policy interventions. In this section, we will explore the key motivations for research in Indian government policy in healthcare. India faces significant challenges in ensuring equitable access to healthcare services, especially for marginalized and rural populations [7]. Research on government policies in healthcare aims to identify barriers to access and evaluate the effectiveness of policy interventions in improving healthcare accessibility. This research motivation recognizes the need to address disparities in healthcare access and develop evidence-based policies that enhance healthcare equity across different regions and socioeconomic groups. Quality of care and patient safety are critical concerns in the Indian healthcare system. Research on government policies in healthcare aims to assess the impact of quality improvement initiatives, regulatory frameworks, and accreditation standards on healthcare quality and patient outcomes. This research motivation seeks to identify gaps in policy implementation, evaluate the effectiveness of existing policies, and recommend evidence-based strategies to enhance healthcare quality and patient safety. India faces numerous public health challenges, including infectious diseases, malnutrition, and non-communicable diseases [8]. Research on government policies in healthcare focuses on evaluating public health initiatives and interventions, such as immunization programs, disease surveillance systems, and public health campaigns. This research motivation aims to assess the effectiveness and efficiency of policies, identify areas for improvement, and provide evidence to guide policymaking for effective public health strategies. Healthcare affordability is a significant concern in India, with out-of-pocket expenses posing a financial burden on individuals and families. Research on government policies in healthcare investigates the impact of health financing models, health insurance schemes, and subsidy programs on healthcare affordability and financial protection [9]. This research motivation aims to identify effective policy interventions that promote financial risk protection, reduce healthcare costs, and ensure affordable access to healthcare services. The Indian government has emphasized the adoption of digital health technologies to improve healthcare delivery and health information management. Research on government policies in healthcare focuses on evaluating the implementation of digital health initiatives, electronic health record systems, telemedicine services, and health information exchange networks. This research motivation aims to assess the impact of digital health policies, identify challenges in implementation, and recommend strategies for effective utilization of digital technologies in healthcare [10]. The availability and distribution of healthcare professionals are crucial for effective healthcare delivery. Research on government policies in healthcare investigates policies related to healthcare workforce planning, training, recruitment, and retention. This research motivation aims to assess the impact of policies on the availability and quality of healthcare professionals, identify gaps in workforce planning, and recommend evidence-based strategies to strengthen the healthcare workforce in India. India has implemented various health insurance schemes and initiatives to achieve universal health coverage. Research on government policies in healthcare focuses on evaluating the impact of health insurance policies, such as Ayushman Bharat, on healthcare access, financial protection, and health outcomes. This research motivation aims to assess the effectiveness of health insurance schemes, identify challenges in implementation, and provide evidence to inform policy decisions for achieving universal health coverage. Research on government policies in healthcare plays a crucial role in promoting evidence-based policymaking. It generates robust evidence on the impact of policies, evaluates policy effectiveness, identifies implementation challenges, and provides recommendations for policy improvement. This research motivation aims to bridge the gap between research and policymaking, ensuring that policy decisions are informed by reliable evidence and have a greater likelihood of achieving their intended outcomes [11]. The research on Indian government policies in healthcare is motivated by the goals of improving healthcare access, enhancing healthcare quality and patient safety, strengthening public health initiatives, addressing healthcare financing and affordability, promoting digital health technologies, strengthening the healthcare workforce, evaluating health insurance schemes, and promoting evidence-based policymaking. By conducting research in these areas, policymakers and stakeholders can make informed decisions, implement effective policies, and continuously improve the Indian healthcare system to meet the evolving needs of the population [12].

4.2 ANALYSIS OF GOVERNMENT POLICIES IN THE IMPLEMENTATION OF SMART HOSPITALS

Implementing smart hospitals, which leverage advanced technologies and data-driven solutions to enhance healthcare delivery, can face challenges due to various government policies. In this section, we will explore the reasons why government policies can act as hindrances in the implementation of smart hospitals. Government policies often have regulatory frameworks in place that govern healthcare practices and technologies. While regulations are necessary to ensure patient safety and quality of care, they can sometimes impede the implementation of smart hospitals. The regulatory approval processes for new technologies and systems can be lengthy and complex, slowing down the adoption of innovative solutions [13]. Additionally, regulations may not be updated or flexible enough to accommodate emerging technologies, hindering their integration into healthcare settings. Smart hospitals rely on the collection, storage, and analysis of large amounts of patient data. Government policies related to privacy and data security can pose challenges to the implementation of smart hospitals. Stringent data protection regulations, such as the General Data Protection Regulation (GDPR) in the European Union, require hospitals to adhere to strict guidelines for handling patient data. Complying with these regulations while utilizing data for smart applications can be a complex task, requiring robust data governance frameworks and security measures. Many countries have fragmented healthcare systems, with multiple stakeholders involved in healthcare delivery [14]. Government policies that fail to address the coordination and interoperability challenges among different healthcare providers and systems can hinder the implementation of smart hospitals. In such scenarios, integrating various technologies and data sources becomes challenging, limiting the effectiveness of smart hospital initiatives. Policies that encourage collaboration, standardization, and interoperability among healthcare providers are crucial for successful implementation. Implementing smart hospitals often requires substantial financial investments. Government policies that do not provide adequate funding or incentives can hinder the implementation of such initiatives [15]. Healthcare budgets may not allocate sufficient resources for acquiring and implementing advanced technologies, which can limit the ability of healthcare organizations to adopt smart hospital solutions. Government policies that promote funding mechanisms, grants, and incentives specifically targeted at smart hospital implementation can help overcome financial barriers. Healthcare systems can be resistant to change, and government policies may inadvertently perpetuate this resistance. Policies that prioritize maintaining the status quo, lack incentives for innovation, or discourage experimentation can hinder the implementation of smart hospitals. Moreover, resistance to change may stem from healthcare professionals who are unfamiliar with or resistant to new technologies [16]. Government policies can play a role in addressing this resistance through educational initiatives, training programs, and incentives that promote technology adoption and change management. Limited Digital Infrastructure: The implementation of smart hospitals requires a robust digital infrastructure, including high-speed internet connectivity, secure networks, and interoperable systems. In regions where digital infrastructure is underdeveloped, government policies that do not prioritize digitalization can hinder the implementation of smart hospitals. Governments need to invest in building and upgrading digital infrastructure to support the seamless integration and functioning of smart hospital technologies. Government policies that lack clear frameworks or guidelines specifically tailored to smart hospital implementation can hinder progress. Without comprehensive policies that address issues such as data governance, cybersecurity, technology procurement, and interoperability, healthcare organizations may face uncertainty and challenges in adopting and integrating smart technologies [17]. Well-defined policies that provide a road map for smart hospital implementation, addressing both technical and governance aspects, are essential to facilitate the adoption of these transformative healthcare solutions. The successful implementation of smart hospitals requires collaboration and engagement from various stakeholders, including healthcare providers, policymakers, technology vendors, and patients. Government policies that do not actively involve and engage these stakeholders in the policymaking process can hinder implementation efforts. Policies that encourage stakeholder participation, establish collaborative platforms, and foster partnerships can overcome barriers and be more inclusive [18].

4.3   INITIATIVE TAKEN BY GOVERNMENT OF INDIA FOR SMART HEALTHCARE

India has recognized the potential of smart hospitals to transform healthcare delivery and improve patient outcomes. The Indian government has implemented various policies and initiatives to promote the implementation of smart hospitals across the country. Below, we will discuss some of the key policies and strategies adopted by India in the implementation of smart hospitals [19–28]:

- National Digital Health Mission (NDHM): Launched in 2020, the NDHM aims to establish a unified digital health ecosystem in India. It focuses on creating a digital health infrastructure that includes electronic health records (EHRs), telemedicine services, health registries, and health information exchange. The NDHM provides a policy framework and guidelines for the implementation of smart hospitals, enabling seamless sharing of patient data and interoperability among healthcare providers.
- Digital India Initiative: The Digital India initiative, launched in 2015, aims to transform India into a digitally empowered society. As part of this initiative, the government has focused on expanding digital infrastructure, promoting digital literacy, and enhancing digital governance. These efforts provide a foundation for the implementation of smart hospitals by ensuring the availability of high-speed internet connectivity, enabling telemedicine services, and facilitating the exchange of digital health information.
- National Health Policy 2017: The National Health Policy 2017 emphasizes the use of technology in healthcare delivery, including the adoption of electronic health records, telemedicine, and mHealth solutions. The policy promotes the integration of digital health technologies in healthcare institutions to improve access, quality, and affordability of healthcare services. It provides a policy framework for the implementation of smart hospitals and encourages their adoption across the country.
- Telemedicine Guidelines: In 2020, the Ministry of Health and Family Welfare released guidelines for telemedicine practices in India. These guidelines provide a regulatory framework for teleconsultations, telemedicine prescriptions, and telemedicine technology standards. By facilitating telemedicine services, the guidelines support the implementation of smart hospitals and promote remote patient monitoring, virtual consultations, and digital healthcare delivery.

- National Digital Health Blueprint: The National Digital Health Blueprint, released in 2019, outlines the strategic road map for digital health in India. It focuses on interoperability, data privacy, and patient consent, laying the foundation for the implementation of smart hospitals. The blueprint envisions the creation of a national health stack, which includes core building blocks such as personal health records, registries, and health analytics. These components are essential for the successful implementation of smart hospitals.
- Atal Innovation Mission (AIM): The AIM, launched by the government in 2016, aims to promote innovation and entrepreneurship in various sectors, including healthcare. It supports the establishment of Atal Incubation Centers (AICs) that provide mentoring, funding, and infrastructure support to start-ups working on innovative healthcare solutions. The AIM encourages the development and implementation of technologies that can contribute to smart hospital initiatives, fostering a culture of innovation in the healthcare sector.
- Make in India and Digital India for Medical Electronics: The Make in India campaign and the Digital India for Medical Electronics initiative promote indigenous manufacturing and innovation in medical electronics. These initiatives encourage the development and production of medical devices, digital health solutions, and smart healthcare technologies within India. By supporting the domestic production of healthcare technologies, these policies contribute to the implementation of smart hospitals.
- Public-Private Partnerships (PPPs): The Indian government recognizes the importance of collaborations between the public and private sectors in implementing smart hospitals. It encourages PPPs to leverage the expertise and resources of both sectors. Through PPPs, the government aims to facilitate the adoption of advanced technologies, develop infrastructure, and enhance healthcare services. These partnerships play a crucial role in implementing and sustaining smart hospitals across the country.

India has taken significant steps to promote the implementation of smart hospitals. Policies and initiatives such as the National Digital Health Mission, Digital India, telemedicine guidelines, and the National Health Policy provide a policy framework, regulatory support, and strategic direction for the adoption of smart hospital technologies. The focus on digital infrastructure, innovation, and public-private collaborations demonstrates India's commitment to leveraging technology for improving healthcare delivery and achieving better patient outcomes.

4.4   INDIAN PENAL CODE (IPC) IN HEALTHCARE

IPC laws are crucial for the implementation and regulation of healthcare facilities in India. These laws are designed to ensure the safety, well-being, and ethical treatment of patients, as well as to hold healthcare providers accountable for any malpractices or misconduct. Let's explore some IPC laws that are particularly relevant to the implementation of healthcare facilities [29–31].

   i. Section 269: This section deals with the negligent act likely to spread infection of disease dangerous to life. It holds individuals accountable for any act that negligently causes the spread of a dangerous disease. In the context of healthcare facilities, this law emphasizes the importance of infection control measures and the responsibility of healthcare providers to prevent the transmission of infectious diseases within the facility.

   ii. Section 270: Section 270 focuses on the malignant act likely to spread infection of disease dangerous to life. It holds individuals accountable for intentionally spreading a dangerous disease. In the healthcare setting, this law is significant in cases where healthcare professionals intentionally endanger the lives of patients or knowingly engage in practices that could lead to the spread of infectious diseases.

   iii. Section 304A: This section deals with causing death by negligence. It holds individuals accountable for causing death due to negligent acts. In the context of healthcare facilities, this law is applicable when a patient dies due to the negligence or misconduct of healthcare professionals or due to the failure of the facility to provide appropriate care.

   iv. Section 336: Section 336 addresses act endangering life or personal safety of others. It holds individuals accountable for acts that endanger the lives or safety of others. In the healthcare setting, this law can be invoked when healthcare professionals or facility staff engage in actions that pose a risk to the well-being or safety of patients, such as administering wrong medication or using faulty medical equipment.

   v. Section 337: This section deals with causing hurt by an act endangering life or personal safety of others. It holds individuals accountable for causing harm to others by endangering their lives or safety. In the context of healthcare facilities, this law is applicable when patients suffer injuries or harm due to the negligence or reckless actions of healthcare providers or facility staff.

   vi. Section 338: Section 338 addresses causing grievous hurt by an act endangering life or personal safety of others. It holds individuals accountable for causing severe injuries or grievous harm to others by endangering their lives or safety. In healthcare facilities, this law is relevant in cases where patients suffer severe injuries or harm due to the negligence or misconduct of healthcare providers or facility staff.

   vii. Section 420: Section 420 deals with cheating and dishonestly inducing delivery of property. In the healthcare context, this law can be applied when healthcare providers or facility staff engage in fraudulent practices, such as misrepresenting treatments, charging exorbitant fees, or providing false information to patients for personal gain.

viii. Section 504: This section addresses intentional insult with intent to provoke a breach of peace. It holds individuals accountable for intentionally insulting or causing provocation to others. In healthcare facilities, this law is significant when healthcare professionals or facility staff engage in behaviour that insults or harasses patients, leading to a breach of peace.

It's important to note that the implementation and interpretation of IPC laws in healthcare facilities require a thorough understanding of the specific circumstances and evidence related to each case. Legal professionals and authorities play a crucial role in ensuring the fair and just implementation of these laws to maintain the integrity and accountability of healthcare facilities.

4.4.1 INDIA CONSTITUTIONAL ARTICLE RELATED TO HEALTHCARE

In India, the implementation of healthcare is governed by several constitutional articles that outline the rights and responsibilities related to health and healthcare. The key constitutional articles that pertain to healthcare implementation in India are as follows [32–37]:

I. Article 21: This article guarantees the protection of life and personal liberty. It has been interpreted by the judiciary to include the right to healthcare as a fundamental right. The state has the obligation to protect and improve the health of its citizens.

II. Article 39(e) and (f): These articles direct the state to ensure the health and well-being of the people. They emphasize the need for equal distribution of resources and opportunities, and the prevention of unjust inequalities.

III. Article 41: This article focuses on the right to public assistance and welfare, including provisions for public health. It emphasizes the importance of providing public health facilities for all citizens, particularly for those who are economically disadvantaged.

IV. Article 42: This article emphasizes the provision of just and humane conditions of work, including maternity relief. It places an obligation on the state to make provisions for securing the health and welfare of workers.

V. Article 47: This article directs the state to improve public health and raise the standard of living. It specifically mentions the prohibition of the consumption of intoxicating substances that are injurious to health.

VI. Article 48: This article highlights the importance of preserving and improving the environment and safeguarding the health and well-being of humans, animals, and plants.

VII. Article 243 G: This article relates to the provision of health services at the grassroots level. It empowers local self-government bodies, such as panchayats (rural local governments) and municipalities (urban local governments), to take initiatives in implementing health programs and services.

VIII. Article 280: While not directly related to healthcare, this article establishes the Finance Commission, which plays a crucial role in the allocation of funds for various sectors, including health, at the central and state levels.

It's important to note that while these constitutional articles lay the foundation for healthcare implementation, the detailed policies, programs, and regulations are formulated by the government through legislative and executive actions.

4.5 IMPACT OF COVID-19 DUE TO SEVERAL CONSTRAINTS IN THE HEALTHCARE POLICY

India faced significant challenges in managing the COVID-19 pandemic, and the lack of adequate healthcare infrastructure was one of the contributing factors to the impact of the virus. Here are some ways in which India's healthcare infrastructure limitations affected its response to COVID-19 [38–40]:

I. Overburdened healthcare system: India's healthcare system, particularly in densely populated urban areas, faced immense pressure due to the sudden surge in COVID-19 cases. Hospitals and healthcare facilities were overwhelmed, leading to a shortage of beds, medical equipment, and healthcare professionals.

II. Insufficient hospital capacity: The surge in COVID-19 cases exposed the limited capacity of hospitals to handle a large number of critically ill patients. Many hospitals faced shortages of Intensive Care Unit (ICU) beds, ventilators, and other critical medical supplies needed for treating severe COVID-19 cases.

III. Inadequate testing facilities: Initially, India faced challenges in scaling up testing facilities to meet the growing demand. Limited testing capacity resulted in delays in identifying and isolating infected individuals, hampering efforts to contain the spread of the virus effectively.

IV. Healthcare workforce shortages: India faced a shortage of healthcare professionals, including doctors, nurses, and paramedics, to handle the increased patient load. The existing healthcare workforce struggled to cope with the overwhelming demand, leading to fatigue and increased risk of infection among healthcare workers.

V. Regional disparities: There were significant disparities in the healthcare infrastructure across different regions in India. Rural areas, in particular, faced challenges in terms of access to healthcare facilities, including hospitals, clinics, and diagnostic centers. This disparity further exacerbated the impact of the pandemic in these areas.

VI. Inadequate public health infrastructure: India's public health infra-structure, including surveillance systems, contact tracing capabilities, and public health emergency response mechanisms, faced limitations. These shortcomings made it challenging to track and contain the spread of the virus effectively.

VII. Vaccine distribution challenges: With the rollout of COVID-19 vac-cines, India faced logistical and distribution challenges due to the vast population size and the need for a large-scale immunization campaign. Ensuring equitable access to vaccines across all regions posed signifi-cant challenges.

It's important to note that the Indian government and healthcare authorities have been working to address these challenges by ramping up healthcare infrastructure, increasing testing capacity, expanding vaccination efforts, and strengthening public health systems.

4.5.1 CHALLENGES FOR ADMINISTRATION IN INDIA POST-PANDEMIC

A well-designed and effectively implemented healthcare policy can have a significant impact on managing and mitigating the impact of COVID-19 in India. Here are some key elements that a good healthcare policy could include to address the challenges posed by the pandemic: A robust healthcare policy should prioritize investments in healthcare infrastructure, including hospitals, clinics, and medical facilities. This involves expanding the number of hospital beds, establishing temporary healthcare facilities, ensuring an adequate supply of medical equipment and essential supplies, and improving healthcare infra-structure in rural areas [41]. A comprehensive healthcare policy should focus on scaling up testing and surveillance efforts. This includes increasing testing capacity, promoting widespread and accessible testing, establishing robust sur-veillance systems for early detection and tracking of COVID-19 cases, and implementing efficient contact tracing mechanisms. Adequate staffing is crucial during a health crisis. The healthcare policy should emphasize measures to strengthen the healthcare workforce by recruiting and training additional doctors, nurses, and other healthcare professionals. Ensuring their safety through the provision of personal protective equipment (PPE) and appropriate working conditions is also important. A healthcare policy should prioritize public health education and awareness campaigns to disseminate accurate information about COVID-19, its transmission, prevention measures, and vaccination. Promoting hygiene practices, wearing masks, maintaining physical distancing, and fol-lowing public health guidelines can help reduce the spread of the virus [42]. A healthcare policy should include a well-planned and efficient vaccination strategy. This involves ensuring an adequate supply of vaccines, prioritizing high-risk populations and vulnerable groups, establishing vaccination centers across the country, and streamlining the vaccination process to maximize cov-erage and minimize wastage. Healthcare policies should support research and development efforts to enhance understanding of the virus, its variants, and potential treatments. Encouraging collaboration between public and private sectors, investing in scientific research, and fostering innovation can contribute to the development of effective therapies and vaccines. A healthcare policy should emphasize the importance of preparedness for future pandemics and public health emergencies [43]. This involves establishing robust emergency response mechanisms, developing contingency plans, stockpiling essential medical supplies, and enhancing coordination between different levels of government and stakeholders [44]. A good healthcare policy should prioritize equitable access to healthcare services, including COVID-19 testing, treatment, and vaccination. Special attention should be given to marginalized and vulnerable populations to ensure they receive adequate healthcare and support. It's important to note that the specifics of healthcare policy implementation may vary based on the evolving nature of the pandemic and scientific understanding of COVID-19. Regular evaluation, monitoring, and adaptation of policies based on emerging evidence and best practices are essential for an effective response to the pandemic [45].

4.6 IMPACT OF INDIA HEALTHCARE POLICY IN THE GLOBAL SCENARIO

The rules and regulations in India can impact the provision of global services in healthcare, depending on the specific context and nature of the services. While India has emerged as a major destination for medical tourism and has a thriving healthcare industry, there are certain regulations and policies that can influence the provision of global healthcare services [46]. Healthcare providers offering services in India, including those catering to international patients, are subject to licensing and accreditation requirements. They need to comply with the regulations set by the Medical Council of India (MCI) and other relevant authorities to ensure the quality and safety of healthcare services. International patients seeking healthcare services in India must adhere to visa and immigration regulations [47]. India offers medical visas specifically designed for individuals seeking medical treatment in the country. These visas have specific requirements and limitations that patients and accompanying individuals need to fulfil. India has regulations regarding data privacy and protection, which can impact the provision of global healthcare services. Healthcare providers and institutions need to ensure compliance with relevant data protection laws to safeguard patient information and maintain confidentiality [48]. The Medical Council of India has guidelines and ethical considerations that healthcare providers must follow. These guidelines ensure that healthcare services are provided ethically and prioritize patient safety, informed consent, and appropriate medical practices. Intellectual property rights, including patents, trademarks, and copyrights, play a role in the provision of healthcare services. Regulations related to intellectual property can impact the availability, accessibility, and affordability of certain medical technologies, treatments, or pharmaceuticals in India [49]. The pricing and payment regulations in India can affect the provision of healthcare services for both domestic and international patients. The government may regulate pricing for certain procedures or treatments to ensure affordability and prevent exploitation. It's important to note that while regulations exist to ensure quality, safety, and ethical practices in healthcare, they can vary and evolve over time. The specific impact of these regulations on global healthcare services in India depends on the nature of the services, the target audience, and compliance with relevant laws and guidelines [50].

4.6.1 IMPACT OF GEOGRAPHICAL CONDITION IN HEALTHCARE INFRASTRUCTURE IN NORTHEAST INDIA

The healthcare system in northeast India differs in certain aspects from the rest of India due to various geographical, socio-cultural, and historical factors. The northeast region is characterized by its hilly terrain, dense forests, and scattered population, which poses challenges in terms of accessibility to healthcare services [51]. The presence of numerous rivers and difficult terrain often leads to limited connectivity and infrastructure, making it harder to reach healthcare facilities. Northeast India is known for its diverse ethnic communities and distinct cultural practices. This diversity influences healthcare-seeking behaviors, traditional healing practices, and the perception of modern healthcare. The healthcare system in the region needs to take into account cultural sensitivities and incorporate traditional healing practices alongside modern medicine [52]. The healthcare infrastructure in northeast India is relatively underdeveloped compared to other parts of the country. There is a shortage of hospitals, clinics, and specialized healthcare facilities in many areas, particularly in remote and rural regions. This lack of infrastructure impacts the accessibility and quality of healthcare services. Historically, northeast India has received comparatively lower resource allocation for healthcare infrastructure and services. This disparity has led to inadequate funding for healthcare facilities, medical education institutions, and public health programs in the region [53]. Northeast India faces certain unique health challenges, such as vector-borne diseases like malaria, dengue, and Japanese encephalitis. Additionally, the region is prone to natural disasters, including floods and landslides, which can disrupt healthcare services and infrastructure. Traditional medicine systems, such as Ayurveda, traditional Chinese medicine, and traditional tribal healing practices, have a significant presence in northeast India. These traditional medicine systems coexist with modern medicine, and efforts are being made to integrate and promote traditional healing practices within the healthcare system. Northeast India shares international borders with countries like Bangladesh, Bhutan, China, and Myanmar. This proximity influences cross-border movement of people, healthcare collaboration, and the need for addressing health issues that transcend national boundaries [54]. However, the efforts are being made to address these disparities and strengthen the healthcare system in northeast India. The government is implementing initiatives to improve healthcare infrastructure, expand access to quality healthcare services, and promote healthcare education and research in the region. Additionally, collaborations with international agencies, NGOs, and private sector involvement are being encouraged to bridge the healthcare gap and improve health outcomes in northeast India.

4.7 CONCLUSION

India faces several constraints in its healthcare policy that hinder the improvement of services. These constraints include inadequate infrastructure, a shortage of healthcare professionals, low public spending on healthcare, and limited access to quality healthcare services, particularly in rural areas. The insufficient healthcare infrastructure in India presents a significant challenge. Many healthcare facilities lack proper equipment, technology, and adequate space to meet the growing healthcare needs of the population. Additionally, the shortage of healthcare professionals, including doctors, nurses, and specialists, further exacerbates the problem. The country needs to invest in training and retaining skilled healthcare workers to bridge this gap. Another critical constraint is the low public spending on healthcare. India's expenditure on healthcare as a percentage of its GDP is significantly lower than the global average. Insufficient funding limits the government's ability to expand healthcare coverage, improve infrastructure, and enhance the quality of services. Moreover, the lack of access to quality healthcare services is a major concern, particularly in rural areas. People residing in remote regions often struggle to reach healthcare facilities due to long distances and inadequate transportation. Additionally, there is a need to focus on improving the quality and affordability of healthcare services to ensure that all citizens can access the care they require. To overcome these constraints, India's healthcare policy should prioritize increased investment in healthcare infrastructure, allocation of more funds to healthcare, and the development of a robust primary healthcare system. Emphasizing preventive care and promoting public-private partnerships can also contribute to improving healthcare services. Additionally, leveraging technology and telemedicine can help overcome geographical barriers and enhance access to quality care, especially in remote areas. Addressing these constraints will require a multi-dimensional approach, involving collaborations between the government, healthcare professionals, non-profit organizations, and the private sector. By recognizing and addressing these challenges, India can strive towards achieving equitable, accessible, and high-quality healthcare services for its population.

REFERENCES

1. Lakshminarayanan S. Role of government in public health: Current scenario in India and future scope. J Family Community Med. 2011 Jan;18(1):26–30. doi: 10.4103/1319-1683.78635. PMID: 21694957; PMCID: PMC3114612.
2. Narayan R, and Narayan T. The voluntary health sector: Some reflections. Health Millions. 1993 Jun;1(3):2–5. PMID: 12318296.
3. Leask, J, Seale, H, Williams, JH, Kaufman, J, Wiley, K, Mahimbo, A, Clark, KK, Danchin, MH, Attwell, K. Policy considerations for mandatory COVID-19 vaccination from the Collaboration on Social Science and Immunisation. Med J Aust. 2021 Dec 13;215(11):499–503. doi: 10.5694/mja2.51269. Epub 2021 Nov 10. PMID: 34510461; PMCID: PMC8661777.
4. Hanney, SR, Gonzalez-Block, MA, Buxton, MJ, Kogan, M. The utilisation of health research in policy-making: Concepts, examples and methods of assessment. Health Res Policy Syst. 2003 Jan 13;1(1):2. doi: 10.1186/1478-4505-1-2. PMID: 12646071; PMCID: PMC151555.

5. Institute of Medicine (US) Committee on the Health Professions Education Summit; Greiner AC, Knebel E, editors. Health Professions Education: A Bridge to Quality. Washington (DC): National Academies Press (US); 2003. Chapter 2, Challenges Facing the Health System and Implications for Educational Reform. Available from: https://www.ncbi.nlm.nih.gov/books/NBK221522/

6. Heller, PS, Hsiao, WC. Chapter 4: Health policy challenges and issues confronting nations. In What Macroeconomists Should Know about Health Care Policy. USA: International Monetary Fund; 2007. Retrieved Jun 23, 2023, from 10.5089/97815 89066182.058.ch004.

7. Lagarde M, Huicho L, Papanicolas I. Motivating provision of high quality care: It is not all about the money. BMJ. 2019 Sep 23;366:l5210. doi: 10.1136/bmj.l5210. PMID: 31548200; PMCID: PMC6753666.

8. Nwobodo-Anyadiegwu, EN, Ditend, MN, Lumbwe, AK. The benefits and challenges of Implementing Smart hospital projects: A systematic review, 2022 IEEE 28th International Conference on Engineering, Technology and Innovation (ICE/ITMC) & 31st International Association For Management of Technology (IAMOT) Joint Conference, Nancy, France, 2022, pp. 1–7, doi: 10.1109/ICE/ITMC-IAMOT55089. 2022.10033238.

9. Tortorella, G, Fogliatto, F, Mac, A, Cawley Vergara, R, Vassolo, R, et al. Healthcare 4.0: Trends challenges and research directions. Production Plan Control. 2019;31(15): 1245–1260.

10. Li and Carayon, P. Health Care 4.0: A vision for smart and connected health care. IISE Transactions on Healthcare Systems Engineering, pp. 1–10, 2021.

11. Kumar, A, Albreem, MA, Gupta, M, Alsharif, MH, Kim, S. Future 5G network based smart hospitals: Hybrid detection technique for latency improvement. IEEE Access. 2020;8:153240–153249, doi: 10.1109/ACCESS.2020.3017625.

12. Al-Jaroodi J, Mohamed N, Abukhousa E. Health 4.0: On the way to realizing the healthcare of the future. IEEE Access. 2020 Nov 18;8:211189–211210. doi: 10.1109/ ACCESS.2020.3038858. PMID: 34976565; PMCID: PMC8675545.

13. Agrawal A. Medical negligence: Indian legal perspective. Ann Indian Acad Neurol. 2016 Oct;19(Suppl 1):S9–S14. doi: 10.4103/0972-2327.192889. PMID: 27891019; PMCID: PMC5109761.

14. Cantor, J, Sood, N, Bravata, DM, Pera, M, Whaley, C. The impact of the COVID-19 pandemic and policy response on health care utilization: Evidence from county-level medical claims and cellphone data. J Health Econ. 2022 Mar;82:102581. doi: 10.1016/j.jhealeco.2022.102581. Epub 2022 Jan 13. PMID: 35067386; PMCID: PMC8755425.

15. Kaye, AD, Okeagu, CN, Pham, AD, Silva, RA, Hurley, JJ, Arron, BL, Sarfraz, N, Lee, HN, Ghali, GE, Gamble, JW, Liu, H, Urman, RD, Cornett, EM. Economic impact of COVID-19 pandemic on healthcare facilities and systems: International perspectives. Best Pract Res Clin Anaesthesiol. 2021 Oct;35(3):293–306. doi: 10.1016/j.bpa.2020. 11.009. Epub 2020 Nov 17. PMID: 34511220; PMCID: PMC7670225.

16. Ghia C, Rambhad G. Implementation of equity and access in Indian healthcare: Current scenario and way forward. J Mark Access Health Policy. 2023 Mar 26;11(1):2194507. doi: 10.1080/20016689.2023.2194507. PMID: 36998432; PMCID: PMC10044314.

17. Bisht R, Pitchforth E, Murray SF. Understanding India, globalisation and health care systems: A mapping of research in the social sciences. Global Health. 2012 Sep 10;8:32. doi: 10.1186/1744-8603-8-32. PMID: 22963264; PMCID: PMC3549840.

18. https://applications.emro.who.int/docs/em_rc53_tech.disc.1_en.pdf.

19. https://www.health.state.mn.us/communities/practice/resources/chsadmin/mnsystem-responsibility.html

20. https://journmed.com/challenges-faced-by-healthcare-policies-in-india/

21. https://www.ey.com/en_us/health/healthpolicy?WT.mc_id=10820879&AA.tsrc=
    paidsearch&gad=1&gclid=Cj0KCQjw4s-kBhDqARIsAN-ipH1SOV44WzMlqbJ0S
    24JQsYxronQDrCaXdGRc93a04MRPxZbV8kXAowaAicCEALw_wcB.
22. https://timesofindia.indiatimes.com/education/news/smart-hospitals-are-future-of-
    public-health-system-in-west-bengal-india-post-pandemic-era-assocham/articleshow/
    99619955.cms.
23. https://www.healthcarefacilitiestoday.com/posts/Roadmap-to-smart-hospital-Step-
    by-step-guide-to-the-future-of-care--23132.
24. https://pib.gov.in/Pressreleaseshare.aspx?PRID=1737184.
25. https://main.mohfw.gov.in/Organisation/departments-health-and-family-welfare/
    e-Health-Telemedicine.
26. https://csc.gov.in/digitalIndia#:~:text=Digital%20India%20is%20a%20flagship,
    Prime%20Minister%20Shri%20Narendra%20Modi.
27. https://ndhm.gov.in/
28. https://www.ibef.org/government-schemes/smart-cities-mission.
29. https://vikaspedia.in/health/nrhm/national-health-policies/national-health-policy-2017
30. https://www.mohfw.gov.in/pdf/Telemedicine.pdf
31. https://abdm.gov.in:8081/uploads/ndhb_1_56ec695bc8.pdf
32. https://aim.gov.in/
33. https://www.makeinindia.com/sector/electronic-systems
34. https://www.legalserviceindia.com/legal/article-6620-right-to-healthcare.html
35. https://www.ima-india.org/ima/archive-page-details.php?pid=207#:~:text=Wrongful
    %20confinement%20(Sec.&text=340%2D342%20of%20IPC.,under%20these%20Sec
    tions%20of%20IPC.
36. https://www.orfonline.org/expert-speak/declaring-the-right-to-health-a-fundamental-
    right/
37. https://www.legalserviceindia.com/legal/article-6107-right-to-health-and-health-care.
    html
38. https://www.constitutionofindia.net/articles/article-39-certain-principles-of-policy-to-
    be-followed-by-the-state/
39. https://www.constitutionofindia.net/articles/article-41-right-to-work-to-education-
    and-to-public-assistance-in-certain-cases/#:~:text=Article%2041%2C%20Constitu
    tion%20of%20India,other%20cases%20of%20undeserved%20want.
40. https://www.latestlaws.com/bare-acts/central-acts-rules/article-243g-constitution-of-
    india-powers-authority-and-responsibilities-of-panchayat
41. https://www.constitutionofindia.net/articles/article-280-finance-commission/
42. https://economictimes.indiatimes.com/news/india/sixty-per-cent-people-delaying-
    treatment-due-to-lack-of-health-cover-survey/articleshow/93904726.cms.
43. https://azimpremjiuniversity.edu.in/faculty-research/understanding-post-covid-19-
    governance-challenges-in-india-a-compendium-of-essays.
44. https://cprindia.org/wp-content/uploads/2022/05/Post-Covid-and-Environment-
    Regulation-Paper-as-published-1.pdf.
45. http://southernvoice.org/indias-bureaucratic-challenge-in-the-post-pandemic-era/
46. https://www.orfonline.org/research/challenges-and-opportunities-for-india-in-the-
    post-pandemic-geopolitical-landscape/
47. https://yourstory.com/socialstory/2022/02/social-sector-india-post-pandemic-challenges-
    oppotunities
48. https://www.commonwealthfund.org/international-health-policy-center/countries/india
49. https://www.brookings.edu/wp-content/uploads/2017/08/mci-impact-series-paper.pdf
50. https://economictimes.indiatimes.com/indian-healthcare-stop-the-brain-drain-of-
    doctors/articleshow/9677156.cms?from=mdr.

51. https://www.researchgate.net/publication/328829755_Status_of_Rural_Health_
Infrastructure_in_the_North-East_India.

52. https://www.academia.edu/8276256/Health_Care_Infrastructure_in_the_Rural_
Areas_of_North_East_India_Current_Status_and_Future_Challenges.

53. https://journals.sagepub.com/doi/abs/10.1177/0973703019870881?journalCode=jhda.

54. https://nehu.ac.in/public/downloads/Journals/Journal_VolXIII_No2_Jul-Dec2015_
A3.pdf

5 Constraints Due to Regularization of Smart Hospitals

To Study the Impact of 5G Technology on the Financial Sector

Arun Gautam
Faculty of Management, JECRC University, Jaipur, Rajasthan, India

Rashid Amin
Department of Computer Sciences, University of Chakwal, Chakwal, Pakistan

Kengne Jacques
Fotso Victor University Institute of Technology (IUT-FV), University of Dschang, Cameroon

5.1 INTRODUCTION

The most recent improvement in mobile technology, known as 5G, is intended to greatly speed up and improve the responsiveness of wireless networks. Mobile phone companies started developing 5G technology globally in 2019, and it will take over the 4G networks that provide connectivity to many current mobile phones in the present scenario. Similar to other cellular networks, fifth-generation technology operates on the same radio waves that your smartphone currently uses, as well as those used by Wi-Fi networks and satellite communications, but it enables considerably more sophisticated technologies.[1] Also, many aspects of our lives will be digitally integrated with this technology [1]. Customers in Germany can now access the 5G network as of September 2019. More bands will be needed for this increased level of communication, and the German Federal Network Agency sold the new spectrum in the spring of 2019. The latest revolution can make an easier and smooth working environment in many sectors. One of the most important sectors of our Indian economy is the banking and financial sector [2]. 5G plays a significant role in it because nowadays 80% of banking services and activities are done through an online mode. In India's banking and financial industry, Motility, a game-changer already, has announced a surge in "all digital" customers who solely use their smartphones, tablets, and personal computers for transactions. Banks are anticipated to reevaluate digital banking for both internal and external operations, as well as for client interaction, as a result of 5G. With operations that extend to him new channels like 5G smartphones, wearables, Internet of Things (IoT) devices, and actual reality, the bank is anticipated to become a channel. Real-time transactions are made possible with 5G connectivity, which also shortens settlement cycles and removes delays [3]. The financial services business has frequently been the fastest developing in terms of digital technology, from ATMs to online and mobile banking. For instance, 81% of financial institutions have changed their technology over time at the corporate and/or branch level, according to research by AT&T and IDG. Many clients are actively looking for new services as the use of mobile phones grows at an increasingly rapid rate. Banks must operate more quickly than ever before to meet these demands. Low procrastination 5G networks' high data capacity and dependability will aid in the development of a new platform for the delivery of banking services [4].

5.1.1 Background

In the 1980s, a new generation of mobile phones launched the first generation. The second generation was first released in the 1990s and buyers were able to do voice calls and send messages. 3G came into use in 2001 and set the path for sharing images, obtaining Bluetooth signals from adjacent phone towers, and using the web on mobile phones. The third generation gave a massive advancement to cellular networks and communications, providing a speed of up to 21.1 Mbps. With 4G, mobile broadband speeds should be at least five times quicker compared to what was offered with 3G [5]. Internet banking emerged in India in the late 1990s; the ICICI bank was the first to offer its customers access to these services in 1996. With the help of digital banking services, customers can make online transitions, submit requests and complaints, and handle their account information and other activities through mobile devices and computers. This significant change is only possible by the technical advancement in network technology. Generation upgrades are very essential for faster growth in the economy, so fifth-generation technology started deploying worldwide in 2019. It has increased the speed of the internet ten times faster than 4G and has improved the experience [6]. The introduction of 5G in South Korea on December 1 marked a first (the fifth-generation mobile wireless standard). Many countries expect to start utilizing 5G by 2020, which is set to drive the Internet of Things (IoT) and big data [7].

5.1.2 Constraints Due to Regularization of Smart Hospitals

The regularization of smart hospitals, which involves the imposition of rules and regulations to ensure compliance and standardization, brings about several constraints that need to be addressed. While smart hospitals offer numerous benefits, such as improved healthcare outcomes, enhanced patient experience, and increased operational efficiency, the process of regularization is necessary to ensure ethical, legal, and secure implementation. Let's delve into the constraints imposed by regularization in smart hospitals. One of the primary concerns in smart hospitals is the protection of patient data privacy and security. The integration of various technologies and data-driven systems collects a vast amount of sensitive information about patients, including their medical records, personal details, and health data. Regularization ensures that adequate safeguards are in place to protect this data from unauthorized access, breaches, or misuse [8]. Compliance with data protection regulations, such as the General Data Protection Regulation (GDPR), Health Insurance Portability and Accountability Act (HIPAA), and relevant local laws, becomes essential. This constraint necessitates the implementation of robust cybersecurity measures, encryption techniques, access controls, and audits to mitigate the risks associated with data breaches. Smart hospitals often rely on multiple devices, systems, and software platforms, each with its own proprietary protocols and data formats. The lack of interoperability and standardization poses a significant constraint to seamless data exchange and integration. Regularization efforts aim to define interoperability standards, such as Health Level Seven International (HL7), Fast Healthcare Interoperability Resources (FHIR), and International Organization for Standardization (ISO) guidelines, to ensure compatibility and harmonization among different healthcare technologies [9]. By adhering to these standards, smart hospitals can facilitate the sharing of patient data, enable collaborative care, and ensure the interoperability of various systems within the healthcare ecosystem. The adoption of advanced technologies in smart hospitals raises ethical concerns that require careful deliberation and regulation. For instance, the use of artificial intelligence (AI) and machine learning (ML) algorithms in decision-making processes should follow ethical guidelines to avoid biases, discrimination, or unfair treatment of patients [10]. Regularization becomes crucial in establishing guidelines and frameworks that govern the development, deployment, and use of AI technologies in healthcare. It involves addressing issues such as transparency, accountability, informed consent, algorithmic fairness, and the ethical handling of patient data. Ethical review boards and regulatory bodies play a vital role in overseeing and enforcing these guidelines. The successful implementation of smart hospital technologies requires a skilled workforce capable of operating and maintaining these complex systems. Regularization efforts should focus on training healthcare professionals, including doctors, nurses, and administrators, to adapt to the changing technological landscape. Training programs should cover aspects such as data analytics, cybersecurity, interoperability, and the effective utilization of smart hospital technologies [11]. Constraints arise from the need to ensure that healthcare professionals are well equipped with the necessary skills and knowledge to maximize the benefits of smart hospitals and deliver quality care. The implementation of smart hospitals necessitates a robust and reliable infrastructure that can support the integration of various technologies, such as Internet of Things (IoT) devices, electronic health records (EHR) systems, and real-time communication platforms. Upgrading the existing infrastructure or building new facilities can be a constraint due to the associated costs and logistical challenges. Regularization efforts should address the allocation of resources, funding mechanisms, and guidelines for infrastructure development to ensure that smart hospitals can function optimally. This includes considerations for network connectivity, data storage, bandwidth requirements, and system scalability. Smart hospitals operate within a regulatory framework that governs healthcare practices, patient safety, and quality standards. Regularization aims to ensure that smart hospitals adhere to these regulations, such as medical device regulations, clinical trial requirements, quality management systems, and accreditation standards [12]. Compliance with these regulations can be challenging due to the rapid advancements in technology and the need to adapt existing regulations to accommodate emerging innovations. Regulatory bodies need to keep pace with technological advancements and provide clear guidelines to address the unique challenges posed by smart hospital implementations. Introducing advanced technologies in healthcare can face resistance and skepticism from patients, healthcare providers, and other stakeholders. User acceptance and trust are essential for the successful implementation of smart hospitals. Regularization efforts should focus on fostering transparency, ensuring the explainability of algorithms, and addressing concerns related to data privacy, security, and the impact on the doctor-patient relationship. Patient education, awareness campaigns, and open dialogues are necessary to build trust and encourage the acceptance of smart hospital technologies. In conclusion, while the regularization of smart hospitals imposes certain constraints, addressing these constraints is crucial for the successful and responsible implementation of these technologies. By ensuring data privacy and security, promoting interoperability, addressing ethical considerations, providing adequate training, managing infrastructure and costs, complying with regulations, and fostering user acceptance, smart hospitals can deliver transformative healthcare while upholding high standards of quality, safety, and patient-centric care [13].

5.1.3 IMPACT OF SMART HEALTHCARE

The constraints imposed by the regularization of smart hospitals can have an impact on the cost of healthcare. While smart hospitals offer potential benefits in terms of improved efficiency and quality of care, the implementation of regulations and standards can introduce additional expenses and considerations. The integration of smart hospital technologies requires significant investment in terms of hardware, software, network infrastructure, and training. Regularization may add additional requirements, such as the need for compliant systems, data security measures, and interoperability standards, which can increase the initial implementation costs. Hospitals and healthcare organizations may need to allocate budgets for acquiring and deploying advanced technologies, upgrading existing systems, and ensuring regulatory compliance [14]. The introduction of new technologies in smart hospitals often necessitates training and skill development programs for healthcare professionals. Regularization efforts may require additional training on data analytics, cybersecurity, interoperability, and the use of smart hospital systems. These training programs come with associated costs, including trainers' fees, educational resources, and time away from clinical duties. The cost of ensuring a skilled workforce proficient in utilizing smart hospital technologies can impact overall healthcare expenditures. Smart hospitals rely on robust and reliable infrastructure to support the seamless integration and functioning of various technologies. Upgrading existing infrastructure or building new facilities to accommodate advanced systems can be costly. Regularization may impose requirements for network connectivity, data storage capabilities, bandwidth, and system scalability. Healthcare organizations may need to invest in infrastructure development to meet these requirements, which can contribute to the overall cost of healthcare [15]. Ensuring regulatory compliance in smart hospitals involves additional administrative and operational efforts. Regularization may require hospitals to invest in resources such as compliance officers, legal counsel, and regulatory consultants to navigate the complex regulatory landscape. Compliance with data protection laws, cybersecurity measures, and quality standards may require ongoing audits, assessments, and certifications, all of which come with associated costs. Adhering to regulatory requirements can add financial burdens to healthcare organizations. Smart hospital technologies require ongoing maintenance, updates, and support to ensure optimal performance. Regularization efforts may introduce requirements for regular system audits, security patches, software updates, and adherence to evolving standards. Healthcare organizations need to allocate resources for monitoring, maintenance contracts, and technical support, which can contribute to the overall cost of healthcare. Smart hospitals often rely on multiple vendors and systems, each with their own proprietary protocols and interfaces [16]. Regularization aims to promote interoperability and adherence to standards, but integration efforts can introduce complexities and costs. Healthcare organizations may face challenges in integrating disparate systems, ensuring smooth data flow, and avoiding vendor lock-in. Integration costs, customization expenses, and ongoing support fees from multiple vendors can impact the overall cost of healthcare. Despite these potential cost implications, it is important to note that the long-term benefits of smart hospitals, such as improved efficiency, streamlined workflows, reduced errors, and better patient outcomes, can offset some of the initial and ongoing costs. Furthermore, as the technology matures and becomes more widespread, economies of scale and market competition can help drive down costs. Balancing the benefits and costs is crucial in making informed decisions regarding the implementation of smart hospitals and ensuring that the potential improvements in healthcare justify the associated expenses [17].

5.2   RESEARCH METHODOLOGY

This review is based upon the secondary data gathered from various sources and a kind of exploratory research for the purpose of analysing the present situation of the 5G technology in telecommunication, AI, and IoT.

5.2.1   APPLICATIONS OF 5G WIRELESS TECHNOLOGY

The fifth-generation mobile communication network (5G) is set to launch in 2020. Research on 5G has been put forward by telecom hardware manufacturers and telecommunication network operators, for example, 700 million euros (via 5G - PPP) from the EU. The term *5G* combines many wireless communication ideas into a credo and describes many ideas, but most ideas have similar concepts in between. Misconceptions about 5G will not be implemented, but the main idea will probably be. It has not yet provided us with the full specification of 5G, but it does provide the ability to understand its main features. The interest in 5G is based on the promises that explain its performance. Through a broad variety of usage scenarios that offer high data-rate instant communication, low latency, and mobile, 5G is fundamentally capable of sparking the formation of new markets, industries, and economic structures as well as the global improvement of living standards. Mass connection, eHealth, autonomous vehicles, smart cities, smart homes, and IoT are necessary for new applications [18].

- **In the business sector**

  The emerging fifth-generation broadband network guarantees at least seven times faster speeds than the average 4G LTE browsing experience. The average 4G browsing speed runs at an average of 56 Mbps, while 5G gets speeds up to 490 Mbps. These increased speeds and powerful connections mean businesses are trying to pull off digital changes. But a wider, faster network also carries more risk. Cybercriminals are always on the lookout for new, sophisticated attack methods, so they naturally use the promise of 5G. The potential risk of 5G does not negate its benefits. But as a business leader, you need to know what 5G brings, how we get there, and how it will benefit your business and get the best out of it$_5$.

- **In the banking sector**

  On the bases of usage, 5G can reduce time, which provides a real-time mobile banking experience. An exciting and innovative small-scale mobile banking utility scenario, such as the capability to instantly purchase an item by scanning its image in a catalog or online, are already more than just concepts. Faster and simpler payments make mobile and digital payments more attractive to the general public and merchants, as well as want to further promote consumption. As the Internet of Things (IoT), and virtual reality (VR) devices grow more prevalent and advanced, many traditional banking processes could be expanded to these new channels. Banks must begin considering how they may seize these new chances in order to leverage this technology.

  On the basis of security – leaving despite the well-known security risks with 5G, businesses may do more to protect end customers. For companies, 5G allows real-time updates without customer interference and usage interruptions. This allows for greater utilization of multi-model biometric security measures that combine the situation where a person owns their mobile phone to verify subtle skills and identity such as user gait. Active fraud protection is greatly enhanced by 5G. Real-time data processing, transaction volume authentication, client geolocation, and merchant IDs are some of the features that limit false positives and errors in fraud detection. Data management, security, and privacy regulations are expanding quickly. The procedures and policies of banks' data collecting and usage must be evaluated by the banks themselves. As data security regulation becomes tougher, banks must strictly adhere to the new regulations in order to successfully bring new 5G-enabled offers to market[6].

- **In healthcare**

    5G will eventually change how health workers and patients interact with data generated during patient travel. Gigabyte imaging files provided in diagnostic animations can be returned to mobile devices on the 5G network using the millimeter wave spectrum or returned to any wired terminal for large files, without the need for doctors to meet for review in seconds to influence the wired network to move everywhere. Physicians are free to move on the 5G + footprint and never lose the quality of the data and views they rely on. The standards of the 5G network and the low latency and ultra-reliable communication built into the structure allow, among other 5G-related technologies and greater granularity of medical data acquisition. These small measurement intervals during a patient visit can show symptoms that take longer to detect and now both health AI systems and therapists are more aware of preventing previous interventions and improving outcomes. For example, there may be subtle gaps and local analysis of ventilator data[7].

5.2.2 THE FUTURE EFFECT OF 5G ON FINANCIAL SERVICES

A stronger framework for a scalable and dependable global connection is brought by 5G. The technology is built for high data rates and quick response times. The speedier real-time flow of data between two or more sites is made possible by these two qualities. You may now use a variety of new applications that were previously impossible thanks to 5G. The term "Internet of Things" (IoT) has gained widespread recognition. It describes intelligent, web-enabled gadgets with more specialized features than a typical smartphone, tablet, or computer. IoT gadgets include connected kitchen appliances, security cameras, door locks, and thermostats. Despite the fact that 5G is only a few years away, it has already become a widely used technology (with many operators anticipated to reach 50% coverage in their regions by 2023–2027) and LTE is used now and impacts the ecosystem of financial services. It should be mentioned that 5G is a technology alternative to think about if you want to improve or change the wired or WLN infrastructure that banks and merchants now utilize in their branches, storefronts, and corporate locations. The list that follows focuses on the novel experiences that "consumers" might expect while using a 5G device to connect to a network [19].

- Drive has spurred the growth of mobile commerce. By 2022, 55% of all digital e-commerce transaction volume will be made up of m-commerce (mobile browser and native app) transactions, overtaking e-commerce for the first time globally. The 5G ultra-low latency offers a better mobile buying experience, which we anticipate will hasten the growth of the mobile share market.

- Shop Deliver on the promise of "shopping videos". Talked about industry efficiency shopping in the video (for example, clicking on a shoe worn by someone and buying it instantly redirects) for at least a decade. 5G can bring these types of high bandwidth and low latency experiences close to actuality.
- Delay banking applications with high priority. 5G has a compelling story for financial applications that aim to reduce rare but expensive transactions. Applications for capacity might include high-frequency trading, cryptocurrency exchanges, and real-time payments. The enhancement of fraud prevention in 5G will advance by enabling more data to travel between parties in real-time
- Using various data sources to test for fraud. It should make it easier for businesses like financial institutions and retailers to implement more reliable data-based risk assessment models with fewer false positives and refunds.
- Facilitate more effective and timely geotargeted offerings. More accurate and timely accountability is provided by 5G's geotargeted capabilities. By informing 56% of customers that they received a personal offer from a store (based on their location or a past purchase), which led to a purchase that wasn't what they had originally intended to make, we estimate great potential.
- Provide opportunities for immersive, online consumer involvement. Merchant banks could develop revolutionary and highly individualized customer care strategies thanks to 5G. Hosted robots in the hotel industry, virtual tellers in the banking industry, and HD digital codes with facial recognition in the retail industry are all possible.

Advantages of the 5G Network

- Faster speed

   The speed of each wireless network generation has increased significantly and the advantages of the 5G cellular network technology, which is the fifth generation, go beyond those of 4G LTE. The 10 Gbps estimated speed represents an increase of 100.1 compared to 4G. In practice, increasing the speed to 4G vs. 5G represents exciting possibilities for consumers. It takes from seven minutes to just six seconds to transfer a high-resolution movie to maximum download speed$_9$.

- Less delay

   The duration of time between a source and your receiver, and then back again, is known as *latency*. Every wireless generation has latency reduction as one of its main objectives. The new 5G network will send data roundtrip in less than five milliseconds and have a delay that is smaller than 4G LTE. Real-time remote device control is now possible thanks to 5G's faster latency than human visual processing. The human reaction time becomes a limiting issue for remote applications using 5G and IoT, and many new applications now use machine-to-machine communication, which doesn't restrict how soon humans can respond. Reductions in delays assist the manufacturing, shipping, and agriculture industries. Gamers are also anxiously anticipating the launch of 5G.

- Increased efficiency

   The pace is exciting, but one question on the minds of analysts and industry leaders is: How can 5G help businesses measure their technology programs? Smart homes and cities will also go a long way in the future of 5G. Using unprecedentedly connected devices, AI Edge can be transported to unprecedented locations with computing. From homes that offer personalized energy-saving tips that increase environmental impact to traffic lights that change their designs based on traffic flow, 5G applications that depend on additional network capacity affect almost everything.
- Wider bandwidth

   A 5G network can transport more data than a 4G LTE network because to its faster speed and higher network capacity. Because 5G networks are built differently than conventional 4G networks, network traffic can be optimised more and utility surges can be handled more easily. Sports fans can now enjoy their experience from any seat on the field thanks to 5G, which has made it easier for crowded stadiums and other venues to deliver smooth connectivity to enormous audiences. Big data is one way that the enhanced bandwidth effect for organizations reverberates across most segments.

   Easy accessibility and coverage. Although consumers and businesses are eager to experience the benefits of 5G for themselves, the availability of 5G coverage is still limited. Today, all major U.S. cellular carriers are expanding their 5G networks in major cities.

Benefits for the Banking Sector

- Worldwide extension of smartphone banking services.
- Capability to gain a huge customer base due to omnipresent services.
- The power to raise the growing popularity of smartphone banking through digital deposit applications.
- Amplify the bank's reputation by providing faster and safer services to its customer smartphone users enlargement.
- Businesses can launch services to attract businesspeople and other tightly scheduled customer pools due to the nature of the businesses.
- Technology improving user reputation of technology 5G technology provides high-quality services [11].

Disadvantages

- Exorbitant price and demanding maintenance

   The installation and maintenance of 5G networks necessitate costly 5G equipment and trained engineers. The price of the 5G rollout and maintenance phase will go up as a result.
- Initial stage

   5G technology is still in process and research is underway.
- Expensive

   5G smartphones are expensive, so it takes time for the common person to use 5G technology. And for 5G, we have to improve our infrastructure facilities, so it is more expensive.

- Connectivity problem in rural areas (limited access)

  Urban regions are the only places where 5G can deliver true connectivity; individuals who live in rural areas will not profit from the connection. As it stands, cell phone coverage is unavailable in the majority of the nation's outlying areas. It's not likely to happen anytime soon, but 5G providers will initially focus on populous metropolitan cities before expanding to the suburbs. Hence, only a small portion of the population will gain from the 5G connection.
- Security

  Security and privacy issues are addressed in 5G.
- Coverage

  Due to larger losses at higher frequencies, coverage distances of 2 m (indoors) and 300 m (outdoors) can be attained (such as millimeter waves). There are numerous losses like this in the 5G mm-wave (penetration damage, attenuation due to rain, damage, etc.).

5.3 SERVICE IMPROVEMENT DUE TO THE SMART HOSPITAL

The regularization of smart hospitals brings about service improvements that can significantly enhance the delivery of healthcare. By implementing regulations and standards, smart hospitals can optimize various aspects of their operations, leading to enhanced patient care, improved efficiency, and better outcomes. The regularization of smart hospitals leads to significant service improvements, including enhanced patient experience, improved diagnostic accuracy, streamlined workflows, proactive and preventive care, data-driven decision making, and adherence to quality and safety measures. These improvements contribute to more efficient healthcare delivery, better patient outcomes, and an overall enhancement in the quality of care provided by smart hospitals [20]. Here are some key service improvements due to the regularization of smart hospitals [21, 22]:

i. Enhanced Patient Experience: Smart hospitals leverage advanced technologies to improve the overall patient experience. Regularization ensures the implementation of patient-centric practices, such as personalized care plans, real-time communication channels, and access to health information. Patients can benefit from streamlined registration processes, reduced wait times, and improved communication with healthcare providers. Smart hospitals can utilize digital platforms and mobile applications to provide convenient appointment scheduling, virtual consultations, and remote monitoring, enhancing convenience and accessibility for patients.

ii. Improved Diagnostic Accuracy: Regularization efforts in smart hospitals emphasize the integration of advanced diagnostic technologies and data analytics. This enables more accurate and timely diagnoses, leading to improved treatment outcomes. Smart hospitals can leverage artificial intelligence (AI) algorithms to analyze medical imaging data, interpret test results, and identify patterns in patient data. This enhances the accuracy and efficiency of diagnostics, aiding healthcare professionals in making informed decisions and providing appropriate treatment plans.

iii. Streamlined Workflows and Efficiency: Smart hospitals optimize workflows and operational processes through the regularization of technological standards and protocols. Interoperability guidelines facilitate seamless data exchange and integration across different systems, enabling healthcare professionals to access patient information and collaborate more effectively. Automation of routine tasks, such as appointment scheduling, billing, and inventory management, reduces administrative burden and allows healthcare providers to focus more on patient care. This streamlining of workflows improves overall efficiency and reduces the likelihood of errors or delays.

iv. Proactive and Preventive Care: Regularization promotes the integration of real-time monitoring and predictive analytics in smart hospitals. By continuously collecting and analyzing patient data, healthcare providers can identify trends, detect early warning signs, and take proactive measures to prevent adverse events. For example, smart hospitals can use wearable devices and remote monitoring systems to track vital signs, activity levels, and medication adherence. This enables healthcare professionals to intervene promptly and provide timely interventions or preventive measures, reducing hospital readmissions and improving patient outcomes.

v. Data-Driven Decision Making: The regularization of smart hospitals emphasizes the utilization of data analytics to support clinical decision making. By analyzing large volumes of patient data, including medical records, treatment history, and population health trends, healthcare providers can gain valuable insights. These insights can inform evidence-based decision making, treatment protocols, and resource allocation. Data-driven decision making enables healthcare professionals to personalize care, identify high-risk patients, optimize treatment plans, and allocate resources efficiently, resulting in improved patient outcomes and cost-effectiveness.

vi. Quality and Safety Measures: Regularization ensures adherence to quality standards and patient safety measures in smart hospitals. By implementing regulatory guidelines and accreditation standards, smart hospitals can improve the quality of care delivered. Regular audits, performance evaluations, and continuous quality improvement initiatives help identify areas for improvement and ensure compliance with best practices. Smart hospitals can also utilize data analytics to identify adverse events, monitor medication errors, and implement strategies to enhance patient safety and reduce medical errors.

5.4 CONCLUSION

There are a lot of advantages of 5G for every sector, despite the challenges, which are related to technology, usage, and adoption. Due to the initial stage, the coverage area of a 5G network is currently very small, at present few countries have been using a 5G network. The US, South Korea, Canada, and China are one of the first adapter countries of the 5G network. Prior to the adoption of remaining countries, there were fears about the cost and security, and complexity of having to adopt devices that could support 5G on a large scale. Issues related to authentication and regulation must also be addressed prior to mass rollout. While the highlighted utility cases are likely to change the field of financial and banking services, this is not going to happen overnight. The banking and finance sector needs to adopt a strategic approach to design 5G-based solutions and implement them on a large scale. It seems that 5G will take time to take over the present network technology. Financial and banking institutions would, therefore, have enough time to build dynamic strategies and execution plans to roll out 5G-enabled services. There is no doubt that 5G technology would lead to better services and results.

REFERENCES

1. Barman, P.P., & Hallur, G. (2022, March). A study on the impact of 5G on the banking industry: An economic impact perspective. In 2022 International Conference on Decision Aid Sciences and Applications (DASA) (pp. 591–600). IEEE.
2. Kumar, A., & Gupta, M. (2018). A review on activities of fifth generation mobile communication system. *Alexandria Engineer. J.*, *57*(2), 1125–1135, 10.1016/j.aej.2017.01.043.
3. Qiu, W. (2021). Enterprise financial risk management platform based on 5 G mobile communication and embedded system. *Microprocessors & Microsyst.*, *80*, 103594.
4. Dash, B., Ansari, M.F., & Sharma, P. (2022). Future ready banking with smart contracts-Cbdc and impact on the Indian economy. *International Journal of Network Security & Its Applications*, *14*, 39–49.
5. Chikermane, G. (2019). 5G infrastructure. *Huawei's techno-economic advantages and India's national security concerns: An analysis. ORF Occasional Paper*, (226), 62.
6. Ganesh, E.N. (2021). Study of 5G technology and its operations and maintenance to improve flexibility, impacts: Review. Recent Trends in Electronics & efficiency and availability. *Although Maintenance Communication Systems, 8*(3), 40–49p.
7. Kesavaraj, S.V., Jakhiya, C.M., & Bhandari, C.N. (2022, October). A study on upcoming central bank digital currency: Opportunities, obstacles, and potential fintech solutions using cryptography in the Indian scenario. In 2022 13th International Conference on Computing Communication and Networking Technologies (ICCCNT) (pp. 1–10). IEEE.
8. Kumar, A., Rajagopal, K., Gugapriya, G., Sharma, H., Gour, N., Masud, M., AlZain, M.A., & Alajmani, S.H. (2022). Reducing PAPR with low complexity filtered NOMA using novel algorithm. *Sustainability, 14*, 9631. 10.3390/su14159631.
9. Whig, P., Velu, A., & Naddikatu, R.R. (2022). The economic impact of AI-enabled blockchain in 6G-based industry. *AI and Blockchain Technology in 6G Wireless Network* (pp. 205–224). Springer, Singapore.
10. Ionescu, C.A., Fülöp, M.T., Topor, D.I., Căpușneanu, S., Breaz, T.O., Stănescu, S.G., & Coman, M.D. (2021). The new era of business digitization through the implementation of 5G technology in Romania. *Sustainability, 13*(23), 13401.
11. Adarsh, A., Kumar, B., Gupta, M., Kumar, A., Singh, A.*, Masud, M. & Alraddady, F.A. (2021). Design of an efficient cooperative spectrum for intra-hospital cognitive radio network. *CMC Journal, 69*(1), 35–4,

12. Lloret, J., Parra, L., Taha, M., & Tomas, J. (2017). An architecture and protocol for smart continuous eHealth monitoring using 5G Comput. *Networking*, *129*(2), 340–351

13. Ramakrishnan, B., Kumar, A., Chakravarty, S., Masud, M., & Baz, M. (2021). Analysis of FBMC waveform for 5G network based smart hospitals. *Appl. Sci.*, *11*(19), 8895. 10.3390/app11198895.

14. Fan, M., Sun, J., Zhou, B., et al. (2016). The smart health initiative in China: The case of Wuhan, Hubei province. *J. Med. Syst.*, *40*(62), 10.1007/s10916-015-0416-y.

15. Sharma, H., Kumar, A., & Albreem, M.A.M. (2021). 5G-driven radio framework for proficient smart health-care institutions. In*Blockchain for 5G Healthcare Applications: Security and Privacy Solutions*, 10.1049/PBHE035E

16. Ahad, A., Tahir, M., & Yau, K.A. (2019). 5G-based smart healthcare network: Architecture, taxonomy, challenges and future research directions. *IEEE Access, 7*, 100747–100762, 10.1109/ACCESS.2019.2930628

17. Kumar, S., Gupta, M., & Kumar, A. (2021a). Breast cancer detection based on antenna data collection and analysis. In: Tanwar S. (eds.) *Fog Computing for Healthcare 4.0 Environments. Signals and Communication Technology.* Springer, Cham. 10.1007/978-3-030-46197-3_19

18. Kuma, A., Bharti, S. & Gupta, M. (2019). FBMC vs OFDM: 5G mobile communication system. *Int. J. Syst. Control Commun.*, *10*(3), 250–264. 10.1504/IJSCC.2019. 100534

19. Ahad, A., Tahir, M., Sheikh, M.A., Ahmed, K.I., Mughees, A., & Numani, A. (2020). Technologies trend towards 5G network for smart health-care using IoT: A review Sensors, *20*(4047), pp. 1–22, 10.3390/s20144047

20. Kumar, A., Dhanagopal, R., Albreem, M.A., & Le, D.-N. (December 2021b). A comprehensive study on the role of advanced technologies in 5G based smart hospital. *Alexandria Engineer. J.*, *60*(6), 5527–5536.

21. Kumar, A., Albreem, M.A., Gupta, M., Alsharif, M.H., & Kim, S. (2020). Future 5G network based smart hospitals: Hybrid detection technique for latency improvement. *IEEE Access*, 8, 153240–153249, 10.1109/ACCESS.2020.3017625.

22. El-hajj, M., Fadlallah, A., Chamoun, M., & Serhrouchni, A. (2019). A survey of Internet of Things (IoT) authentication schemes. *Sensors.*, *19*(5), 1141. 10.3390/s19051141

6 Integrating the Vertical and Horizontal Dimension of Medical and Technology for Brain Tumour Segmentation in Medical Image Processing

Mukesh Chand
Poornima University, Jaipur, Rajasthan, India

Garima Mathur
Department of Electronics & Communication Engineering,
Poornima University, Jaipur, Rajasthan, India

Prashant Jamwal
Department of Electrical and Computer Engineering,
Nazarbayev University, Republic of Kazakhstan

6.1 INTRODUCTION

A human life is at stake and the need for high accuracy when dealing with medical images drives the development of automated classification and detection of tumours. As a result, medical institutions demand computer assistance because it can improve human performance in a field where the rate of false negatives has to be extremely low [1]. Double-reading medical images have been shown to improve the detection of tumours. Double-reading costs a lot of money, which is why medical institutions are interested in good software that can assist humans in their work. A human observer is required to detect the presence of specific features in order to monitor and diagnose the diseases [2].

DOI: 10.1201/9781003403678-6

6.1.1 IMAGE SEGMENTATION

In order to extract, measure, and render objects from multi-dimensional images, segmentation problems must be overcome. Using local pixel-neighbourhood classification as a starting point, simple segmentation techniques can be developed quickly. The failure of these methods is that they only work for local appearances, not global objects, and they frequently necessitate extensive manual intervention. Because an object's "logic" does not always follow its local image representation, this is the reason [3]. It is not always the case that local properties, such as roughness, edginess, and ridges, are indicative of the object as a whole.

Division of images results in a large number of fragments dispersed throughout the image or a variety of new forms derived from the original (see edge detection). Colour, brightness, and surface properties are all considered for each specific location within the image. It's remarkable to find two places that share many of the same characteristics. Threshold: The quest to cross the border. There are two ways to think about mathematics: In mathematics, gray-value morphology is studied. When looking into the things in pictures, it's critical to distinguish between "the rest" and "the premium" artefacts. "The base" is often used as a synonym for the final meeting. Segmentation techniques are commonly used to distinguish between the foreground and background in intrigue artefact detection systems.

6.2 K-MEANS SEGMENTATION

K-means segmentation is a popular and simplest clustering algorithm for brain tumour segmentation. A prearranged number of clusters (assume k clusters) is used to categorise the data in this procedure. Any cluster is characterised by a single k-centroid. The placement of these centroids must be done carefully so that each location has a different effect. The next step is to locate the nearest centroids for each point in a given data set. The first stage has been accomplished and an early age has been established. k new centroids are needed here to represent the clusters formed in the previous step, so we need to recalculate k new centroids here [4]. Once we have these k new centroids, we need to redo the binding between the original data points and the new centroids that are closest. There is now a loop in the system. To see how the k centroids change over time, we need to look at the loop in which the k points change location. In other words, the centres of the universe have ceased to shift. At the end, the K-means algorithm aims to minimise a specific objective function, which is the squared error [5].

6.2.1 THRESHOLDING

Thresholding is a simple segmentation method and is based on a level clipping (or level threshold) to convert a gray-scale image into a bit image. The main advantage of the thresholding is selecting the clipping level (or the values of its multiple-threshold levels are selected). The other most common image segmentation methods are medical is the max method.

The scheme relies on a fundamental concept. The brilliance limit is chosen for a parameter and added as follows to the picture [m, n]:
If

$$x[a, b] \geq \theta$$

then

$$x[a, b] = object = 1 \tag{6.1}$$

(Brightness in two-dimensional pixel picture expresses) Else

$$[a, b] = background = 0 \tag{6.2}$$

(Brightness in two-dimensional pixels of the image set to zero if value is below the threshold)
This algorithm version assumes that we want illumination objects from uni-lluminated background. We will use the following for unilluminated objects on an illumination background:
If

$$x(a, b) < \theta$$

then

$$x(a, b) = object = 1 \tag{6.3}$$

(The two-dimensional pixel of the dark image communicates brightness) Else

$$x[a, b] = background = 0 \tag{6.4}$$

The yields are the mark 'books' or 'foundations,' which can be referred to as Boolean variable '1' or '0' because of its dichotomy. The test condition can, at a fundamental level, be built on a different property than the basic splendour (e.g., If (Redness {x[a, b]} > = θ red), but the principle is simple.
Then it turns out that the emphasis of the thresholding is: how do we select the limit? Although there is no all-inclusive restricting approach for dealing with all images, a number of options are offered.
Fixed edge: One choice is to use a rim freely collected from the information on the image. When it is understood that highly differentiated images are handled where artefacts are especially dull and the base is homogenous and very light, a clear 128 border with a size of 0 to 255 may at this time be reasonably accurate. By precision, we mean that a minimum number of pixels should be held in an unequivocal order.

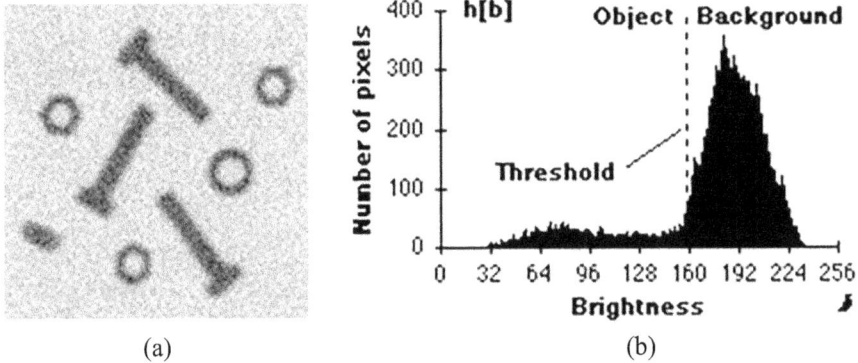

FIGURE 6.1   (a) Image to be threshold. (b) Histogram of the brightness image.

Histogram-inferred limits: In many cases, the edge of the region or image that we want to segment is presented over the brilliance histograms. Figure 6.1 displays an image and its corresponding histogram of brightness.

Threshold (x [a, b] < θ) of pixel object will be labelled as pixel artefacts, those of the background pixel above the threshold.

A number of methods were designed to naturally select a {h[b], 1, 2^{b-1}} limit starting at the dim value histogram. The most popular ones are possibly introduced below. Smoothing of the crude histogram information will benefit a large number of these calculations in order to expel little variance, but the smoothing calculations should not move the positions of the spine. This translates into a zero-stage calculation of smoothing under which the average quality of W is 3 or 5.

6.3   DESIGN STEPS OF THRESHOLDING

6.3.1   PRINCIPAL COMPONENT ANALYSIS

Principle components, which are sets of values that are not linearly connected but may still be used to estimate the prospective correlation between two sets of observations, are one method that principal component analysis (PCA) accomplishes this. Less or an equivalent number of major components exist for the original variables. This conversion is defined in a way to give the first primary component as much variance as possible while still accounting for as much variability in the data as possible. While remaining orthogonal (uncorrelated with) to the preceding components, each following component has the maximum variance. if the data are evenly distributed, it might be possible to guarantee the autonomy of the main components. Performance of PCA is impacted by the original variables' relative scale [6].

Drawbacks

• Poor discriminatory
• High load computational

6.3.2 DISCRETE WAVELET TRANSFORM

A wavelet series is an Ortho-normal series generated by wavelets that can be represents by a square integral (real/complex function valued) function. Ortho-normal wavelets and integral wavelet transforms are defined in this article using a formal, mathematical definition.

6.3.2.1 Definition

A function $\varphi \epsilon L^2(R)$ known as an Ortho-normal wavelet can be implemented to define a Hilbert function, that may be a complete Ortho-normal system, for the Hilbert $L^2(R)$ of square integral functions.

The Hilbert basis function is constructed by the family of functions for j, $k \in Z$ integers.

This family is an Ortho-normal system if it is Ortho-normal under the inner product where $\delta_{j\ l}$ is the Kronecker delta and [f, g] is the standard inner product on $L^2(R)$.

The basic requirement of every function that must fulfil the thoroughness criterion is that every function $f \epsilon L^2(R)$ may be expanded in the basis as

$$f(x) = \sum_{j,k=-\infty}^{\infty} (c_{jk} \varphi_{jk}(x)) \tag{6.5}$$

with the series convergence being considered to be the convergence of the norm. A wavelet series is a variant of such function representation. This shows that an orthonormal wavelet is dual in both directions.

6.3.3 K-NN CLASSIFIER

The K-nearest neighbours algorithms (K-NN) in pattern recognition are used to classify the objects based on the adjacent training sets in the feature space. In K-NN, all computation is delayed until classification and the function is only locally approximated. Instance-based learning, commonly referred to as lazy learning, is demonstrated here. The majority of machine learning algorithms employ the K-nearest neighbour algorithm, which categories objects into classes according to the percentage of their K-nearest neighbours who agree with that classification (K is a positive type integer, typically small). When determining an object's closest neighbour, K must match 1.

The same approach can be used to do regression, which averages the values of the object's nearest neighbours to get the property value of the object. It might be advantageous to weight the neighbours' contributions so that those who are closest to you make larger average contributions. A weight of 1/d, where d is the separation between the neighbours, is assigned to each neighbour. Here, linear interpolation is applied in a general context [7].

An accurate diagnosis relies on the acquisition and comprehension of images. Over the past few years, picture acquisition devices have advanced greatly; for example, we now have radiological images (X-ray, CT, and MRI examinations, and so forth) with much higher goals. It doesn't matter, though, because automated picture translation is already paying dividends [8]. Traditional AI computations for picture understanding rely heavily on master-made highlights, such as lung tumour detection, which necessitates the extraction of structure highlights. Conventional learning methods are unreliable because of the wide range of information from patient to silence. By its ability to sift through complex and large amounts of data, AI has evolved in recent years [9].

As of right now, deep learning is a hot topic in every industry, but it's expected to take over the $300 million medical imaging business by 2021. As a result, by 2021, the medical imaging sector will have received more investments than the entire examination industry did in 2016. It's the most efficient and targeted AI method out there right now. Using models of deep neural networks, which are advanced models of neural networks, this method employs models of deep neural networks, which are advanced models of neural networks. The use of a deep neural network is referred to as "deep learning." There are many different types of neurons in a neural network, each of which accepts a variety of input signals, combines them, and then passes the combined flags through nonlinear tasks to produce output signals, inspired by the study of the human brain.

6.4 FEATURE EXTRACTION

Using the dyadic scales and locations, the DWT (discrete wavelet transform) is a potent version of the wavelet transform. The following is an insight to DWT's fundamentals. Let x(t) be a function that can be square-integrated and then the cont. WT of x (t) relative to a given wavelet ψ (t) is defined as:

$$(a, b) = \int_{-\infty}^{-\infty} (t), (t)dt \qquad (6.6)$$

The wavelet ψa,b(t) is calculated by translation and dilation from the mother wavelet ψ(t) and is the dilation factor, and b is the translation parameter (both real positive numbers). Wavelets come in a variety of shapes and sizes, and have grown in prominence as wavelet analysis has progressed. The Harr wavelet, which is the most fundamental and generally applied, is the most significant wavelet.

The DWT is applied to each dimension independently in 2D images. The schematic diagram of 2D DWT is shown in Figure 4.1. As a result, at each scale, there are four sub-band pictures (LL, LH, HH, and HL). For the next 2D DWT, the sub-band LL is used (Figure 6.2).

The gray-level co-occurrence matrix (GLCM) approach is frequently utilised in medical image analysis and categorisation. This approach tells us the relative position of two pixels in relation to one another. The GLCM is then generated by counting the number of pixel pairings that occur at a given distance. A distance vector d=(x, y) is defined to compute the GLCM matrix for an image f I j).

6.5 PRE-PROCESSING ALGORITHM

Pre-processing of brain tumour MRI images consists of the following steps:

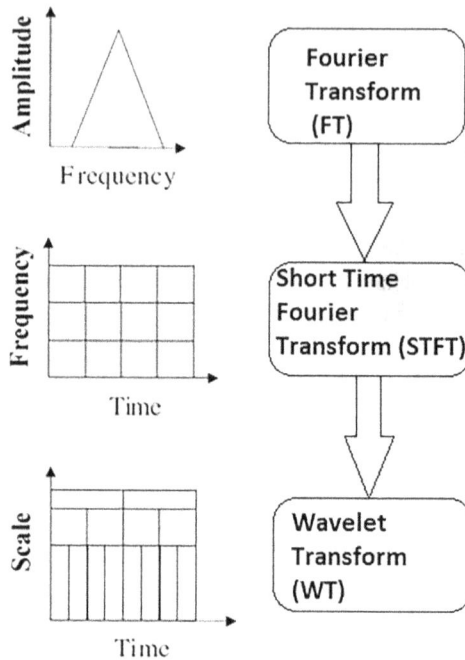

FIGURE 6.2 Discrete wavelet transform.

A. Pre-processing – In this step, the output of the brain tumour MRI image is extracted and reduces the feature of MRI images.
B. After the pre-processing of the MRI image, we trained the kernel SVM.
C. After training the kernel SVM, we added new MRI brain images into the SVM and compared both images to get the output in the form of normal or abnormal.

As shown in Figure 6.3, this block diagram is a standard method of brain tumour classification. We will explain the details of the pre-processing in the following sub-sections.

6.6 IMPROVED KERNEL-BASED SUPPORT VECTOR MACHINE

Support vector machines (SVMs), a subset of supervised learning models, can be used to categorise data by locating patterns in the input data. The SVM, a non-probability binary linear classifier, predicts two possible outputs, malignant or benign, for each given input, using a set of input data. An SVM training technique builds a model that automatically classifies incoming instances into one of two groups based on a set of previously labelled examples. Modelling the examples as points in space, an SVM model maps the examples into several categories, separating them by a significant distance [10]. New instances are then added to it, and their projected category membership is determined by where they fall on the spectrum.

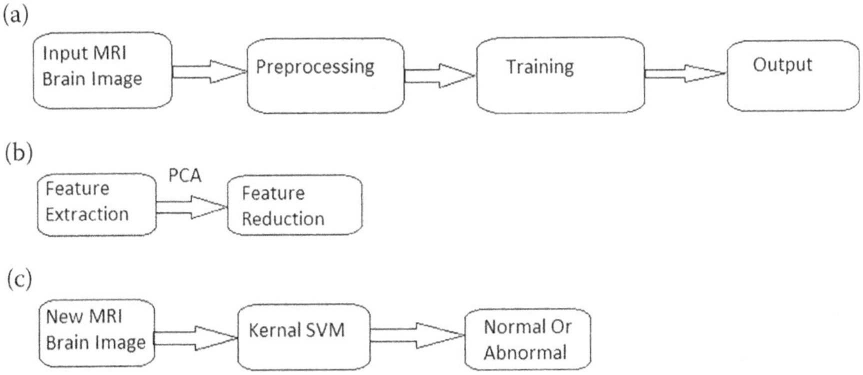

(a)

(b)

PCA

(c)

FIGURE 6.3 (a) Preprocessing. (b) Training the kernel SVM. (c) Output of proposed method, overview of proposed methodology.

If you want to get more technical, an SVM builds an infinite or high-dimensional space filled with hyper-planes, which can be used to classify data and do regression analysis. The functional margin (the distance between a class's nearest training data point to the hyper-plane's closest training data point) is a good indicator of a good separation between hyper-planes.

Given an N-size p-dimensional training data set, we can construct the following model:

$$\{(x_n, y_n | x_n \in R_p, y_n \in \{-1, +1\}\}, n = 1, \ldots \ldots \ldots, N \ldots \ldots \ldots \ldots \quad (6.7)$$

where y_n is either -1 or 1 and corresponds to the class 1 or 2. Each x_n is a p-dimensional vector. The support vector machine we desire is the maximum-margin hyper-plane that separates classes 1 and 2.

Given that each hyper-plane may be expressed in terms of

$$w. x - b = 0 \quad (6.8)$$

where the normal vector to the hyper-plane and the dot product are indicated. As much as possible while still maintaining the data's separation, we wish to choose and maximise the margin between the two parallel hyper-planes. As a result, the equations that define the two parallel hyper-planes are as follows:

$$w. x - b = \pm1 \quad (6.9)$$

As a result, the problem can be reduced to an optimisation problem, in which we wish to maximise the distance between two parallel hyper-planes while avoiding data dropping into the margin. The problem can be expressed as follows using basic mathematical knowledge:

$$min\|w\|$$

$$w, \ s. \ t. \ (w. \ x_n - b) \geq 1, \ n = 1, \ \ldots \ldots, N$$

In practical situations, the $\|w\|$ is usually replaced by

$$min \ \|w\|^2 \tag{6.10}$$

$$(w. \ x_n - b) \geq 1, \ n = 1, \ \ldots \ldots \ldots, N$$

An SVM takes a set of feature vectors as input; scales, selects, and validates a training model; and outputs a training model.

6.7 VISUALISATION OF RESULTS

With the aid of the suggested technique, the simulation results for the classification and detecting brain tumours using MRI images are shown in this part. The result demonstrates the creation of a graphical user interface (GUI) using the suggested technique, as well as a comparative analysis of the findings using a review of the literature. The method for visualising the outcome has been described in detail as follows (Figures 6.4–6.7).

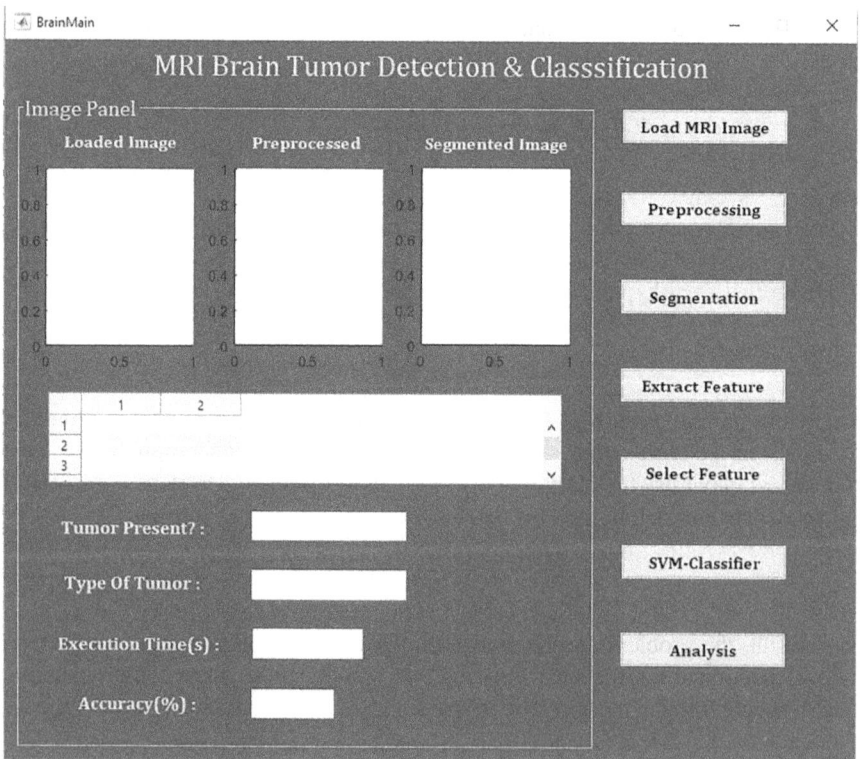

FIGURE 6.4 GUI for the proposed work.

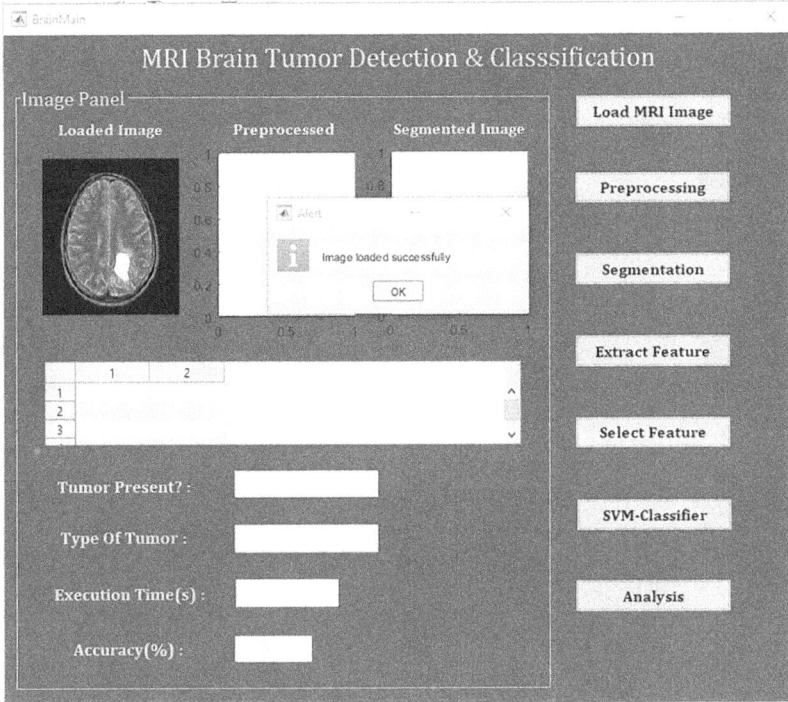

FIGURE 6.5 Image loading in GUI.

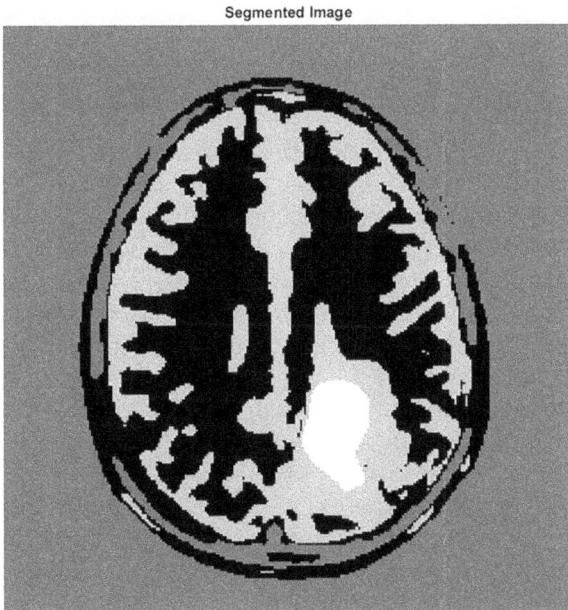

FIGURE 6.6 Snapshot of segmented image.

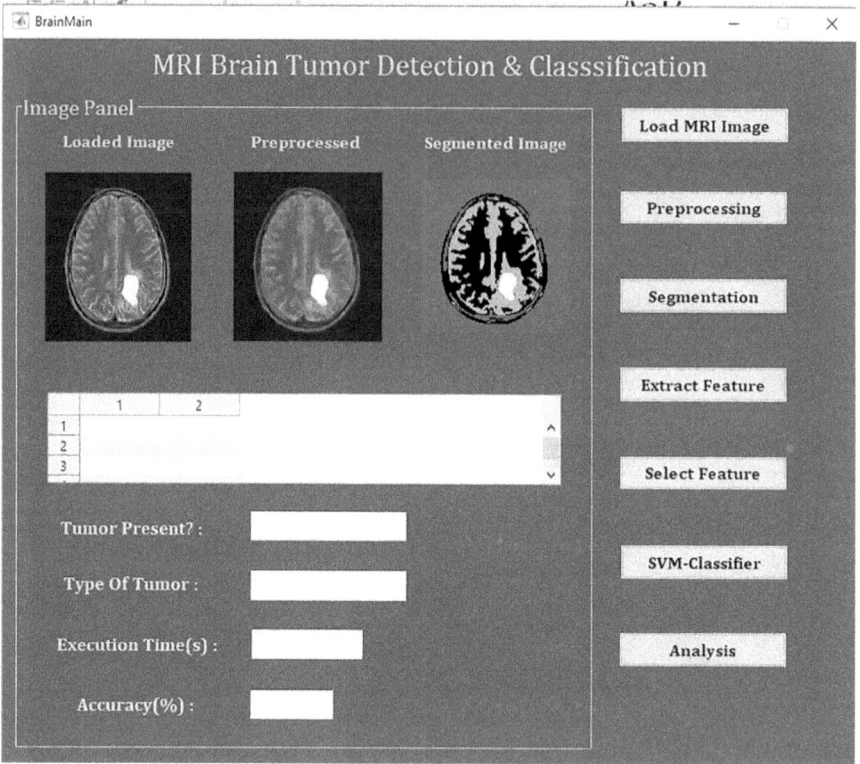

FIGURE 6.7   Feature extraction from the processed image.

6.8   CONCLUSION

In this paper, we improved the method of tumour detection and localisation using MRI brain image segmentation. We developed a new hybrid brain tumour detection clustering algorithm for reducing computation time and a binarization method for calculating the area in terms of millimetres squared. After determining the tumour's location and computing time, we ran simulations using the proposed shaft algorithm and compared the results. Last but not least, the new algorithm has outperformed the existing ones while requiring significantly less computational time. One of the most lethal forms of cancer, brain tumours can save lives if detected early enough. It is possible that cancer has already spread and is more difficult to treat by the time symptoms begin to appear. It is possible to divide the screening process into two main tasks (the process of MRI or CT scans in order to detect tumours). A doctor's first task is to determine the type of brain tumour that has been diagnosed. Meningioma, pituitary, and glioma are the three main types of brain tumours. It is possible to tell how aggressive a tumour is based on its type, but in order to accurately measure its size and spread, an expert must first segment the tumour into its various parts. Because of this, the second and more time-consuming task of segmenting brain tumours was required, which required doctors to label each pixel on the scan in order to separate infected tissues from healthy ones. Cancer is the most dangerous disease in the world, accounting for approximate 9.6 million deaths each year. Men and women have a 34% and 36% 5-year survival rate, respectively, from brain cancer. Radio-therapy is a mostly used in the treatment for brain tumours that uses high-energy radioactive particles to target and kill the tumour cells while sparing the surrounding tissues. The infected cells must be separated from the healthy ones in order to perform radiation treatment on the segmented tissues. Automating the laborious, costly, time-consuming, and error-prone process of creating an accurate segmentation map is a major step forward. Deep learning researchers are working on semantic segmentation. Numerous new counts have been proposed in the last decade to segment and request the psyche in MR/CT images.

REFERENCES

1. Bhandari, A., Koppen, J., & Agzarian, M. Convolutional Neural Networks for Brain Tumour Segmentation. *Insights Imaging* 11 (2020): 77. 10.1186/s13244-020-00869-4
2. Jin, K. H., McCann, M. T., Froustey, E., & Unser, M. Deep Convolutional Neural Network for Inverse Problems in imaging. *IEEE Trans Image Process* 26 (2017): 4509–4522
3. Kumar, A., Dhana, G. R., Albreem, M., & Le, D. A Comprehensive Study on the Role of Advanced Technologies in 5G Based Smart Hospital. *Alexandria Engineering Journal* 2021 (2021), (60): 5527–5536.
4. Ramakrishnan, B., Kumar, A., Chakravarty, S., Masud, M., & Baz, M. Analysis of FBMC Waveform for 5G Network Based Smart Hospitals. *Applied Sciences.* 11 (2021) (19): 8895. 10.3390/app11198895, Suwalka Isha, and Navneet Agrawal. "An improved unsupervised mapping technique using AMSOM for neuro-degenerative disease detection." *International Journal of Computational Systems Engineering* 4, no. 2–3 (2018): 185–194.
5. Saraswathi, D., Lakshmi Priya, B., & Punitha Lakshmi, R. Brain Tumor Segmentation and Classification Using Self Organizing Map. In *2019 IEEE international conference on system, computation, automation and networking (ICSCAN)*, pp. 1–5. IEEE, 2019.
6. Mapari, R. M. & Virani, H. G. Automated Technique for Segmentation of Brain Tumor in MR Images. In 2019 3rd International Conference on Trends in Electronics and Informatics (ICOEI), pp. 867–870. IEEE, 2019.
7. Madhupriya, G., Guru, N. M., Praveen, S., & Nivetha, B. Brain Tumor Segmentation with Deep Learning Technique. In *2019 3rd International Conference on Trends in Electronics and Informatics (ICOEI)*, pp. 758–763. IEEE, 2019.
8. Sunila, Verma, A. & Godara Analysis of Various Clustering Algorithms. *International Journal of Innovative Technology and Exploring Engineering* 3(2013) (1): 186–189.
9. Sarwar, B., Karypis, G., Konstan, J., & Riedl, J. Item-based Collaborative Filtering Recommendation Algorithms, ACM International Conference on World Wide Web, 2001, pp. 285–295
10. Kumar, A. & Gupta, M. A Review on Activities of Fifth Generation Mobile Communication System. *Alexandria Engineering Journal* 57(2017) (2): 1125–1135. https://www.sciencedirect.com/science/article/pii/S1110016817300601

7 Analysis and Design of a Next-Generation Wearable Antenna
Case Study in Wearable Device Health Systems

Ira Joshi
Department of ECE, JECRC University, Jaipur,
Rajasthan, India

Mohammed H. Alsharif
Department of Electrical Engineering, College of Electronics
and Information Engineering, Sejong University, Seoul,
Republic of Korea

Sifeu Takougang Kingni
Department of Mechanical, Petroleum and Gas Engineering,
National Advanced School of Mines and Petroleum
Industries, University of Maroua, Maroua, Cameroon

Nishant Gaur
Department of Physics, JECRC University, Jaipur,
Rajasthan, India

Arun Kumar
Department of Electronics and Communication Engineering,
New Horizon College of Engineering, Bengaluru, India

7.1 INTRODUCTION

To monitor our health and send a biological signal, wearable gadgets are crucial to biological communication. The specifications for these gadgets are small in size, flexible in design, robust, reliable, cheap, and have low maintenance requirements. Antennas in these devices play a vital role. To achieve these requirements, much research work has been done to minimize the size using

DOI: 10.1201/9781003403678-7

various techniques in designing these antennas. Wearable antennas have a great future as wireless technologies are emerging in our day-to-day life very efficiently. This wireless biological antenna system has the potential to take a medical facility to the next level as it creates the opportunity for a real-time healthcare and fitness monitoring system. With the development of wearable antennas, a patch antenna is designed, using flexible substrate for all such reasons that textile substrates are widely used day by day [1]. The permittivity and height of the substrate are responsible for the gain and effectiveness of the planar antenna [2]. The textile substrate consists of a polymer thread and metal thread that have little dielectric value due to the reduced surface wave losses and increased antenna impedance bandwidth [3]. Other technology like electromagnetic bandgap structure, artificial magnetic conductor, and high impedance structure design also give good results as a wearable antenna [4]. Metamaterial also improves the radiation properties of antennas and reduces the size of antennas [5]. A wearable antenna is a device that can be attached to or embedded in clothing, jewelry, or other accessories worn by a person, to transmit or receive radio frequency signals. These wearable wires can be utilized in a variety of applications, including healthcare, sports and fitness, communication, and location tracking. Wearable antennas may be extremely helpful in the healthcare industry by monitoring patients' vital signs including heart rate, blood pressure, and temperature and sending this information to medical specialists in real time. This can improve patient outcomes by allowing for early detection of health problems and more timely interventions. However, developing and implementing wearable antennas in healthcare has some difficulties, such as ensuring that the antennas are small, comfortable, and reliable enough for patients to wear for extended periods of time, while also providing accurate and secure data transmission. Despite these challenges, the utilization of wearable antennas in healthcare is expected to continue to grow, as advancements in technology enhance the performance of the framework. As a result, wearable antennas have the capabilities to transform the way healthcare is delivered and enhanced service standard for patients around the world. In this work, we will focus on several antenna designs, their performance, and different material used as substrates. The design of the proposed antenna is given in Figure 7.1.

7.2 WIRELESS BODY AREA NETWORK

As seen in Figure 7.1, these antennas are now often utilized in medical applications for the detection and treatment of different diseases [6]. Nuclear magnetic resonance signals—which carry information about changes in the structure of nuclei—are produced when an antenna used in body area networks radiates electromagnetic waves into the body and then receives those electromagnetic waves back after colliding with nuclei. We compare those signals with nuclear magnetic resonance (NMR) signals from healthy bodies to make a diagnosis. The information pertaining to the interior body is to be provided to the server system by healthcare monitoring systems. Figure 7.2 depicts the various components of the health monitoring system.

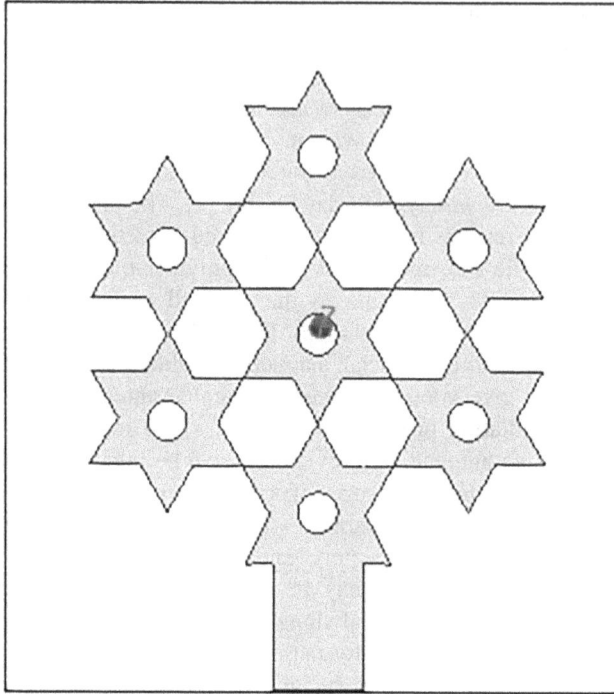

FIGURE 7.1 Antenna design.

In this figure, the base station consists of a control system, a receiver system, and internet to communicate with other devices, channel for the propagation of signal, human body, insulators that support to diminish the adverse effects of EM waves on body tissue, implantable antennas that help in diagnosis and treatment although we have different kind of antenna used in these field as shown in Figure 7.3, electronics system and power supply to helps in communication and signal conversion process and health care monitoring system [7–10].

The requirement for the wearable antenna is as follows:

- Must have high bandwidth to transmit good quality of signal.
- Efficiency of antenna should have a fast data rate transmission.
- The antenna's dielectric constant needs to be high for the performance to adapt to the electrical properties of the body.
- The capture antenna should be compact in size.

7.3 DESIGN METHODOLOGY OF WEARABLE ANTENNA

New technologies are created daily and put to use to make wearable antennas more effective and smaller, to reduce adverse effects of these antennas on the body and to achieve the required features of the wearable antenna. Let's discuss the various design technology used in wearable antennas and their features in brief.

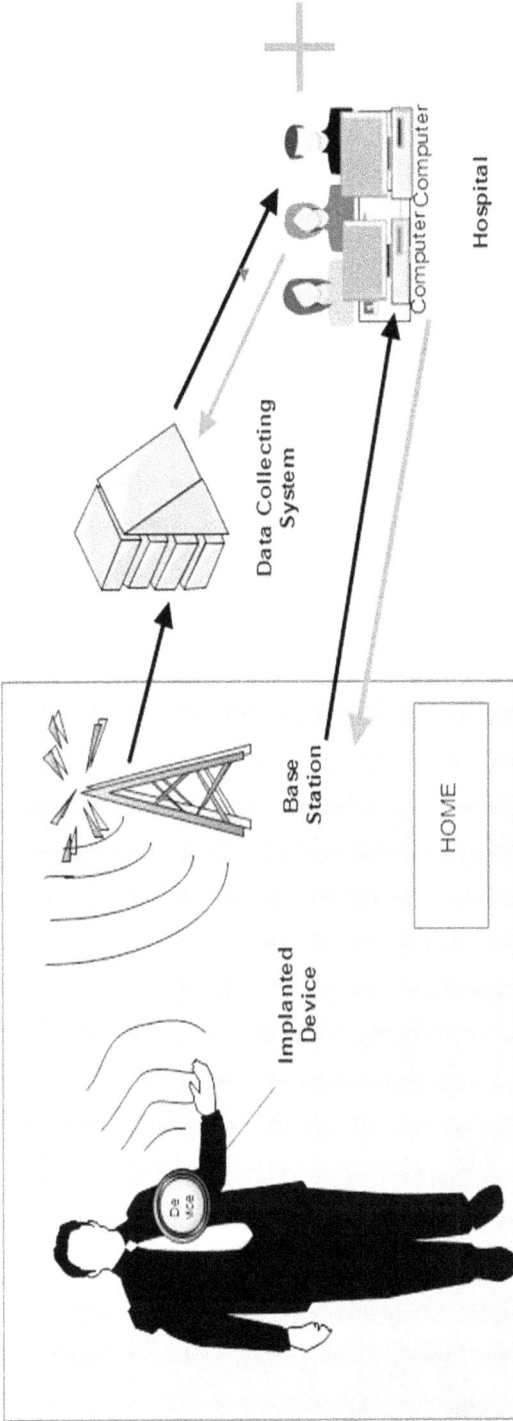

FIGURE 7.2   A general healthcare system that uses an implantable device and a wireless body area network.

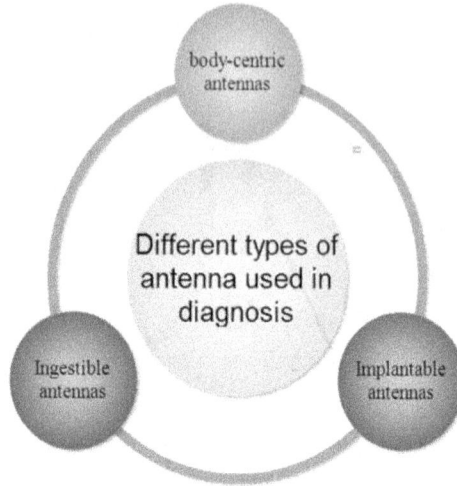

FIGURE 7.3 Different kinds of antennas for diagnosis.

A small-sized antenna was created by Karacolak et al. in their study [11] for glucose monitoring purposes, which is operated in MICS and ISM bands. Using the simulation code and swarm optimization algorithm, this antenna was made to operate in the dual band. The real-time measurement is done in gel, which shows the same electrical properties as the human body. Kim et al. [12] presented a low-profile antenna and measured the effects of EM waves on the human body, mainly on the head and shoulder. They applied the DGF expansion and FDTD to calculate its effects on the human body and it is operated in MICS bands. Kumar and Shanmuganantham in their paper [13] presented an antenna operated in ISM bands and designed using IE3D software with FR4 substrate. It is V-shaped and it may be used in human tissues, including skin, fat, and muscle. In their paper, Duan et al. [14] designed an implantable antenna of size 27 mm × 14 mm × 1.27 mm. It can be used for neural recording with a high data rate. It resonates at two frequencies that are near to the MICS bands of 402–405 MHz, 433.9 MHz, and 542.4 MHz, respectively. The measurement is done in tissue to mimic a solution. Hatmi et al. in their studies [15] presented a magnetic induction link system with the human body. They designed the transmitter and receiver module separately and then combined them properly to form a system. A magnetic antenna seems less fussy than electrical antennas and their battery life also increases by less power consumption. In their article [16], Lee et al. presented an ingestible capsule endoscope device. A thick arm of the spiral structure was implemented to achieve a wide band. They are utilized to deliver the internal body's high-quality biological image. The measurement was carried out by employing a phantom human. A tiny antenna that worked in the medical device radio communication services (MedRadio) band (401–406 MHz) was proposed by Psathas et al. in their study [17]. Ingestible capsule endoscopy is intended to use it. The FE simulation is done with the assumption that the capsule is surrounded by human tissues. M. E. Jalil et al. [18] presented the antenna mentioned in Figure 7.4(a).

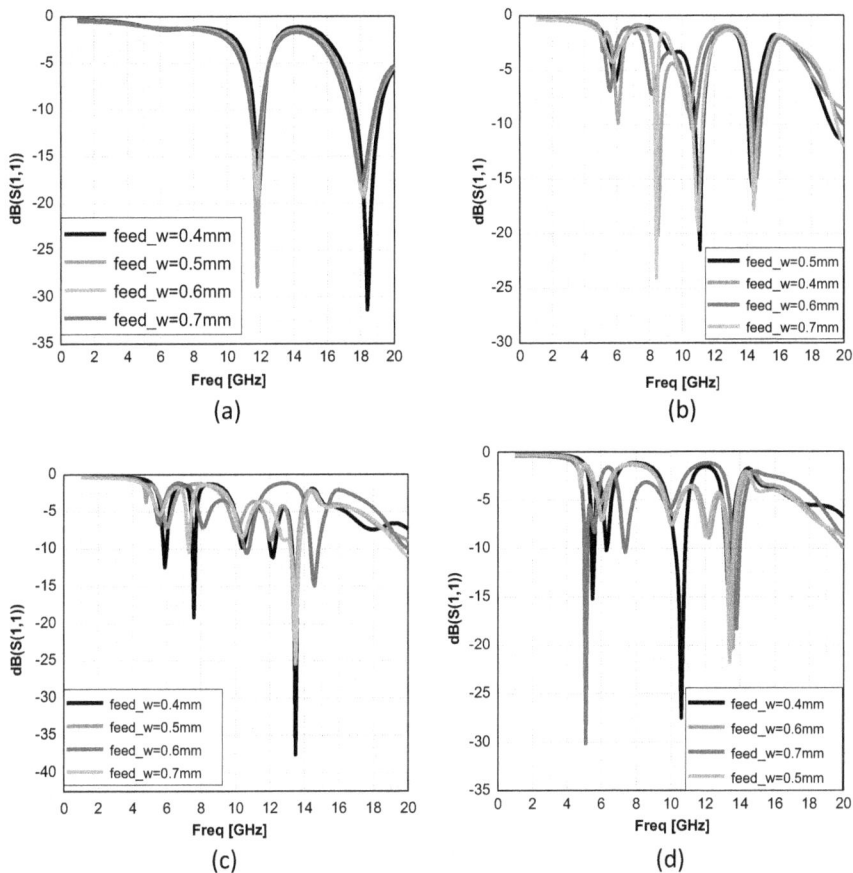

FIGURE 7.4 Simulated return loss for a hexagonal microstrip patch antenna at (a) first iteration, (b) second iteration, (c) third iteration, (d) proposed hexagonal circular slot.

They have used copper tape and ground and jean fabric as the substrate. The dielectric constant of jean material is 1.68, loss tangent is 0.01, and thickness is 1 mm. High bandwidth is achieved using slits in the design. H Gidden et al. [19] presented a dipole antenna designed in a diamond shape. The proposed structure is implemented on the textile to provide the flexibility. E. F. Sundarsingh et al. [20] presented a polygon structure with a circular slot in between the structure. It is operated in GSM 900 and GSM 1800 bands. The substrate has a loss tangent of 0.025 and a dielectric constant of 1.7. M. A. R. Osman et al. [21] presented a wearable antenna that is small in size and displays a wide bandwidth. The wire is premeditated using a patch of copper tape. In W. A. M. Alashwal et al. [22], a portion of human arm is placed at antenna location and phantom section is chosen wisely for the simulation in CST software. This antenna shows an enhanced performance. A. M. Al Ashwal et al. [23] proposed a flexible conformal antenna using jeans as a substrate and copper tape as a metallic radiator. In these antennas, the slot and truncation techniques are introduced in the design to improve bandwidth characteristics; 1.76 for the dielectric constant and 0.078

for the loss tangent. The outcome is simulated in the presence of a human body with muscles, fat, and skin that moves often. The increases are 2.74 dB at 3.0 GHz, 4.17 dB, and 4.07 dB, respectively, at 7.0 GHz and 9.0 GHz. S. Velan et al. [24] designed an antenna using jeans substrate and copper tape. It's a monopole structure operated at GSM and ISM bands. The antenna is stacked with $3 \times 3 \times 3$ EBG array of dimension 150×150 mm^2. The antenna's reflection coefficient plot, both with and without EBG, is measured in free space.

7.4 RESULTS

The return loss of the first iteration antenna is obtained in Figure 7.4(a). The feed (w) is varied to obtain a return loss. For w = 0.5, 0.4, the resonant frequency is 12 GHz, 18.2 GHz with return loss −28 dB, and −19 dB with operating spectrum ranges from 11.8 GHz to 18.2 GHz. The return loss of the second iteration antenna is obtained in Figure 7.4(b). The feed (w) is varied to obtain a return loss. For w = 0.7, the resonant frequency is 8.4 GHz, 11 GHz, and 14.4 GHz with return loss −24dB, −20 dB, and −18 dB with operating spectrum ranges from 6.5 GHz to 15 GHz. The proposed structure operates in the triple band as compared to Figure 7.4(a). The return loss of the third iteration antenna is obtained in Figure 7.4(c). The feed (w) is varied to obtain a return loss. For w = 0.4, the resonant frequencies are 5.9 GHz, 7.6 GHz, and 13.5 GHz, with return losses of −12 dB, −19 dB, and −37 dB, with an operating spectrum ranging from 4.2 GHz to 13 GHz. The proposed structure operates in three different bands, as compared in Figure 7.4(c). The return loss of the final proposed antenna is obtained in Figure 7.4(d). The feed (w) is varied to obtain a return loss. For w = 0.7, the resonant frequency is 5.1 GHz, 7.4 GHz, and 13.8 GHz with return loss −30 dB, −11 dB, and −18 dB with operating spectrum ranges from 3.2 GHz to 15 GHz. The radiation pattern of the proposed antenna is obtained at different frequencies, as given in Figure 7.5(a),(b), and (c). From the simulation, we can say it is an ideal pattern for wireless applications. The group delay measures the noise of the pulse signal. The group delay graph for a fractal hexagonal circularly slotted antenna is indicated in Figure 7.6. The Smith chart is shown in Figure 7.7. It is utilized to demonstrate authentic aerial impedance. The simulated surface current distribution for a proposed antenna is shown in Figure 7.6. At 5.1 GHz, impedance matching can

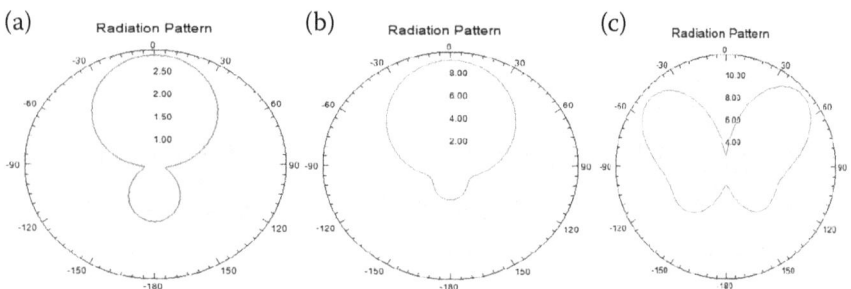

FIGURE 7.5 Radiation pattern of final hexagonal circular slot microstrip patch antenna: (a) E-plane at f = 5.1 GHz, (b) f = 7.4 GHz, (c) f = 13.8 GHz.

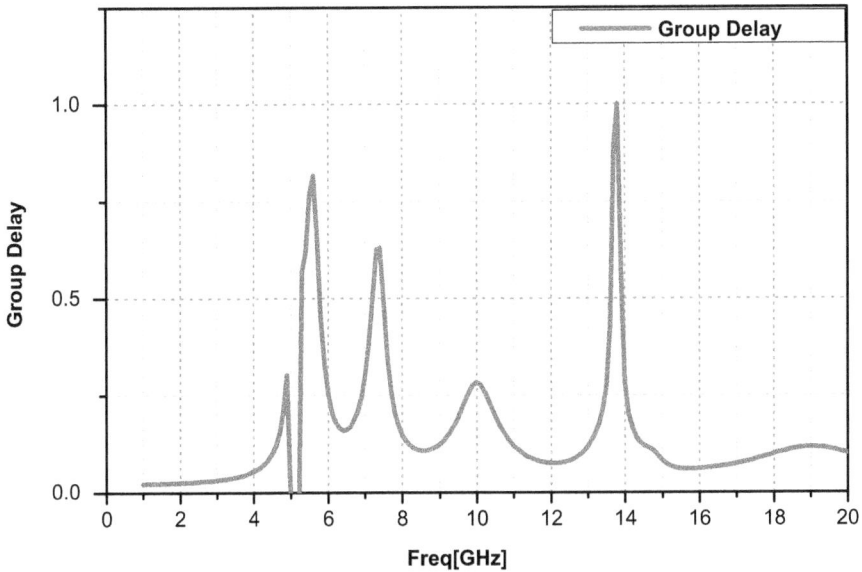

FIGURE 7.6 Group delay.

Name	Freq	Ang	Mag	RX
m1	5.1000	-87.9618	0.5073	0.6081 - 0.8302i
m2	7.4000	-1.8371	0.5239	3.1933 - 0.1479i
m3	13.8000	-34.5826	0.6062	1.7128 - 1.8634i

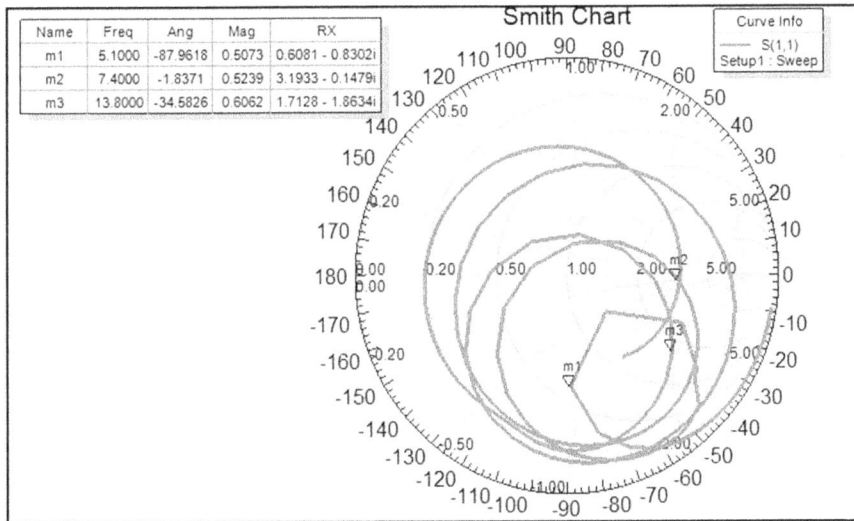

FIGURE 7.7 Simulated Smith chart.

be analyzed from Figure 7.8(a). In this case, the current distribution is mainly at the edges of the patch and on the ground. At 7.4 GHz, the current distribution is shown in Figure 7.8(b). At 13.8 GHz, the current variation is shown in Figure 7.8(c), at the fractal boundaries of feed and ground. The measured and simulated VSWR (voltage standing wave ratio) is given in Figure 7.9. Figure 7.10 indicates the measured and simulated return loss.

(a)

(b)

(c)

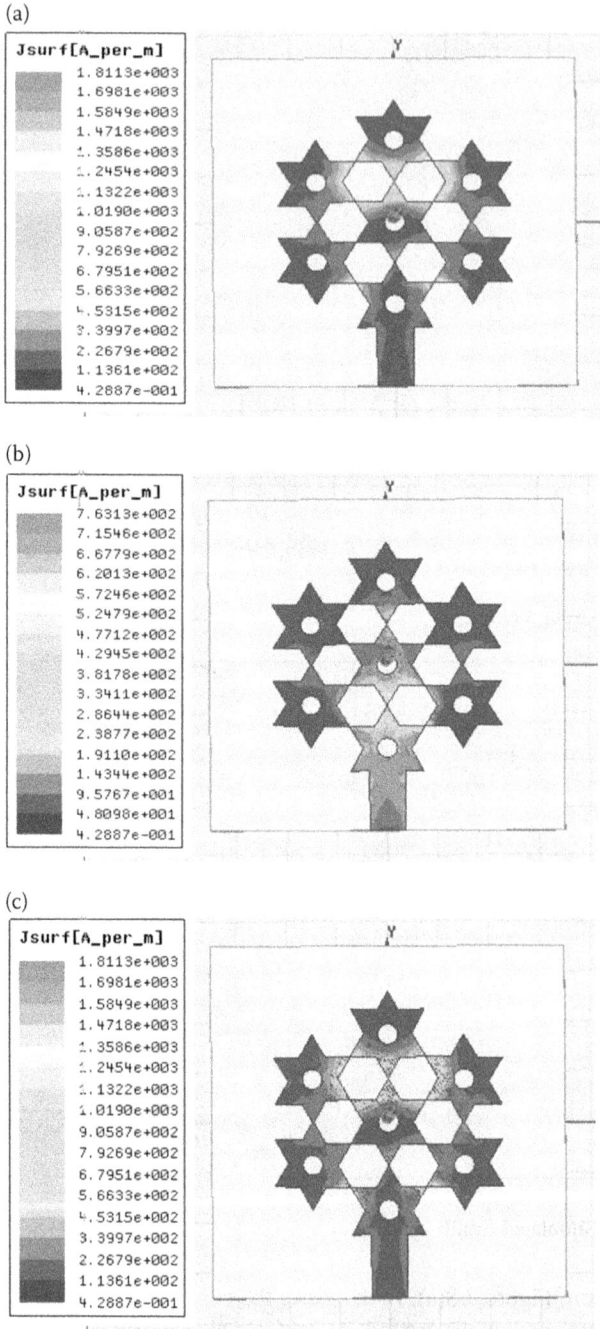

FIGURE 7.8 Surface current distribution for final hexagonal circular slot microstrip patch antenna: (a) f = 5.1 GHz, (b) f = 7.4 GHz, (c) f = 13.8 GHz.

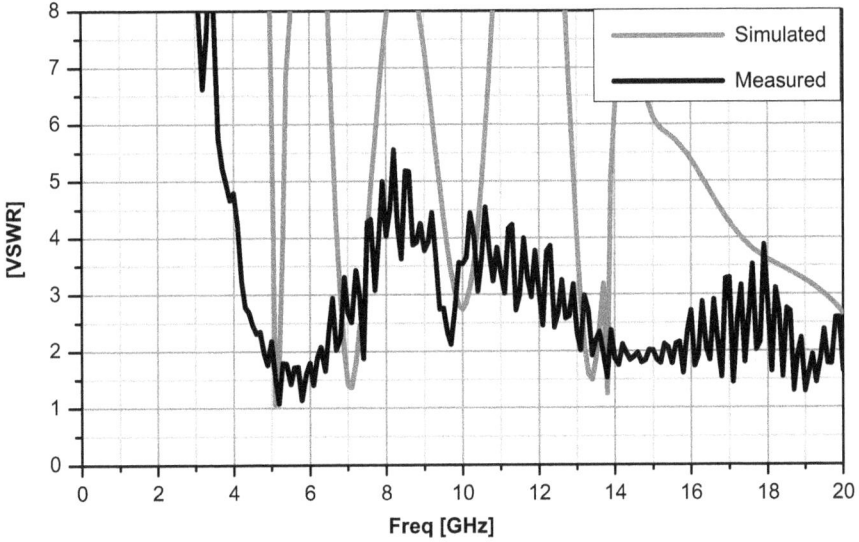

FIGURE 7.9 Simulated and measured VSWR.

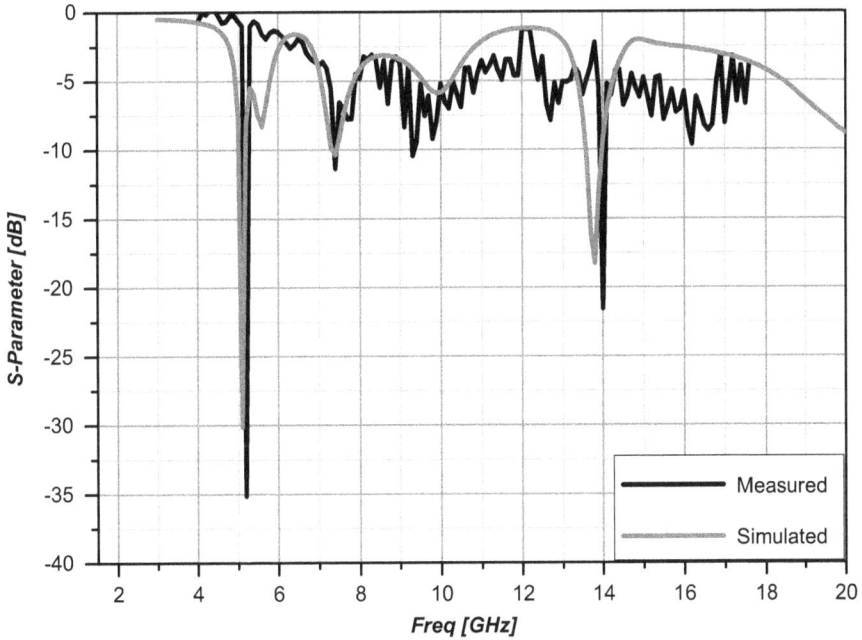

FIGURE 7.10 Simulated and measured S-parameter.

7.5   CERTAIN DIFFICULTIES AND CONSIDERATIONS

The low profile and easy fabrication of the planar patch antenna make it an ideal choice for designing wearable technology. In addition to this, the jean substrate added advantages with its design to be flexible and conformal. When these are put on the human body, it shows adverse effects on human tissue that lead to health risks. So, it's a challenge to minimize the SAR.

With the metamaterial concept, the SAR can be improved at the cost of size and complexity of the antenna structures. The antenna performance its robustness and deformation like wrinkling, wetting, and bending in practical simulation is also challenge for the researchers. We have to investigate more to fulfill it's all requirements [25].

7.6   CHALLENGES IN WEARABLE ANTENNAS

Wearable antennas in healthcare can offer a range of benefits, such as improved patient monitoring, more accurate data collection, and increased mobility. Here are some of the key challenges [26]:

   I. Size and comfort: Wearable antennas need to be small and comfortable enough for patients to wear for extended periods of time. This can be challenging since antennas need to be large enough to operate effectively.
  II. Interference: Affected by electromagnetic interference from other devices are wearable antennas, such as medical equipment, smartphones, and other wireless devices. This will cause inaccurate data and other issues.
 III. Power consumption: Wearable antennas need to be low power to extend the battery life and reduce the need for frequent recharging.
  IV. Signal strength and range: Wearable antennas need to be able to transmit and receive signals with sufficient strength and range to provide reliable data. This can be challenging in areas with weak signal strength that can block signals.
   V. Security and privacy: Wearable antennas can transmit sensitive health data, so it is essential to ensure that the data is secure and protected from unauthorized access or interception.
  VI. Standardization: To ensure compatibility and interoperability between various devices and systems, wearable antenna design and implementation in the healthcare industry need to be standardized.

Overall, even if there are numerous advantages to adopting wearable antennas in healthcare, overcoming these difficulties will be crucial for their effective adoption and application.

7.7   INTEGRATION OF WEARABLE ANTENNAS WITH 5G

The integration of wearable antennas with 5G technology can deliver plentiful paybacks, with faster data transfer speeds, higher bandwidth, lower latency, and improved connectivity. Wearable antennas equipped with 5G technology can enable real-time remote monitoring and diagnostics, leading to improved patient outcomes and reduced healthcare costs. 5G provides several benefits for wearable antennas in healthcare applications, as it can support large amounts of data transmission and communication with low latency. This implies that wearable antennas can provide real-time data to healthcare specialists, enabling rapid and precise diagnosis and treatment [27]. In addition, 5G technology can provide improved connectivity in areas with weak signals, making it simple to transmit and receive data from remote locations. Wearable antennas can be equipped with 5G technology combined with other gadgets, such as smartphones, to enable remote control and monitoring. However, the integration of wearable antennas with 5G technology also poses some challenges, adding the high efficiency and miniaturization to ensure that the antennas can be comfortably worn by patients for extended periods of time. Overall, the integration of wearable antennas with 5G technology can transform healthcare delivery and improve patient outcomes, but it will require careful consideration of the technical challenges and the expansion of advanced solutions to overcome them [27, 28].

7.8   CASE STUDY OF WEARABLE ANTENNAS IN SMART HOSPITAL

Modern healthcare facilities, known as "smart hospitals," make use of a variety of technology to improve the standard of healthcare provided. A vital part of the Internet of Things (IoT) ecosystem in smart hospitals are wearable antennas. They are discreet, lightweight, and readily fit into clothes or medical equipment to wirelessly communicate information to the hospital's main computer system. In this case study, we'll look at how a smart hospital uses wearable antennas. Wearable antennas in healthcare have gained significant attention due to their potential for monitoring and transmitting vital signs and health-related data wirelessly. However, several concerns and challenges need to be addressed to ensure the effective and safe use of wearable antennas in healthcare settings. One of the primary concerns is designing wearable antennas that are compact, lightweight, and flexible enough to be integrated into wearable devices comfortably. Achieving efficient radiation performance, such as high gain and wide bandwidth, while considering the size and form factor constraints of the wearable device is a significant challenge. The design process must also account for factors like the proximity of the antenna to the human body, which can affect antenna performance due to body absorption, reflection, and interference. Wearable antennas are susceptible to signal interference from various sources, including other electronic devices, nearby antennas, and the human body itself. These interferences can degrade the quality of the transmitted or received signals, leading to errors in data transmission and compromised accuracy of healthcare monitoring. Mitigating interference and ensuring reliable signal quality are crucial to maintain the integrity of the healthcare data being collected or transmitted. The proximity of wearable antennas to the human body raises concerns about the absorption of electromagnetic energy by the body tissues. Excessive absorption can lead to thermal effects, causing discomfort or potential harm to the wearer. Therefore, wearable antenna designs must adhere to specific safety guidelines and regulations to minimize the absorption of electromagnetic radiation by the body and ensure user safety. Wearable antennas often rely on battery-powered devices. Balancing the power consumption of the antenna with the need for long battery life is a critical concern. Energy-efficient antenna designs, low-power wireless communication protocols, and optimized data transmission techniques are essential to prolong the battery life of wearable devices, allowing for continuous monitoring and reducing the need for frequent recharging or battery replacement. Wearable antennas must be designed with materials that are bio-compatible and safe for prolonged contact with the skin. Some individuals may have skin sensitivities or allergies to certain materials or adhesives used in wearable devices. Therefore, careful material selection and thorough testing are necessary to ensure the comfort and safety of users, minimizing the risk of skin irritation or adverse reactions. As wearable antennas collect and transmit sensitive healthcare data, ensuring data security and privacy is paramount. Measures must be taken to protect the confidentiality and integrity of the transmitted data, prevent unauthorized access or data breaches, and comply with privacy regulations. Encryption techniques, secure communication protocols, and robust data storage practices should be implemented to safeguard the healthcare data collected by wearable antennas. Wide-scale adoption of wearable antennas in healthcare relies on user acceptance and satisfaction. Factors such as user comfort, ease of use, reliability, and perceived benefits play a crucial role in determining the acceptance and adoption of wearable healthcare devices. Addressing user concerns, providing clear instructions and support, and continuously improving the user experience are vital for ensuring the widespread utilization of wearable antennas in healthcare settings.

7.8.1 BACKGROUND

A smart hospital in a large city has adopted a number of cutting-edge technologies to enhance healthcare offerings. The management staff of the hospital strives to offer top-notch medical treatment while maintaining the convenience and comfort of patients. Wearable antennas are a crucial part of the hospital's technological environment.

7.8.2 DIFFICULTIES

In order to adopt wearable antennas, the hospital's management team had to overcome a number of obstacles. Designing and implementing antennas that could function dependably in a hospital setting were the main problems. Small, lightweight antennas that could wirelessly transfer data to the hospital's main system were required. The antennas also have to be strong and able to tolerate adverse environmental factors, such as contact with chemicals, moisture, and physical strain.

7.8.3 REMEDY

The administrative team of the hospital collaborated with a group of wearable antenna technology specialists to address these issues. The group created a wearable antenna that was compact, light, and capable of wireless data transmission. Doctors and nurses were able to keep an eye on patients' vital signs in real-time because of the antenna's integration with the hospital's patient monitoring system. The wearable antenna was built to last and tolerate challenging climatic conditions. The antenna was constructed with premium components that could withstand physical stress, chemicals, and dampness. For the convenience of both patients and healthcare professionals, the antenna was also made to be readily incorporated into clothes and medical equipment.

7.8.4 RESULTS

There were various advantages of using wearable antennas in the smart hospital. In order to enable early diagnosis and intervention of any medical difficulties, healthcare personnel were able to monitor patients' vital signs in real time using wearable antennas. This resulted in better patient outcomes, shorter hospital stays, and lower medical expenses. Wearable antenna technology also increased patient convenience and comfort. Patients could walk around freely and take part in activities that would hasten their recovery since they were no longer attached to monitoring equipment.

7.8.5 CHOICE

Wearable antennas were successfully implemented in the smart hospital. These antennas allowed medical professionals to keep an eye on patients' vital signs in real time, improving patient outcomes and lowering expenses. Patients also reported more comfort and convenience, which raised their level of satisfaction overall. As healthcare facilities continue to adopt cutting-edge technology, wearable antennas will likely become an even more important part of the IoT ecosystem in smart hospitals.

7.9 CONCLUSION AND FUTURE SCOPE

We may infer from the review that the wearable technology is a miracle in the area of medical applications. The flexibility of the antenna construction is increased by the cloth antenna. The antenna's structure offers certain benefits and drawbacks depending on the textile substrate used. It is simpler and more comfortable to use these wireless antennas in the medical area for illness diagnosis and treatment. As these antennas are essential in the treatment of many diseases in our digital age, research in these sectors is constantly improving. By enabling real-time remote monitoring, better data accuracy, and lower healthcare costs, the use of wearable antennas in smart hospitals has the potential to completely change the way healthcare is provided. Even further benefits, including faster data transfer rates, larger bandwidth, reduced latency, and enhanced connection, may be provided by wearable antennas that use 5G technology. However, there are significant difficulties in integrating wearable antennas into smart hospitals, such as the requirement for higher power efficiency, miniaturization, and design standardization. For wearable antennas to be dependable, safe, and secure, it is crucial to solve these issues through creative solutions and industry stakeholder engagement. The integration of wearable antennas into smart hospitals has the potential to significantly enhance patient outcomes, lower healthcare costs, and increase access to healthcare services despite these obstacles. Wearable antennas will become more prevalent in healthcare as technology develops, and smart hospitals will rely on them more and more to give patients high-quality treatment. The future scope of wearable antennas in healthcare is incredibly promising, with the potential to revolutionize the way we monitor and deliver healthcare services. Wearable antennas can enable continuous monitoring of vital signs and health parameters, allowing healthcare providers to remotely track patients' health in real time. This technology can be particularly useful for patients with chronic conditions, elderly individuals, or those recovering from surgeries. Wearable antennas can collect and transmit data such as heart rate, blood pressure, respiratory rate, body temperature, and activity levels, enabling timely intervention and personalized care without the need for frequent hospital visits. Wearable antennas can play a crucial role in telemedicine and telehealth services by facilitating remote consultations and diagnostics. By transmitting data wirelessly, healthcare professionals can remotely assess patients' conditions, provide medical advice, and make informed decisions about further treatment or intervention. Wearable antennas can enable the integration of sensors, cameras, and microphones, allowing for comprehensive telehealth consultations and remote examinations. Wearable antennas can aid in disease management and prevention by monitoring patients' health and lifestyle habits. For instance, wearable antennas can track physical activity levels, sleep patterns, and nutrition, providing valuable insights for personalized disease management plans. By analyzing long-term data trends, healthcare providers can identify risk factors, predict health deterioration, and implement preventive measures to improve overall health outcomes. Wearable antennas can be integrated into rehabilitation devices or wearable exoskeletons to monitor and analyze movements during physical therapy sessions. By accurately tracking joint angles, muscle activity, and range of motion, wearable antennas can provide real-time feedback to both patients and therapists, ensuring proper technique and progress monitoring. This technology can enhance rehabilitation outcomes, assist in gait analysis, and optimize the delivery of personalized therapy. Wearable antennas can be utilized in devices such as smart watches or wearable pendants to monitor the well-being of elderly individuals. By detecting changes in movement patterns, deviations from regular activity levels, or sudden falls, wearable antennas can automatically alert caregivers or emergency services, ensuring timely assistance and reducing the risks associated with falls or medical emergencies.

REFERENCES

1. Ramakrishnan, B., Kumar, A., Chakravarty, S., Masud, M., Baz, M. Analysis of FBMC Waveform for 5G Network Based Smart Hospitals. *Appl. Sci.* 2021; 11:8895. 10.3390/app11198895.
2. Grupta, B., Sankaralingam, S., Dhar, S. Development of Wearable and Implantable Antennas in the Last Decade: A Review. In Proceedings of Mediterranean Microwave Symposium (MMS), Guzelyurt, Turkey, 25–27 August 2010, pp. 251–267

3. George, G., Nagarjun, R., Thiripurasundari, D., Poonkuzhali, R., Alex, Z. C. Design of Meander Line Wearable Antenna, IEEE Conference on Information and Communication Technologies, 2013, pp. 1190–1193.

4. Erentok, A., Ziolkowski, R. W., "Metmaterial-Inspired Efficient Electrically Small Antennas, *IEEE Trans. Antennas Propagat.* 2008; 56(3):691–707.

5. Soontornpipit, P., Furse, C. M., Chung, Y. C. Design of Implantable Microstrip Antenna for Communication with Medical Implants. *IEEE T. Mircrow. Theory.* 2004; 52(8):1944–1951.

6. Kiziltas, G., Psychoudakis, D., Volakis, J. L., Kikuchi, N. Topology Design Optimization of Dielectric Substrates for Bandwidth Improvement of a Patch Antenna. *IEEE T. Antennas Propag.* 2003; 10:2732–2743.

7. Zhou, Y., Chen, C. C., Volakis, J. L. Dual Band Proximity-fed Stacked Patch Antenna for Tri-Band GPS Applications. *IEEE T. Antennas Propag.* 2007; 1:220–223.

8. Tang, Z., Smith, B., Schild, J. H., Peckham, P. H. Data Transmission from an Implantable Biotelemeter by Load-Shift Keying Using Circuit Configuration Modulator. *IEEE T. Bio-Med Eng.* 1995; 42(5):524–528.

9. Valdastri, P., Menciassi, A., Arena, A., Caccamo, C., Dario, P. An Implantable Telemetry Platform System for In Vivo Monitoring of Physiological Parameters. *IEEE T. Inf. Technol. B.* 2004; 8(3):271–278.

10. Kumar, A., Albreem, M. A., Gupta, M., Alsharif, M. H., Kim, S. Future 5G Network Based Smart Hospitals: Hybrid Detection Technique for Latency Improvement. *IEEE Access.* 2020; 8:153240–153249, 10.1109/ACCESS.2020.3017625.

11. Zimmerman, T. G. Personal Area Networks: Near-Field Intra-body Communication. *IBM Syst. J.* 1996; 35(3-4):609–617.

12. Kim, J., Rahmat-Samii, Y. Implanted Antennas Inside a Human Body: Simulations, Designs, and Characterizations. *IEEE T. Microw. Theory.* 2004; 52:1934–1943.

13. Kumar, S., Gupta, M., Kumar, A. (2021). Breast Cancer Detection Based on Antenna Data Collection and Analysis. In: Tanwar, S. (eds.), *Fog Computing for Healthcare 4.0 Environments. Signals and Communication Technology.* Springer, Cham. 10.1007/ 978-3-030-46197-3_19.

14. Duan, Z., Guo, Y. X., Xue, R. F., Je, M., Kwong, D. L. Differentially Fed Dual-Band Implantable Antenna for Biomedical Applications. *IEEE T. Antenn. Propag.* 2012; 60:5587–5595.

15. Hatmi, F. E., Grzeskowiak, M., Protat, S., Picon, O. Link Budget of Magnetic Antennas for Ingestible Capsule at 40 MHz. 6th European Conference on Antennas and Propagation (EUCAP), Prague, March 2012. pp. 1–5.

16. Lee, S. H., Lee, J., Yoon, Y. J., Cheon, C., Kim, K., Nam, S. A Wideband Spiral Antenna for Ingestible Capsule Endoscope Systems: Experimental Results in a Human Phantom and a Pig. *IEEE T. Bio-med Eng.* 2011; 58:1734–1741.

17. Kumar, A., Singh, M. K. Band-Notched Planar UWB Microstrip Antenna with T-Shaped Slot. *Radio Electron. Commun. Systems.* 2018; 61(8):371–376.

18. Jalil, M. E., Rahim, M. K. A., Samsuri, N. A., Murad, N. A., Othman, N., Majid, H. A. On-Body Investigation of Dual Band Diamond Textile Antenna for Wearable Applications at 2.45 GHz and 5.8 GHz. 7th European Conference on Antennas and Propagation, 2013, pp. 414–417.

19. Gidden, H., Paul, D. L., Hilton, G. S., McGeehan, J. P. Influence of Body Proximity on the Efficiency of Wearable Textile Patch Antenna. The 6th European Conference on Antennas and Propagation (EUCAP), Prague, 2012, pp. 1353–1357.

20. Kumar, A., Choudhary, M. Dual Band Modified Split-Ring Resonator Microstrip Antenna for Wireless Applications. *Natl. Acad. Sci. Lett.* 2020; 43 (3): 237–240. 10.1007/s40009-019-00845-7.

21. Osman, M. A. R., Rahim, M. K. A., Azfar, M., Samsuri, N. A., Zubir, F., Kamardin, K. Design, Implementation and Performance of Ultrawideband Textile Antenna. *Prog. Electromagn. Res. B*. 2011; 27:307–327.
22. Alashwal, W. A. M., Ramli, K. N. Small Planar Monopole UWB Wearable Antenna with Low SAR. IEEE Region 10 Symposium, 2014, pp. 235–239.
23. Kumar A., Gupta M. (2016) Design, Development of MC-CDMA, and Reduction of ISI for Different Modulation Techniques. In: Afzalpulkar, N., Srivastava, V., Singh, G., Bhatnagar, D. (eds.), *Proceedings of the International Conference on Recent Cognizance in Wireless Communication & Image Processing*. Springer, New Delhi. 10.1007/978-81-322-2638-3_9.
24. Bansal, G., Toshniwal, S., Kumar, A. Cognitive Radio System with OFDM and Beamforming Technique for Data Communication. 2016 IEEE 1st International Conference on Power Electronics, Intelligent Control and Energy Systems (ICPEICES), Delhi, 2016, pp. 1–3. https://ieeexplore.ieee.org/document/7853719.
25. Al Ashwal, W. A. M., Ramli, K. N. Compact UWB Wearable Antenna with Improved Bandwidth and Low SAR. IEEE International RF and Microwave Conference, 2013, pp. 90–94.
26. Velan, S., Sundarsingh, E. F., Kanagasabai, M., Sarma, A. K., Raviteja, C., Sivasamy, R., Pakkathillam, J. K. Dual-Band EBG Integrated Monopole Antenna Deploying Fractal Geometry for Wearable Applications. *IEEE Antennas Wireless Propag. Lett.* 2015; 14:249–252.
27. Kumar, A. Singh, M. K. Band Notched Planar UWB Microstrip Antenna with T-Shaped Slot. *Radio Electron. Commun. Systems*. 2018; *61*(8):371–376. https://link.springer.com/article/10.3103/S0735272718080058.
28. Kumar, A., Rathore, H. Design and Implementation of OFDM System Using QPSK & QAM. *J Optic. Commun.* (2018), 10.1515/joc-2018-0128.

8 A Smart Multimodal Biomedical Diagnosis Based on Patient's Medical Questions and Symptoms

Dr Vijaya Gunturu
Department of ECE, School of Engineering, SR University,
Warangal, Telangana

R. Krishnamoorthy
Centre for Advanced Wireless Integrated Technology,
Chennai Institute of Technology, Chennai, India

M. Amina Begum
Department of ECE, Oxford College of Engineering,
Venmani, Thiruvannamalai District, India

Dr R. Jayakarthik
Department of Computer Science, Saveetha College of
Liberal Arts and Sciences SIMATS, India

Kazuaki Tanaka
Kyushu Institute of Technology, Japan

Janjhyam Venkata Naga Ramesh
Department of Computer Science and Engineering, Koneru
Lakshmaiah Education Foundation, Vaddeswaram, Guntur
District, Andhra Pradesh, India

8.1 INTRODUCTION

In the recent decade, developments in portable and wearable sensor technologies, IoT-based medical tools, and big data analytics via artificial intelligence and machine learning have fueled a meteoric rise in the area of smart health [1].

Big data service platforms, which offer the infrastructure for large-scale data space and processing, have helped to speed up the industry as well [2]. Constant multi-modal monitoring of physiological conditions is just one aspect of the patient-generated health data (PGHD) that has been made possible by the widespread availability and use of wearable wireless sensor tools. Healthcare can be shifted toward prevention and early disease diagnosis with the help of digital health because of the big data analytical technologies used, especially ML and DL [3].

While smart-health technologies have made it easier to keep tabs on a wide range of physiological states, one issue that has arisen is how to ensure that all of the devices involved in monitoring a patient's health are in sync with one another. The accuracy of the timing of physiological signals is crucial to their subsequent applications [4]. To begin with, it is the backbone of comparing new technology to industry standards. The digital health toolkit is always being updated with new features and data modalities. Comparisons with data obtained at the same time from gold-standard medical devices are used in validation studies to verify their accuracy [5]. The core of the validation is the ability to precisely match the time stamps of various signals. Second, an increasing number research uses supplementary data from multimodal physiological signals to uncover novel insights and enhance system performance across a range of tasks. Again, precise time alignment is the bedrock upon which such synchronous multimodal data sets are constructed [6].

It is tricky to determine the likeness metric for the time-matching techniques when synchronizing multimodal signals since their morphology may differ. In addition, there is no universal truth available to verify the efficacy of the algorithm while dealing with signals from various devices [7]. In an effort to develop a time alliance key for multimodal physiological signals, numerous investigations have been conducted. To identify the best temporal alignment between two signals, they utilized ML models. When two time-series are calculated with diverse sample rates, the DTW algorithm is known to experience the singularity problem. By exploiting local knowledge in the signal from the prescribed actions, the authors ease this problem and show superior performance compared to two previous classical DTW algorithms [8]. Another unique method developed by Liu et al., dubbed Phyio2Video, turns the signal alignment problem into a video frame configuration task by extracting spectral features from various physiological data. Using a DCNN to achieve nonlinear encoding of the feature films, the authors were able to handle the video frame alignment task and utilize a canonical correlation loss to calculate the final alliance of two signals [9].

There are a number of different prediction-related learning methods that can be loosely categorized as model-based or data-based. The former rely on preconceived notions of how the data should evolve, while the latter make use of the plethora of digital resources at their disposal and the ever-improving performance of AI strategies to train from the data itself [10]. From an artificial intelligence standpoint, the three basic fusion strategies that combine information from several modalities are early fusion, joint fusion, and late fusion. The first method combines the features from each modality into a single feature vector before presenting it to the learner; the next method combines the modalities at the hidden and entrenched levels; and the third method aggregates the predictions from the various modalities [11].

To aid in the clinical diagnosis and evaluation of the efficacy of a wide range of major diseases, DL offers exact strategies for processing massive data. Since medical image analysis is a crucial part of current medical imaging technology [12], it is imperative that this long-standing scientific challenge be resolved as soon as possible. The utilization of DL for multi-modal medicinal image fusion has the potential to greatly enhance the diagnostic and evaluative utility of medical images. Videos, for instance, can be broken down into its component parts, which include static text, static images, and static speech [13]. Evidence from the field suggests that multi-model approaches to processing data outperform their single-model counterparts [14]. To enhance image quality while keeping certain details intact, medical professionals often resort to multi-modal medical image fusion [15]. Because of the many fascinating disciplines involved, medical image fusion has found widespread use in clinical practice. These disciplines include image processing, computer vision, pattern recognition, ML, and AI. Medicinal image fusion provides doctors with new perspectives on lesions.

Most current uses of AI in healthcare have focused on solving specific problems with a single data modality, such as a computed tomography (CT) scan or an image of the retina. When making a diagnosis, prognosis assessment, or treatment plan, however, professionals interpret data from a wide variety of sources and modalities [16]. Furthermore, present AI assessments are often one-off snapshots, depending on a moment in time when the appraisal is performed, and therefore not seeing health as an unremitting condition. However, AI models should be capable to exploit any and all datasources, including ones that are occupied to most doctors [17]. We analyze the potential benefits of such multimodal data sets in healthcare, along with the major obstacles they provide, and some possible approaches to overcoming them in this review. The fundamentals of artificial intelligence and machine learning will not be covered here, but they are extensively covered elsewhere (Figure 8.1).

The issue and its impetus are depicted in Figure 8.2. In this chapter, we use a multimodal classification strategy based on ML techniques to the issue of detecting potential diagnoses. This paradigm is projected to have a number of benefits, including, first, facilitating accurate identification at an early stage, which is difficult because symptoms at this time are often vague or inconsistent [18]. Next, the capacity to assimilate vital information such as a patient's medicinal history or an allergy, the absence of which complicate the diagnostic procedure and sometimes leads to an incorrect illness differentiation [19]. Third, it helps with the time-consuming and error-prone process of mapping clinical notes to diagnoses according to the International Classification of Diseases (ICD) [20]. The suggested classification scheme integrates several different approaches. As a result, it integrates data, features, scores, and decisions from different sources, each of which contributes something unique. The effectiveness of the learning algorithm can be enhanced by combining data from several modalities. Integrating data from a person's facial signs, speech, behavior, and physiological signals can help a machine learning model better understand that person's emotions [21]. Patients' inquiries and doctors' descriptions of symptoms form the basis for the proposed multimodal machine learning system. In this setup, two ML strategies are

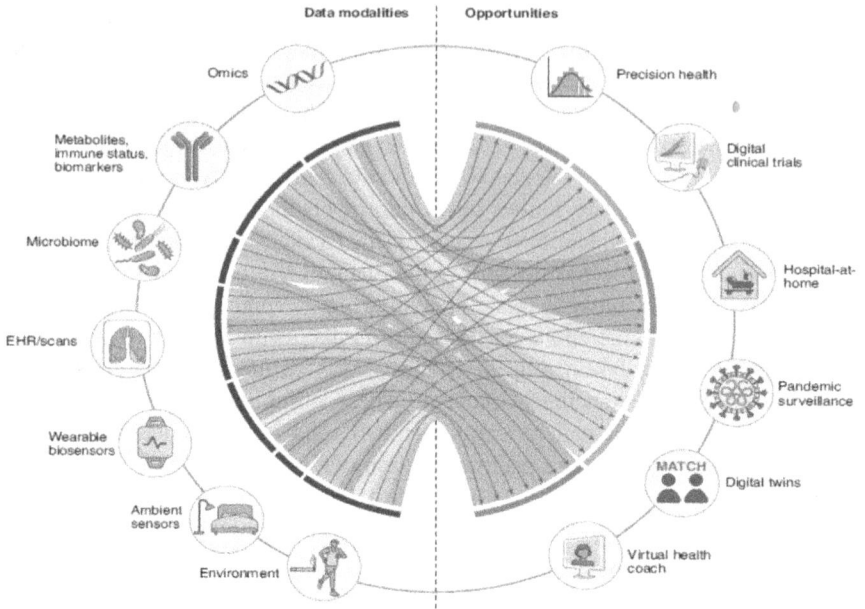

FIGURE 8.1 Data modalities and opportunities for multimodal biomedical AI.

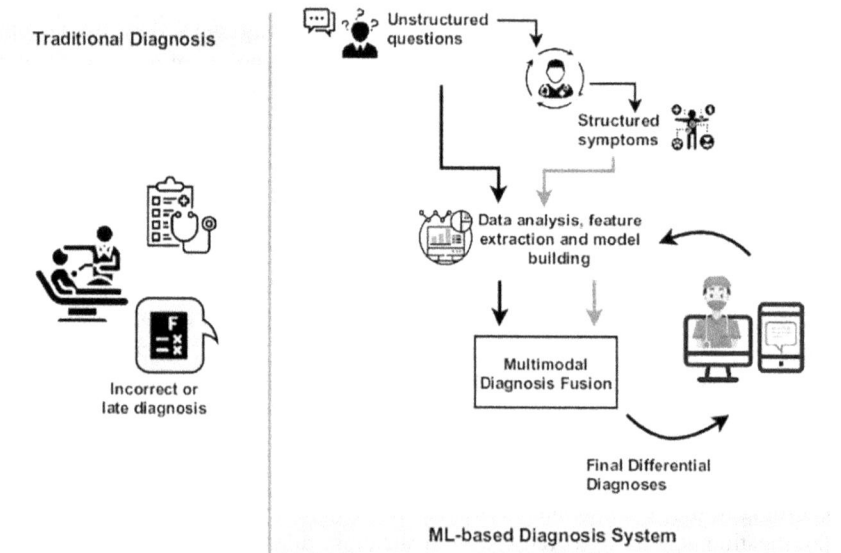

FIGURE 8.2 The conventional and ML-based discrepancy diagnosis structure.

constructed separately for every modality, and then their output is integrated to form a whole.

Text vectorization methods, which convert words in a document into numerical values, process the patients' inquiries. The TF-IDF and the hashing vectorizer are two such methods that focus mostly on syntactical aspects of a document. Also, the embedding models (like Doc2vec embedding) can be used to glean the documents' hidden meanings [22]. On the other hand, doctors' notations of ICD-10 codes for patients' symptoms constitute organized data. The One-Versus-Rest (OVR) method is used to map consultations to their accurate diagnosis, which is formulated as a multi-class classification. In order to solve multi-class classification issues, OVR employs a heuristic method that generalizes the capabilities of binary-based machine learning techniques. Experiments have been conducted using several machine learning classifiers and comparing them separately according to each modality [23]. The LR, RF, SGD classifier, and MLP classifiers were utilized, and their details are provided later in the paper. Various methods, including ranking, summing, and multiplication, are used to merge the two models' final results. The suggested model is tested for precision, efficiency in inference and loading, and manageability in terms of classification model size. The designed diagnosis approach accomplished an impressively high rate of accuracy (84.9%) in its categorization results.

The suggested method's primary contributions are:

- Combining organized clinical data with unstructured free-text consultations to create a diagnosis decision support system.
- The formidable difficulty of designing a system to accommodate the wide variety of Arabic dialects spoken today. To further aid physicians in making sound diagnoses, the suggested technology will be integrated into the digital health platform.

The rest parts of the chapter are structured as pursues. Section 8.2 presents recent relevant work in DL- and ML-based differential diagnosis systems. In Section 8.3, we discuss the technique, which includes the data gathering, pre-processing, features-extraction, proposed QSDM architecture, and assessment criteria. Section 8.4 offered the investigational conditions, the actual trials, and an argument of the outcomes. Section 8.5 concludes with the results and recommendations for further research.

8.2 RELATED WORKS

A thing's way of existence, experience, or expression is its modality. A multi-modal research challenge is one that involves more than one possible solution. At the same time, modes can be defined in a wide variety of ways. Data collected in two languages or fewer than two different conditions, for instance, can be considered two modes [24]. One of the keys to understanding the world around us is picking up on several signals at once. Images typically have accompanying labels and explanatory text, and articles frequently include visuals to help convey the article's main point. Since each mode has its own set of statistical characteristics, MMDLM can be utilized to interpret and comprehend multi-source modal information through the lens of deep learning. Figure 8.3 shows the variety of existing models [25].

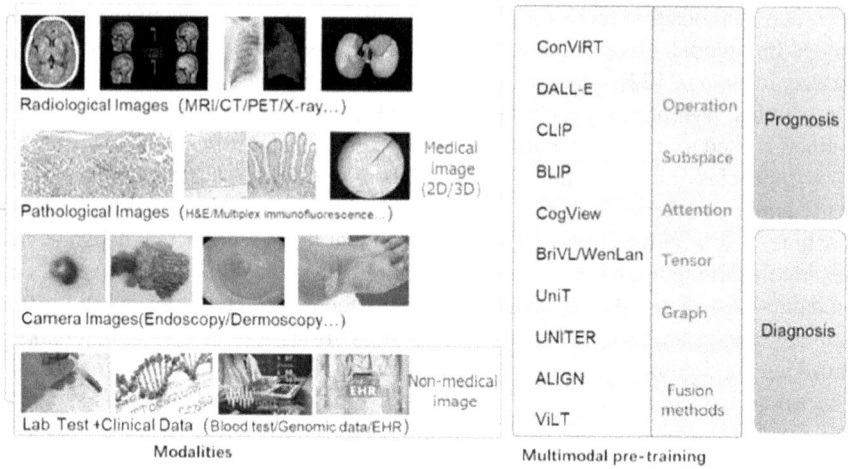

FIGURE 8.3   Structure of the related works.

At the moment, researchers are digging deep into multi-modal learning for pictures, videos, sounds, and words [26]. For the purpose of learning multi-layer displayers and the pensiveness of data prior to its conversion into high-level intangible properties of the system, a lot of focus is currently on deep neural networks. Classification, segmentation, detection, and localization are just a few of the medical applications that have benefited greatly from research into image analysis [27]. Segmentation, anomaly detection, illness categorization, computer-aided analysis, and picture rescue are just few of the medical image processing tasks that have seen widespread application of deep convolutional networks. Clinical applications have relied on medical imaging as a diagnostic tool for quite some time. The field of medicinal imaging has profited greatly from modern expansions in device design, security software, computer power, and data-storage capacity [28]. Findings demonstrated that the interpretable AI-aided analysis greatly enhanced the diagnostic accuracy of doctors, enhanced the irrefutable use of its supplementary verdict, and generated novel hypotheses for future studies of clinical translation. As medical IT and tools have advanced, so too has the volume and variety of medical data that has been available [29]. Based on its content and structure, medical data can be divided into three primary groups:

1. Clinical text data is mostly structured test data like hemoglobin and urine routine and unstructured text data like patient complaints and clinician-recorded pathologic texts.
2. Imaging data (ultrasound, CT, MRI) and waveform data (ECG, EEG) are examples of images and waveforms.
3. Biomics data, which can be further categorized at the molecular level into genomic, transcriptomic, proteomic, and other types.

In [30], the authors used MIMIC-III to create a NN-based approach for clinical note diagnosis. The top ten classification was 80% more accurate than the top 50. Ref [31]. automated clinical document ICD-10 mapping. BOW, TF-IDF, Word2Vec, LSTM, and CNN were combined into the SVM algorithm. The deep learning classifier outperformed. In [32], they presented an automated pathology report diagnosis classification. TF-IDF extracted features for linear SVM, XGBoost, and LR. XGBoost had the highest f1-score (92%). In [33], the authors used emergency department data to automate mental state detection. SVM, NB, RF, and CNN were compared. DL performed best with 98.1% accuracy. In [34], the authors created a web-based ML system for mental disease analysis. The tool matches symptoms to an ICD-10 disorder. The TF-IDF feature vectorizer was used to train the KNN classifier to diagnose Alzheimer's and vascular dementia using machine learning. Adaptive neuro-fuzzy inference has 84% accuracy.

In [35], the researchers created a ML strategy to diagnose and predict major depressive and bipolar disorder. The model scored 97% area under the curve for a limited data set. They constructed a ML approach to predict schizophrenia bipolar disorder. It incorporates multi-domain immune indicators from 513 diseases. Based on 16,114 instances, the authors [36] developed a deep CNN for disparity skin disease investigation. It predicted 419 skin disorders and recognized 26. It has 73% top-one precision, whereas three professional dermatologists had 63%. In [37], the creators applied DL to ultrasound images to differentially diagnose COVID-19. The model classified COVID-19, pneumonia, and healthy pictures with almost 90% accuracy. The previous investigations showed possible efforts to apply discrepancy analysis to improve physician decision making. They showed that Arabic has no such mechanisms. MENA clinical diagnosis decision support systems need more research [38].

Multi-modal DL uses deep learning to combine many data kinds. Imaging aids medical diagnosis. Since clinical diagnosis requires processing significant volumes of data, single-mode medical images provide limited information. Deep learning–based multi-modal medical image fusion may extract and combine feature information from multiple modalities, improving medical image diagnostics and evaluation. It has gained popularity due to its benefits.

This study addressed these literature gaps:

1. Insufficient medical imaging multi-modal data fusion literature to organize and summarize studies.
2. Lack of clinical expertise and data scientists and data analysis algorithm knowledge.
3. Lack of multi-modal DL bibliometric analysis in medicinal imaging.

8.3 PROPOSED METHODOLOGY

The methodology includes data collection and pre-processing, feature extraction for questions, classification model creation, and model evaluation. Figure 8.4 summarizes the process.

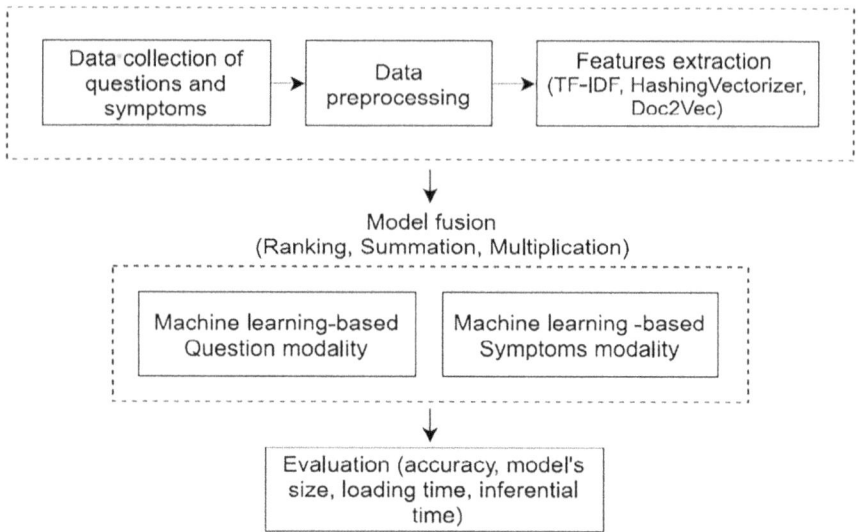

FIGURE 8.4 Proposed approach concept diagram.

8.3.1 DATA COLLECTION AND PRE-PROCESSING

The total amount of information obtained through Altibbi consists of 263,867 questions (consultations), each of which is escorted by symptoms and queries. The overall quantity of diagnoses is 8,410, whereas the number of symptoms comes in at 7,324. Each appointment is accompanied by a number of symptoms and a number of diagnoses, despite the fact that some of these conditions only appear seldom. In the first place, we got rid of the diagnoses that came up less than 20 times throughout all of the consultations [39]. After that, the consultations that had resulted in a lack of a diagnosis were eliminated. As a result, the total amount of diagnoses was 2,368, while the quantity of consultations came to a total of 246,814. A comparison of the number of diagnoses with the total number of consultations is presented in Figure 8.5. It is quite obvious that the majority of consultations concern a single diagnosis. During this time, a number of pre-processing activities are carried out in order to spot and organize the data in preparation for the predictive approach [40].

8.3.2 FEATURE EXTRACTION

Vectorization is the primary method utilized in the process of extracting features from the textual material. The practice of translating textual records into arithmetical feature vectors is referred to as "vectorization." Several methods, such as TF-IDF, the hashing vectorizer, and word embeddings, have been suggested in research that has been published so far [41].

8.3.3 QUESTION-SYMPTOM-DIAGNOSIS MODEL (QSDM)

This primary focus is on outlining the process that went into designing the QSDM strategy. It is a combination of two diagnostic approaches: examines the symptoms

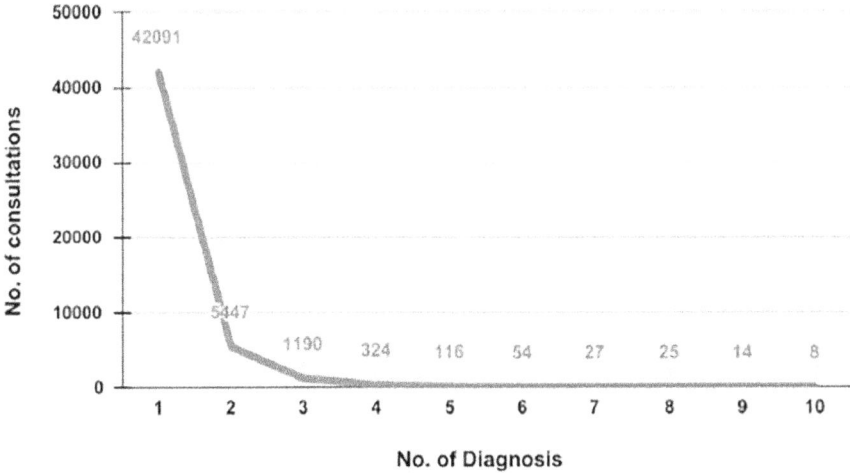

FIGURE 8.5   The association amid the quantity of consultations and investigation.

and organizes them into four distinct diagnoses based on their characteristics. Because offering more than potential scrutiny is likely to be confusing to the patient, we have decided to limit the number of diagnoses that can be suggested to only four. The second modality is called the question categorization modality, and it forecasts a maximum of four possible diagnoses. The final forecast is determined by integrating the results of the first and second modalities.

8.3.4   SYSTEM ARCHITECTURE

As can be seen in Figure 8.6, the QSDM is essentially the result of the combination of two distinct models: the symptom finding and the questions model. The output of the questions design are intended to be improved by merging the results of the symptoms model with the questions model in order to aggregate informative elements from the symptoms design. It takes into account all symptoms as binary features; hence, it takes into account the complete collection of distinctive symptoms gleaned from the queries (7,324 features in total). The suite of labels (2,368), each of which is showed by a binary value, is what constitutes the individual diagnoses. Eighty percent of the symptom data will be used for training, and 20% will be used for testing. The information is then processed by a number of different ML strategies. The learning models are constructed with the help of the training set, while the testing set is utilized in order to evaluate how well the models have performed. When it comes to dealing with multi-class categorization, the developed models use the OVR approach as their foundation. Each model undergoes training and testing on an individual basis. However, the final anticipated diagnoses are derived from the component of this submodel that has the highest classification accuracy. The TF-IDF algorithm, the hashing vectorizer, and document embedding were the feature extraction methods that were used individually for the questions model. The document embedding was

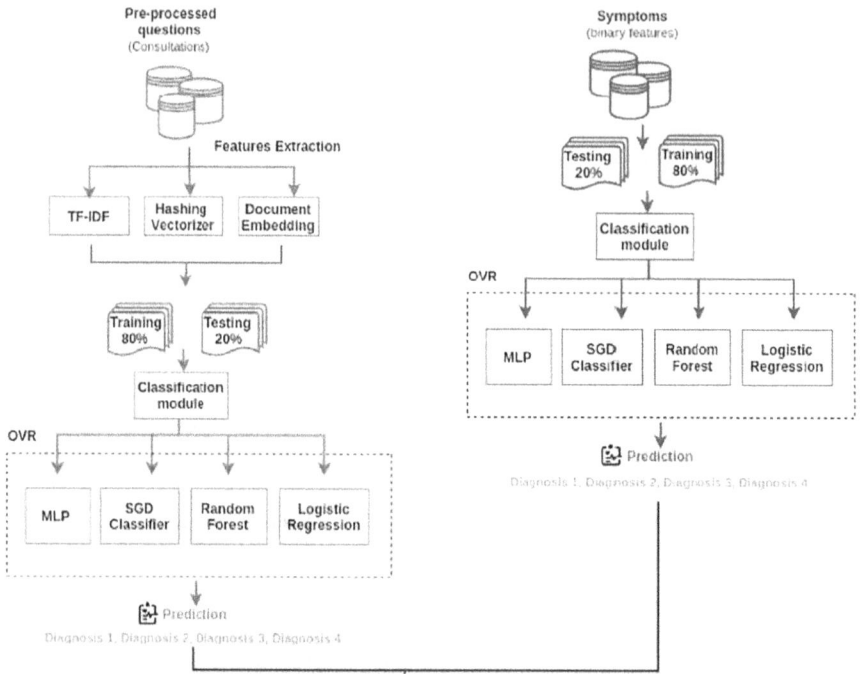

FIGURE 8.6 Architecture of the QSDM model.

accomplished with the help of the Doc2Vec program. The three data sets that were generated are then split into training data sets consisting of 80% and testing data sets consisting of 20%, respectively. During this time, they are being sent through OVR and into the four classifiers. Next, the results of the classifier that had the best overall performance are chosen to serve as the ultimate predictions of the question model.

8.3.5 EVALUATION CRITERIA

The accuracy at varying degrees of precision, the size of the technique, the loading, and inferential time were the four quantitative assessment variables examined while measuring the performance of the QSDM model. According to Equations (8.1) and (8.2), accuracy is the proportion of correct diagnoses relative to the number of diagnoses (m). Probabilities of all possible diagnosis are represented by Px in Equation (8.1), where X = [x1, x2,..xn], and n is the total number of possible diagnoses. Consultation actual diagnosis (y) is substituted for the expected diagnostic (x) in Equation (8.2), where (m) is the total number of potential diagnoses, in this case 4. Probabilities of all diagnoses are denoted by P, and indexes of diagnoses are denoted by j.

$$\text{Argmax } P_x = \{x| \text{ } if \text{ } v > z\} \tag{8.1}$$

$$\text{Accuracy (Acc)} = \frac{1}{m} \sum_i^m \left\{ f(y) = 1 | yargmax(p_a) \right\} \tag{8.2}$$

The precision (P) is how the accuracy is demonstrated to the audience. For instance, the accuracy at precision one indicates how well the algorithm is able to get at least one true diagnosis out of the truth diagnoses that are available. This is what is known as P_1, if you were wondering. P_2 refers to the ability of the model to identify at least two right diagnoses, while P_3 represents the ability to identify at least three diagnoses. The size of the model is a significant metric, particularly in light of the fact that increasing the size of the model would invariably lead to an improvement in the model's overall performance. Nevertheless, it is essential since, in circumstances in which there is a limited amount of infrastructure, it may reduce the effectiveness. Additionally, the loading time and the inferential time are two relevant measures that indicate the effectiveness of the model in delivering real-time predictions. The amount of time required to load the model onto the web is referred to as the loading time, while the amount of time required making a prediction is referred to as the inferential time.

8.4   RESULTS AND DISCUSSIONS

With regard to the questions module, this part presents a contrast of the classifiers at various feature-extraction approaches. These techniques include the TF-IDF, hashing vectorizer, and the record embeddings. It is abundantly obvious from the data presented that all strategies produced superior outcomes when they properly anticipated a minimum of one diagnosis (P_1). According to the results presented in the table, the LR approach was the top performing classifier overall (53.7%). Even while the MLP (10) showed a minor decrease in exactness as compared with LR, it still managed to attain a very respectable 45.2% accuracy. Both the MLP (20) and the MLP (30), however, were able to attain pretty respectable results (44.0% and 41.4%, respectively). On the other hand, the SGDClassifier had the worst performance (33.5%). In terms of the scenario to forecast a minimum of two correct diagnoses (P_2), the LR fared the finest with a percentage of 40.4%, followed by the MLP (10) and the MLP (20) with percentages of 36.7% and 38%, correspondingly. In the same vein, the LR obtained the highest accuracy (39%) when it came to predicting at least three right diagnoses (P_3), followed by MLP (10), which had an accuracy of 37.9%, and MLP(20), which had an exactness of 39%, correspondingly. When constructing a machine learning model, some of the most significant factors to take into consideration are the model's size, the amount of time necessary to install it on the web, and the amount of time required to execute an inferential anticipation. Incidentally, the MLP (10) had the smallest size, at 5.2MB, in terms of the M.S., while RF had the largest size, at 17,300 MB. When taking into account the amount of time required to load, the MLP required only 0.35 seconds. However, when it came to making a forecast, the two algorithms that were the quickest were the LR and the SGDClassifier. Both of these desired only 0.06 seconds to make a prediction. In spite of the fact that the MLP classifiers had the smallest design sizes and the quickest loading times, the LR was still

50-60%   70-80%   ● 80-90%   ● 100%

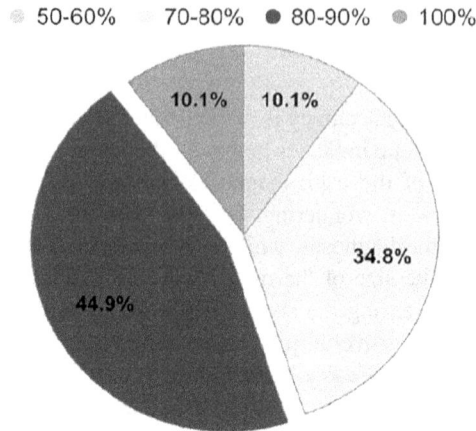

FIGURE 8.7   Qualitative investigation dependent on expert doctors.

capable of achieving a higher accuracy score. On the other hand, because of this, MLP classifiers are preferred for a decision maker that places a higher priority on the size and the amount of time than they do on the accuracy.

Figure 8.7 is a pie chart showing the qualitative assessment of the proposed component. According to the data, over half (44.9%) of the anticipated diagnoses are accurate to within (80–90)%, while nearly a third (34.8%) are accurate to within (70–80)%. Additionally, the first 10% is correct between (50–60)% of the time, and the final 10% is correct 100% of the time. The results of the suggested module's quantitative analysis agree strikingly with those of the experts' qualitative analysis, demonstrating the model's sturdiness and the reliability of projected diagnoses. Another example: one of Dr. Altibbi's patients came in with a runny nose and needed an appointment. Two applicable diagnoses and two irrelevant diagnoses were indicated by the created model. In the meantime, the doctor decided that a simple cold was to blame. According to Altibbi's doctors' qualitative assessment, however, the established QSDM model has certain drawbacks. For one, the indicated diagnosis may include duplication on occasion, such as diagnosing the common cold twice. Second, the model may miss the possibility that a patient's symptoms are caused by a fairly common disease. The common cold is an example of a symptom that might not be considered at first. These constraints could slow down the diagnostic process or prevent clinicians from making the best decision possible. Consequently, addressing these constraints is crucial for enhancing the established QSDM model.

In Table 8.1 and Figure 8.8, we see how well the final fused models perform with respect to four fusion criteria (R-I, R-II, Sum, & Multiply), as measured by correctness scores for anticipating 20%, 40%, and 80% of the diagnoses (depicted by P_1, P_2, and P_3, respectively). It is evident that P_1 produced the highest degree of precision. Multiplication-based fusion, on the other hand, achieved a 94.9% accuracy; this was followed by summation's 84.6%; then R-I's 92.8%; and R-II's 91.3%. There is a distinct and significant difference between P_3 and P_1, despite the fact that P_2 and P_3 behave similarly.

TABLE 8.1
Performance of Models

	Acc			
	R_I	R_II	Sum	Multiply
P_1	91.3	83.2	93.5	94.9
P_2	73.2	81.7	79.2	83.2
P_3	76.1	76.5	77.	79.6

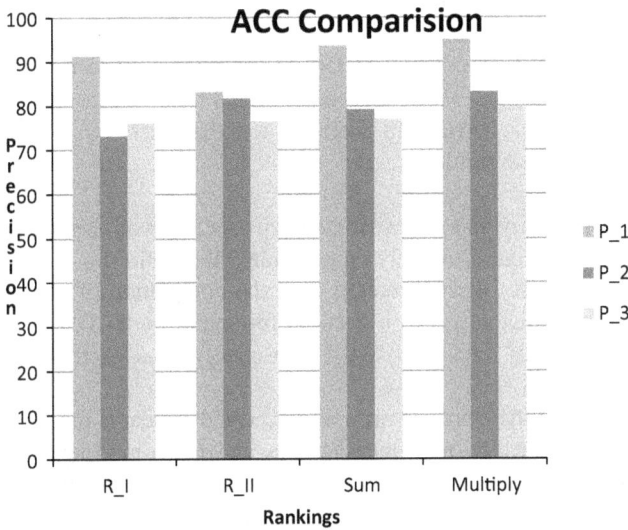

FIGURE 8.8 Performance comparison of models.

8.4.1 CHALLENGES OF THE MULTIMODEL DL IN HEALTHCARE

The use of data, models, and the completion of complex tasks all provide difficulties that must be overcome for multi-modal DL to proceed successfully in the area of medicine [42]. The primary obstacles are outlined below.

1. The heterogeneity and diversity of participants, the sample size, the depth of phenotypic analysis, the level of data consistency and synchronization, and the scale of association amid data sources all combine to create a challenge that is greater than that posed by a single-mode DLM in the medical field. Therefore, it is important to take into account the difficulty of working with the vastly varied data seen in real-world medical databases.
2. The gathering, connecting, and cost-effective footnote of multi-dimensional medical data presents problems with respect to cost and speed in the development of multi-modal medical research and clinical applications.

3. Good feature extraction and accurate data type association are pre-requisites for multi-modal medical fusion. However, there are several obstacles to overcome, such as the prevalence of small and partial datasets and non-standardized data structures.
4. In some domains, such as three-dimensional imaging and genomics, dis-pensation of even a single instant of data necessitates a substantial total of computational capacity. Therefore, it is a key problem to construct models that can rapidly and simultaneously process massive amounts of data such as tumor pathology slides, genomes, or medical text.
5. Patients and doctors may be concerned about their privacy when their health and clinical data is collected for study. It is crucial to set up a reliable process to monitor and address these problems, and this calls on researchers to propose and investigate further solutions.
6. Clinicians and doctors need to collaborate frequently to design research schemes in the field of multi-modal medical data fusion psychoanalysis. There are many barriers to working together that make this kind of communication difficult.

The medical community and AI researchers will need to work together to build and validate new models and ultimately demonstrate their ability to improve diagnosis and treatment. The use of data, models, and the completion of complex tasks all provide difficulties that must be overcome for multi-modal DL to proceed suc-cessfully in the field of medicine [43]. The primary obstacles are outlined below.

1. Problem is that there aren't universally accepted standards for collecting and annotating data, which might introduce bias and reduce model generalizability.
2. It is currently difficult to interpret the results of multi-modal deep learning models, which could limit their use in clinical settings.
3. Data heterogeneity across modalities, which may necessitate a variety of pre-processing and integration strategies.
4. The accessibility and availability of multi-modal data, as the collection and integration of data from numerous sources, may necessitate cooperation between different institutions and data sharing agreements.
5. Model overfitting, which is especially troublesome in medical applications because it can escort to pitiable performance on new data.

Impact on patient privacy and autonomy, as well as other potential ethical concerns related to the use of deep learning models in medical decision making.

8.4.1.1 Few Visions

1. The capacity to generate more accurate and tailored predictions using MMDL shows significant potential for enhancing medical investigation and treatment.
2. Multi-modal data integration can aid in the accurate scrutiny and predic-tion of diseases like cancer and Alzheimer's, as well as in the prediction of disease risk and the individualization of treatment.

3. MMDL can improve clinical decision making by providing more precise and quicker diagnoses and treatment suggestions.

Finally, MMDL shows considerable promise for enhancing healthcare outcomes and individualized treatment when applied in medical research and clinical practice. However, there are problems with these models that must be solved. These include things like data heterogeneity, interpretability, and ethical concerns. Together, we can overcome these obstacles and realize the full promise of MMDL in healthcare, leading to better patient diagnosis, care, and outcomes.

8.5 CONCLUSIONS AND FUTURE WORKS

Early on in the progression of a disease, symptoms are often vague and can easily be mistaken for those of another condition, making it difficult to provide a previous, correct differential diagnosis. It is crucial to create a computer-aided diagnosis system that would aid doctors in building accurate diagnoses. Differential scrutiny decisions made during consultations at Altibbi can be aided by the MMDL investigative system suggested in this study. The proposed method integrates the use of symptoms and queries. Differential diagnosis between the two modalities has been accomplished using a wide variety of machine learning methods. There have been a number of feature extraction techniques used in the questions module, including term frequency, a hashing vectorizer, and document embeddings. The final model is the result of a late fusion of two models; this fusion is accomplished in a number of different ways, including via ranking, summing, and multiplying. The best results in terms of accuracy (84.9%) were found using the fusion method that relied on multiplication. As a result, this design may hold promise as the basis for a differential diagnosis-capable decision-support system. However, boosting the model's precision is crucial. The growing number of Altibbi consultations is a great commodity that may be used to improve the model's effectiveness. In addition, this causes the structural symptoms to worsen. In order to improve accuracy, modern computing techniques like deep learning and transformer approaches can be applied to enormous amounts of data. The model's weaknesses can be addressed and improved upon by incorporating a third modality, such as diagnostic test and laboratory findings, into the categorization process.

Beyond the scope of this article, the potential uses of multimodal medical AI in healthcare are vast. Many activities in the realm of drug discovery, such as target classification and confirmation, anticipation of drug interactions, and prediction of adverse effects, could benefit from the use of multidimensional data. Although we covered a lot of ground in this analysis, there are still significant obstacles to the widespread adoption of multimodal AI, such as the possibility of false positives and how physicians should evaluate and convey the dangers to patients.

REFERENCES

1. Faris, H., Habib, M., Faris, M., Elayan, H. and Alomari, A., 2021. An intelligent multimodal medical diagnosis system based on patients' medical questions and structured symptoms for telemedicine. *Informatics in Medicine Unlocked*, 23, p.100513.

2. Lim, A., Hoek, H. W. and Blom, J. D., 2015. The attribution of psychotic symptoms to jinn in Islamic patients. *Transcultural Psychiatry, 52*(1), pp.18–32.

3. Acosta, J. N., Falcone, G. J., Rajpurkar, P. and Topol, E. J., 2022. Multimodal biomedical AI. *Nature Medicine, 28*(9), pp.1773–1784.

4. Reddy, P. C. S., Pradeepa, M., Venkatakiran, S., Walia, R. and Saravanan, M., 2021. Image and signal processing in the underwater environment. *Journal of Nuclear Energy Science and Power Generation Technology, 10*(9), p.2.

5. Alberdi, A., Aztiria, A. and Basarab, A., 2016. On the early diagnosis of Alzheimer's disease from multimodal signals: A survey. *Artificial Intelligence in Medicine, 71*, pp.1–29.

6. Kumar, A., Albreem, D. G. R. M. and Le, D., 2021. A comprehensive study on the role of advanced technologies in 5G based Smart hospital. *Alexandria Engineering Journal, 2021*(60), pp.5527–5536.

7. Ramakrishnan, B., Kumar, A., Chakravart, S., Masud, M. and Baz, M., 2021. Analysis of FBMC waveform for 5G network based smart hospitals. *Applied Sciences, 11*(19), p.8895. 10.3390/app11198895

8. Maurya, A. K., Lokesh, K., Kumar, S. R. and Krishnamoorthy, R., 2022. Deep neuro-fuzzy logic technique for brain meningiomasa prediction, *7th International Conference on Communication and Electronics Systems (ICCES)*, pp.1244–1248. 10.1109/ICCES54183.2022.9836008

9. Shams, A. B., Raihan, M., Khan, M., Preo, R. and Monjur, O., 2021. Telehealthcare and Covid-19: A noninvasive & low cost invasive, scalable and multimodal real-time smartphone application for early diagnosis of SARS-CoV-2 infection. *arXiv preprint arXiv:2109.07846.*

10. Kumar, A. and Gupta, M., 2017. A review on activities of fifth generation mobile communication system. *Alexandria Engineering Journal, 57*(2), pp.1125–1135. https://www.sciencedirect.com/science/article/pii/S1110016817300601

11. Kumar, A., Albreem, M. A., Gupta, M., Alsharif, M. H. and Kim, S., 2020. Future 5G network based smart hospitals: Hybrid detection technique for latency improvement. *IEEE Access, 8*, pp.153240–153249. 10.1109/ACCESS.2020.3017625.

12. Cai, Q., Wang, H., Li, Z. and Liu, X., 2019. A survey on multimodal data-driven smart healthcare systems: Approaches and applications. *IEEE Access, 7*, pp.133583–133599.

13. Reddy, P. C. S., Sucharitha, Y. and Narayana, G. S., 2021b. Forecasting of Covid-19 virus spread using machine learning algorithm. *International Journal of Biology and Biomedicine, 6*, pp. 32–39.

14. Guohou, S., Lina, Z. and Dongsong, Z., 2020. What reveals about depression level? The role of multimodal features at the level of interview questions. *Information & Management, 57*(7), p.103349.

15. Shanmugaraja, P., Bhardwaj, M., Mehbodniya, A., Vali, S. and Reddy, P. C. S., 2023. An efficient clustered m-path sinkhole attack detection (MSAD) algorithm for wireless sensor networks. *Adhoc & Sensor Wireless Networks, 55*, pp. 1–21.

16. Zheng, G., Zhang, D. and Zhao, W., 2021. Guest editorial multi-modal computing for biomedical intelligence systems. *IEEE Journal of Biomedical and Health Informatics, 25*(9), pp.3256–3257.

17. Sucharitha, Y., Reddy, P. C. S. and Suryanarayana, G., 2023. Network intrusion detection of drones using recurrent neural networks. *Drone Technology: Future Trends and Practical Applications*, pp.375–392.

18. Vásquez-Correa, J. C., Arias-Vergara, T., Orozco-Arroyave, J. R., Eskofier, B., Klucken, J. and Nöth, E., 2018. Multimodal assessment of Parkinson's disease: A deep learning approach. *IEEE Journal of Biomedical and Health Informatics, 23*(4), pp.1618–1630.

19. Dhanalakshmi, R., Bhavani, N. P. G., Raju, S. S., Shaker Reddy, P. C., Marvaluru, D., Singh, D. P. and Batu, A., 2022. Onboard pointing error detection and estimation of observation satellite data using extended Kalman filter. *Computational Intelligence and Neuroscience, 2022*, pp. 1–8.

20. Van Abbema, R., Van Wilgen, C. P., Van Der Schans, C. P. and Van Ittersum, M. W., 2011. Patients with more severe symptoms benefit the most from an intensive multimodal programme in patients with fibromyalgia. *Disability and Rehabilitation, 33*(9), pp.743–750.

21. Rahman, T., Ibtehaz, N., Khandakar, A., Hossain, M. S. A., Mekki, Y. M. S., Ezeddin, M., Bhuiyan, E. H., Ayari, M. A., Tahir, A., Qiblawey, Y. and Mahmud, S., 2022. QUCoughScope: An intelligent application to detect COVID-19 patients using cough and breath sounds. *Diagnostics, 12*(4), p.920.

22. Singh, B., Somasekhar, K., Anand, K., Gopikrishnan, M. and Krishnamoorthy, R., 2022. Machine learning based predictive modeling of plasma treatment in biomedical surfaces. *Second International Conference on Artificial Intelligence and Smart Energy (ICAIS)*, pp.1043–1046. 10.1109/ICAIS53314.2022.9743031

23. Wang, C., Wang, H., Zhuang, H., Li, W., Han, S., Zhang, H. and Zhuang, L., 2020. Chinese medical named entity recognition based on multi-granularity semantic dictionary and multimodal tree. *Journal of Biomedical Informatics, 111*, p.103583.

24. Prasath, A. S. S., Lokesh, S., Krishnakumar, N. J., Vandarkuzhali, T., Sahu, D. N. and Reddy, P. C. S., 2022. Classification of EEG signals using machine learning and deep learning techniques. *International Journal of Health Sciences, 2022*, pp.10794–10807.

25. Kline, A., Wang, H., Li, Y., Dennis, S., Hutch, M., Xu, Z., Wang, F., Cheng, F. and Luo, Y., 2022. Multimodal machine learning in precision health: A scoping review. *NPJ Digital Medicine, 5*(1), p.171.

26. Muthappa, K. A., Nisha, A. S. A., Shastri, R., Avasthi, V. and Reddy, P. C. S., 2023. Design of high-speed, low-power non-volatile master slave flip flop (NVMSFF) for memory registers designs. *Applied Nanoscience*, pp.1–10.

27. Al Bassam, N., Hussain, S. A., Al Qaraghuli, A., Khan, J., Sumesh, E. P. and Lavanya, V., 2021. IoT based wearable device to monitor the signs of quarantined remote patients of COVID-19. *Informatics in Medicine Unlocked, 24*, p.100588.

28. Cavalcanti, T. C., Lew, H. M., Lee, K., Lee, S. Y., Park, M. K. and Hwang, J. Y., 2021. Intelligent smartphone-based multimode imaging otoscope for the mobile diagnosis of otitis media. *Biomedical Optics Express, 12*(12), pp.7765–7779.

29. Sabitha, R., Shukla, A. P., Mehbodniya, A., Shakkeera, L. and Reddy, P. C. S., 2022. A fuzzy trust evaluation of cloud collaboration outlier detection in wireless sensor networks. *Adhoc & Sensor Wireless Networks 53*, pp. 165–188.

30. Yang, G., Ye, Q. and Xia, J., 2022. Unbox the black-box for the medical explainable AI via multi-modal and multi-centre data fusion: A mini-review, two showcases and beyond. *Information Fusion, 77*, pp.29–52.

31. Ashok, K., Boddu, R., Syed, S. A., Sonawane, V. R., Dabhade, R. G. and Reddy, P. C. S., 2022. GAN Base feedback analysis system for industrial IOT networks. *Automatika*, pp.1–9.

32. Shams, A. B., Raihan, M., Sarker, M., Khan, M., Uddin, M., Monjur, O. and Preo, R. B., 2021. Telehealthcare and telepathology in pandemic: A noninvasive, low-cost micro-invasive and multimodal real-time online application for early diagnosis of COVID-19 infection. *arXiv preprint arXiv:2109.07846.*

33. Shaker Reddy, P. C. and Sucharitha, Y., 2022. IoT-enabled energy-efficient multipath power control for underwater sensor networks. *International Journal of Sensors Wireless Communications and Control, 12*(6), pp.478–494.

34. Roy, S., Meena, T. and Lim, S. J., 2022. Demystifying supervised learning in healthcare 4.0: A new reality of transforming diagnostic medicine. *Diagnostics*, *12*(10), p.2549.
35. Lokesh, S., Priya, A., Sakhare, D. T., Devi, R. M., Sahu, D. N. and Reddy, P. C. S., 2022. CNN based deep learning methods for precise analysis of cardiac arrhythmias. *International Journal of Health Sciences*, 6, pp. 10808–10819.
36. Gyrard, A., Jaimini, U., Gaur, M., Shekharpour, S., Thirunarayan, K. and Sheth, A., 2022. Reasoning over personalized healthcare knowledge graph: A case study of patients with allergies and symptoms. *Semantic Models in IoT and Ehealth Applications* (pp.199–225). Academic Press.
37. Albreem, M. A., Kumar, A. et al., 2021. Low complexity linear detectors for massive MIMO: A comparative study. *IEEE Access*, 9, pp.45740–45753. 10.1109/ACCESS.2021.3065923
38. Chakravarty, S. and Kumar, A., 2023. PAPR reduction of GFDM signals using encoder-decoder neural network (autoencoder). *National Academy of Science Letters.* 10.1007/s40009-023-01230-1
39. Liu, L., Shafiq, M., Sonawane, V. R., Murthy, M. Y. B., Reddy, P. C. S. and Kumar Reddy, K. C., 2022. Spectrum trading and sharing in unmanned aerial vehicles based on distributed blockchain consortium system. *Computers and Electrical Engineering*, *103*, p.108255.
40. Kumar, A., Venkatesh, J., Gaur, N., Alsharif, M. H., 2023. Peerapong Uthansakul and Monthippa Uthansakul, "Cyclostationary and energy detection spectrum sensing beyond 5G. *Electronic Research Archive*, *31*(6), pp.3400–3416. 10.3934/era.2023172
41. Faris, H., Faris, M., Habib, M. and Alomari, A., 2022. Automatic symptoms identification from a massive volume of unstructured medical consultations using deep neural and BERT models. *Heliyon*, *8*(6), p.e09683.
42. Reddy, P. C. S., Suryanarayana, G. and Yadala, S., 2022. November. Data analytics in farming: Rice price prediction in Andhra Pradesh. In *2022 5th International Conference on Multimedia, Signal Processing and Communication Technologies (IMPACT)* (pp.1–5). IEEE.
43. Palliya Guruge, C., Oviatt, S., Delir Haghighi, P. and Pritchard, E., 2021. October. Advances in multimodal behavioral analytics for early dementia diagnosis: A review. In *Proceedings of the 2021 International Conference on Multimodal Interaction* (pp.328–340).

9 Sliding Window Adaptive Filter for Denoising PCG Signals Used in Healthcare Systems

Vishwanath Madhava Shervegar
Department of Electronics & Communication Engineering,
Mangalore Institute of Technology & Engineering, India

Jagadish Nayak
Department of Electronics & Electrical Engineering,
Birla Institute of Technology and Science, UAE

9.1 INTRODUCTION

Cardiovascular diseases (CVDs) are the prime cause of high death rates worldwide. Various methods like electrocardiogram (ECG) [1], phonocardiogram (PCG) [2], and photoplethysmogram (PPG) [3] are many times used for detection and diagnosis of CVD. PCG signal is the only one that provides acoustic information about the working of the heart. The electronic stethoscope is the most versatile tool that is often used tool to record the PCG. However, recording of the PCG is challenging in the presence of other biological signals and nearby acoustic disturbances and noises using an electronic stethoscope [4, 5]. Phonocardiography using PCG signals is difficult because the PCGs are corrupted by various noise signals such as lung sounds, environmental noise, stethoscope movement, etc. This leads to incorrect diagnosis of the pathological heart sound. So, it is very necessary and important to denoise PCG signals [6] before conducting further signal processing. Denoising a PCG signal is done in order to improve signal quality by reducing background noise. Clinical evaluation [7] of the PCG should be performed to test the quality of the cardiac signal. The accuracy of the methods used to denoise PCGs decides the performance. This performance is dependent on the noise level [8]. There are various types of time-domain PCG denoising methods available in the literature [9]. The time domain approach provides the occurrence of the various events in the time domain.

DOI: 10.1201/9781003403678-9

The time domain denoising algorithms are the traditional Chebyshev IIR filters [10] and adaptive noise cancellers (ANCs) [11, 12]. In this work, we have investigated the feasibility of adopting the Sliding Window Adaptive Noise Cancellation approach, commonly used for very large signal denoising of PCG signal denoising in this study. The proposed filter model employs the adapted Sliding Window LMS algorithm, which requires a minimum number of computations for denoising of the PCG signals. We use a single module of the Adaptive Noise Canceller so that, firstly, a Sliding Window of fixed duration slides over the PCG signal. The estimate of the clean signal is obtained from each of the Sliding Windows by using the LMS Adaptive algorithm on each of the windowed signals. As the window slides over the signal, the signal gets denoised by virtue of the LMS Adaptive filter that removes the noise in each window. A completely denoised signal results from the noisy signal in a very short duration. The materials and methods are described in Section 9.2. Section 9.3 contains the MATLAB® simulation results, demonstrating the usefulness of the proposed approach. Section 9.4 presents the discussion of the results comparatively, and Section 9.5 concludes with future scope.

9.2 MATERIALS AND METHODS

9.2.1 DATA

This study used experimental PCG raw data available at PhysioNet/PhysioBank to evaluate the proposed filter's denoising capability.

9.2.2 EXPERIMENTAL DATA

PCG data for analysis (both normal and pathological) are obtained from the PhysioNet database. The data set has sounds from both healthy subjects and pathological patients, including children and adults. Each subject/patient may have contributed between one and six heart sound recordings. The recordings last from several seconds to more than 100 seconds. All recordings in .wav format and have been resampled to 2,000 Hz. Each recording contains just only a single PCG lead. The heart sound recordings were extracted from different locations on the body. The typical four locations are the aortic, pulmonic, tricuspid, and mitral, but they could be one of nine different locations. A healthy PCG signal (a0007) and a pathological PCG signal (a0001) of a duration of 2 s that are sampled at 8 kHz have been used in this study.

9.2.3 PROPOSED ROBUST SLIDING WINDOW ADAPTIVE FILTER CONFIGURATION

ANCs that use LMS adaptive filters are simple to construct and provide reliable performance, but the steady-state MSE takes a long time to converge [13, 14]. We propose a robust Sliding Window LMS adaptive filter model to obtain a faster denoising speed. Figure 9.1 shows that the proposed filter architecture has two modules. A Sliding Window structure is employed in the first module. In the second module, the signal windowed signal is passed through the conventional LMS

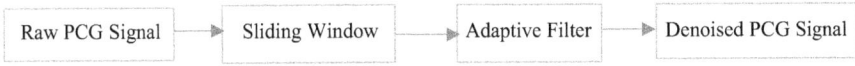

FIGURE 9.1 Block diagram of the proposed filter structure.

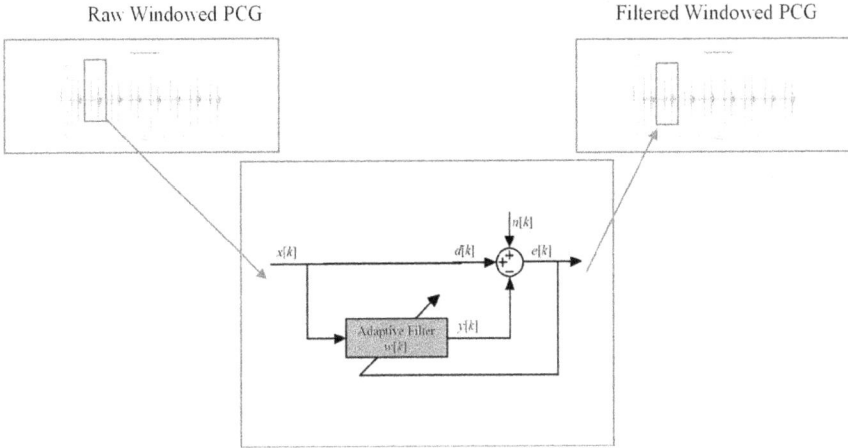

FIGURE 9.2 Single-stage LMS filter structure.

adaptive filter to obtain an accurate estimate of the original signal [15, 16]. The robust Sliding Window adaptive filter structure is shown in Figure 9.2.

The windowed signal $x(n)$ is the product of the original signal $x_0(n)$ and the time-domain window $w(n)$.

$$x(n) = x_0(n) \times w(n) \tag{9.1}$$

The noisy signal $x_1(n)$ is obtained when the noise $n(n)$ adds to the original signal $x(n)$.

$$x_1(n) = x(n) + n(n) \tag{9.2}$$

The output of the LMS adaptive filter stage $e(n)$ is the difference of $x_1(n)$ and $y(n)$, where

$$y(n) = w_1^T(n) \times x_1(n) \tag{9.3}$$

$$e(n) = x_1(n) - y(n) \tag{9.4}$$

The weights are updated as

$$w_1(n + 1) = w_1(n) \times \mu_{LMS} \times x_1(n) \tag{9.5}$$

where the filter weights are $w_1(n) = [w_0, w_2, \ldots w_{L-1}]^T$ and filter inputs are $x_1(n) = [x_0(n), x_1(n)\ldots x_{L-1}(n - L + 1)]^T$ with L being the filter order.

Step size is an important parameter that is used in the LMS adaptive algorithm. Large step sizes result in excessive mean square error (MSE). This results in loss of stability. A too small step size causes delayed convergence. The upper bound for the step size is determined by

$$0 < \mu < \frac{2}{\lambda_{max}} \tag{9.6}$$

where μ and λ_{max} represent the step size and the greatest eigen value of the input signals autocorrelation matrix. The step size in the proposed model is determined automatically from the minimum correlation between the windowed original signal $x(n)$ and the windowed noisy signal $x_1(n)$.

$$\mu_{LMS} = E\left(|x(n)x_1(n)|\right) \tag{9.7}$$

9.2.4 STATISTICAL ANALYSIS

The performance of the robust Sliding Window adaptive filter model is analyzed with the PCG signal that is corrupted with Gaussian and pink noise with both high and low input SNR levels. The algorithm's performance is described by various metrics shown in Eqs. (9.8)–(9.11).

Mean square error (MSE) is given by

$$MSE = \frac{1}{N} \sum_{i=1}^{N} \left(|x(n)| - |y(n)|\right)^2 \tag{9.8}$$

Signal to noise ratio (SNR) (in dB) is given by

$$SNR = 10\log_{10} \frac{\sum_{i=1}^{N} (x(n))^2}{\sum_{i=1}^{N} (x(n) - y(n))^2} \tag{9.9}$$

Peak signal to noise ratio (PSNR) (in dB) is given by

$$PSNR = \frac{\max(x[n])^2}{MSE} \tag{9.10}$$

Correlation coefficient (CC) is given by

$$CC = \frac{N\left(\sum_{i=1}^{N} x(n)y(n)\right) - \left(\sum_{i=1}^{N} x(n)\right)\left(\sum_{i=1}^{N} y(n)\right)}{\left[\sqrt{N\sum_{i=1}^{N} (x(n))^2 - \left(\sum_{i=1}^{N} x(n)\right)^2}\right]\left[N\sum_{i=1}^{N} (y(n))^2 - \left(\sum_{i=1}^{N} y(n)\right)^2\right]} \tag{9.11}$$

In Eqs. (9.8)–(9.11), $x(n)$ represents the clean signal, $y(n)$ is the filtered signal, and N is the number of samples.

9.3   RESULT

The performance of the Robust Sliding Window Adaptive Filter method was measured by testing it against the sounds taken from PhysioNet database. The sounds were of 2-s duration and were sampled at a Nyquist rate of 8 kHz. Different levels of additive white Gaussian noise (AWGN) were considered for corrupting the sounds from the database. These noisy sounds were then evaluated using the proposed method. The simulation software that is used for the purpose is MATLAB R2022A. The fixed parameter for the simulation was the window width w and the filter length L. The step size μ_{LMS} was chosen as the minimum correlation value between the windowed original signal and the windowed noisy signal.

9.3.1   QUALITATIVE ASSESSMENT

The quality of the output signal obtained by virtue of denoising the noisy PCG by the proposed method is analyzed through subjective evaluation. We have considered the sounds from the PhysioNet database and additive white Gaussian noise of different levels for the purpose of evaluation. Figure 9.3(a) and (b) show the original PCG and the AWGN of +4 dB. Figure 9.3(c) and (d) show the noise-corrupted PCG and the recovered PCG. The aberrant PCG a007 was distorted with an AWGN of +4 dB, as seen in Figure 9.4, and the suggested solution successfully gets rid of the noise and recovers the signal. The diagram explicitly shows that the proposed method effectively removes noise and recovers the signal. Figure 9.5(a) and (b) show the original PCG and the AWGN of −4 dB. It is evident from Figure 9.5(c) and (d) that the original signal can be recovered even in the presence of higher levels of noises.

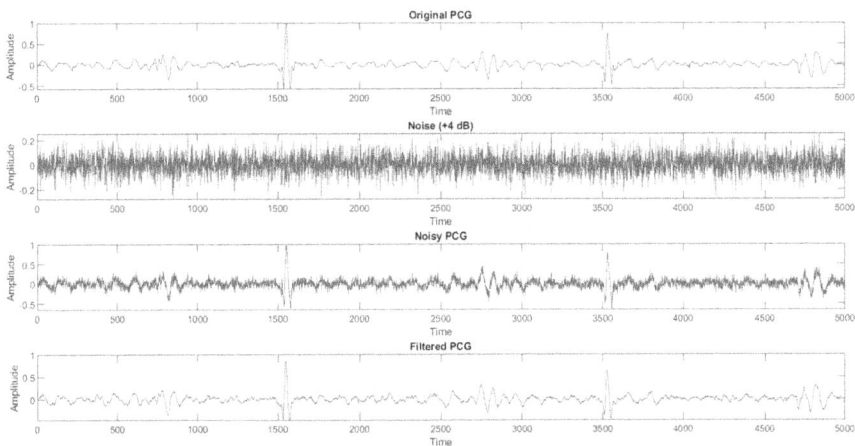

FIGURE 9.3 Proposed robust Sliding Window adaptive filter denoising performance for Gaussian noise-corrupted normal PCG signal: (a) noise-free signal, (b) additive Gaussian noise input signal to noise level of +4 dB, (c) signal with noise, (d) proposed robust Sliding Window adaptive filter output.

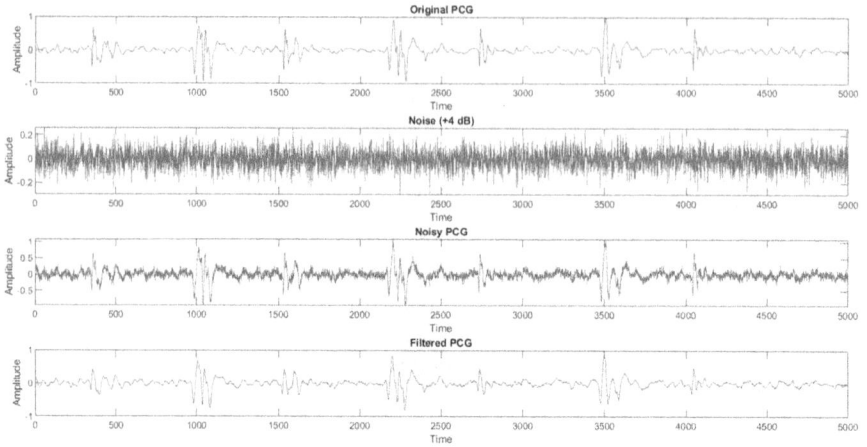

FIGURE 9.4 Proposed robust Sliding Window adaptive filter denoising performance for Gaussian noise-corrupted abnormal PCG signal: (a) noise-free signal, (b) additive Gaussian noise input signal to noise level of +4 dB, (c) signal with noise, (d) proposed robust Sliding Window adaptive filter output.

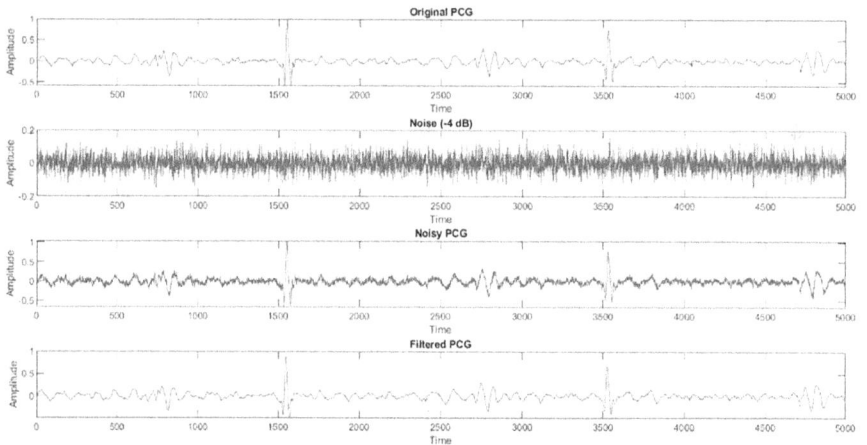

FIGURE 9.5 Proposed robust Sliding Window adaptive filter denoising performance for Gaussian noise-corrupted normal PCG signal: (a) noise-free signal, (b) additive Gaussian noise input signal to noise level of −4 dB, (c) signal with noise, (d) proposed robust Sliding Window adaptive filter output.

In Figure 9.4, it is shown that the abnormal PCG a007 was corrupted with AWGN of +4 dB and the proposed method removes the noise and recovers the signal. In Figure 9.6, it is shown that the same abnormal PCG a007 was corrupted with higher-order noise levels of −4 dB and the proposed method removes this noise as well.

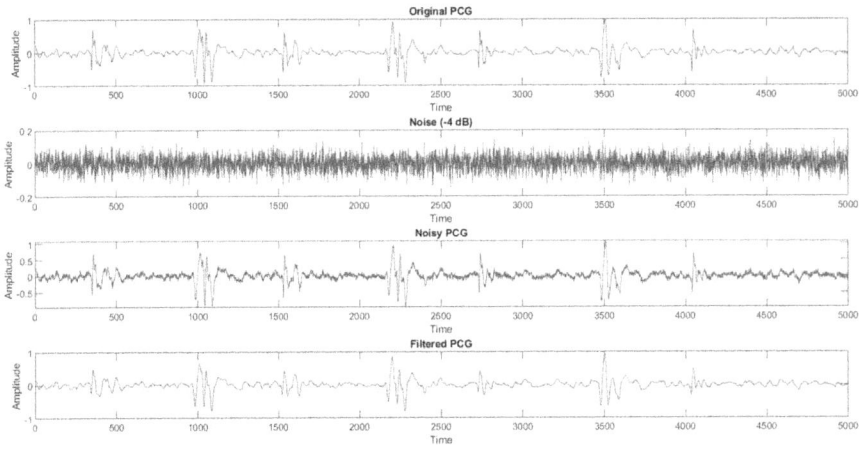

FIGURE 9.6 Proposed robust Sliding Window adaptive filter denoising performance for Gaussian noise-corrupted abnormal PCG signal: (a) noise-free signal, (b) additive Gaussian noise input signal to noise level of −4 dB, (c) signal with noise, (d) proposed robust Sliding Window adaptive filter output.

The aualitative analysis was also carried out by considering the pink noise. The pink noise of level +4 dB was used to corrupt the normal PCG signal, as shown in Figure 9.7. The proposed method successfully removes the noise to produce a clean signal. Figure 9.8 shows the noise analysis of an abnormal PCG signal corrupted by +4 dB noise. The proposed method denoises the abnormal PCG effectively and produces a clean signal. Figure 9.9 shows that pink noise of higher noise levels,

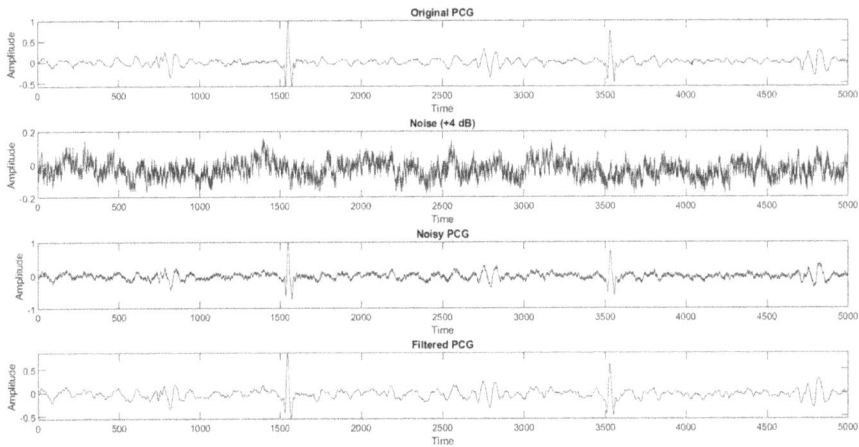

FIGURE 9.7 Proposed robust Sliding Window adaptive filter denoising performance for pink noise corrupted normal PCG signal: (a) noise-free signal, (b) pink noise input signal to noise level of +4 dB, (c) signal with noise, (d) proposed robust Sliding Window adaptive filter output.

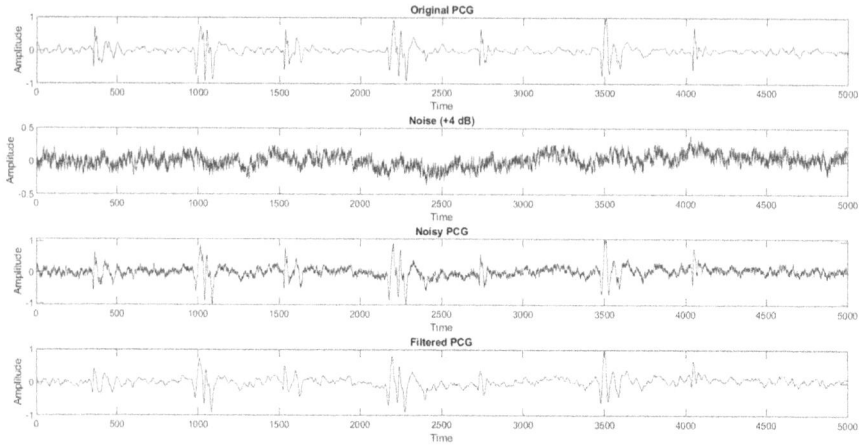

FIGURE 9.8 Proposed robust Sliding Window adaptive filter denoising performance for pink noise-corrupted abnormal PCG signal: (a) noise-free signal, (b) pink noise input signal to noise level of +4 dB, (c) signal with noise, (d) proposed robust Sliding Window adaptive filter output.

namely −4 dB, was used to corrupt the original PCG. Even in the presence of higher noise levels, the method successfully removes the redundant noise. Experiments were also carried out with respect to abnormal PCG, as shown in Figure 9.10. The method was able to reduce the noise to the lowest level and produce the signal that was a close approximate of the original signal.

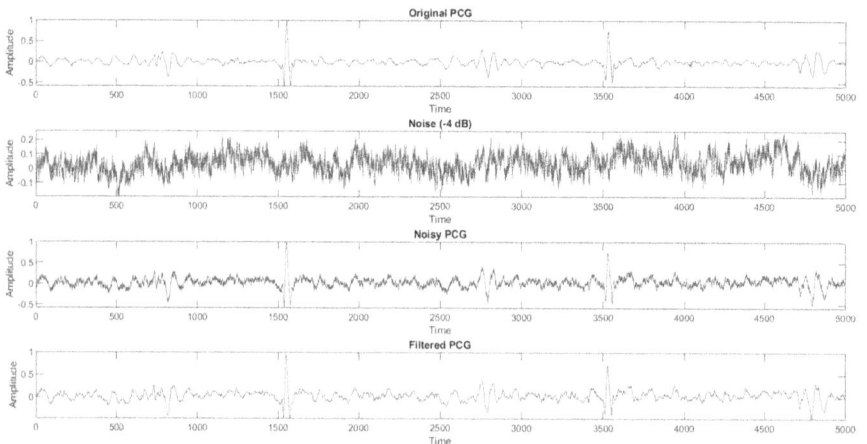

FIGURE 9.9 Proposed robust Sliding Window adaptive filter denoising performance for pink noise-corrupted normal PCG signal: (a) noise-free signal, (b) pink noise input signal to noise level of −4 dB, (c) signal with noise, (d) proposed robust Sliding Window adaptive filter output.

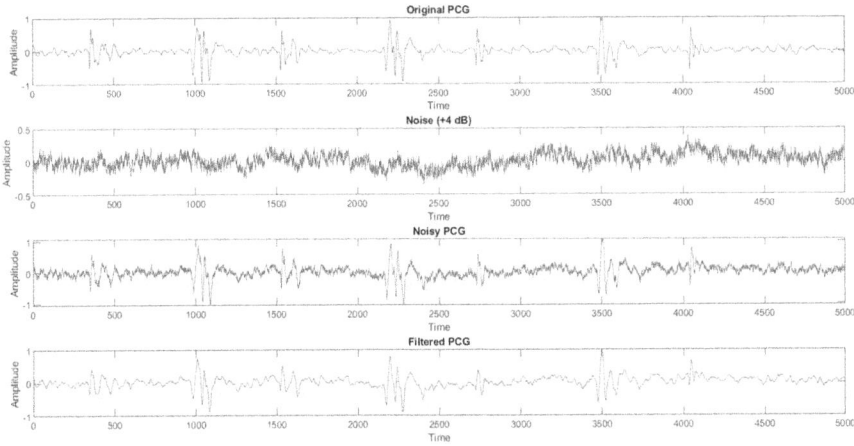

FIGURE 9.10 Proposed robust Sliding Window adaptive filter denoising performance for pink noise-corrupted abnormal PCG signal: (a) noise-free signal, (b) pink noise input signal to noise level of +4 dB, (c) signal with noise, (d) proposed robust Sliding Window adaptive filter output.

9.4 DISCUSSION

Findings of the comparative study on the robust Sliding Window Adaptive Filter with the state-of-the-art traditional LMS filter are presented below. Evaluation of the proposed method is assessed with the state-of-the-art method mentioned in literature using the obtained accuracy. The performance of the proposed algorithm is evaluated based on the denoising ability of the method. Tables 9.1 and 9.2 compare the performance measures in terms of SNR, MSE, PSNR, and CC for the proposed method as against the state-of-the-art LMS adaptive filter model for both normal and abnormal sounds with various induced AWGN noise levels. The table shows that in case of the proposed method, the MSE reduced by ten times, the SNR

TABLE 9.1
Performance Metrics of Sliding Window LMS Filter and the State-of-the-Art LMS Filter for AWGN Corrupted Signal

Signal Type	Input SNR	Adaptive Filter Configuration	MSE	SNR	PSNR	CC
Normal	+4 dB	LMS	0.0025	6.2899	25.9982	0.8963
		Sliding Window LMS	**0.00046**	**13.3042**	**33.0125**	**0.9754**
	−4 dB	LMS	0.0025	6.2528	25.9611	0.8956
		Sliding Window LMS	**0.00023**	**16.4753**	**36.1456**	**0.9866**
Abnormal	+4 dB	LMS	0.0039	8.4532	23.8702	0.9299
		Sliding Window LMS	**0.0010**	**14.1053**	**29.5224**	**0.9805**
	−4 dB	LMS	0.0039	8.4507	23.8677	0.9302
		Sliding Window LMS	**0.00075**	**15.4884**	**30.9055**	**0.9858**

TABLE 9.2

Performance Metrics of Sliding Window LMS Filter and the State-of-the-Art LMS Filter for Pink Noise-Corrupted Signal

Signal Type	Input SNR	Adaptive Filter Configuration	MSE	SNR	PSNR	CC
Normal	+4 dB	LMS	0.0025	6.26	26.9683	0.8958
		Sliding Window LMS	**0.0012**	**8.66**	**28.3683**	**0.9302**
	−4 dB	LMS	0.0025	6.2432	25.9515	0.8954
		Sliding Window LMS	**0.0013**	**8.5441**	**28.2524**	**0.9290**
Abnormal	+4 dB	LMS	0.0039	8.4592	23.8762	0.9303
		Sliding Window LMS	**0.0015**	**12.3321**	**27.7491**	**0.9704**
	−4 dB	LMS	0.0039	8.5975	23.8812	0.9302
		Sliding Window LMS	**0.0015**	**12.2816**	**27.6986**	**0.9701**

improved by at least three times, and the PSNR improved by 25% compared to the state-of-the-art traditional LMS filter. The CC for the proposed filter was more than 0.97 in all cases. Considering pink noise analysis, the proposed method reduced MSE by two times, improved PSNR by 33%, and increased SNR by 4% compared to the traditional LMS algorithm. Using the proposed method the correlation between original and denoised signal was at least 0.92. Based on these results, it can be summarized that the robust Sliding Window Adaptive filter outperforms the traditional LMS filter in terms of performance metrics.

9.4.1 SELECTION OF STEP SIZE

The selection of step size is important for accurate denoising of the PCG. In the proposed method, the step size is automatically adjusted based on the minimum

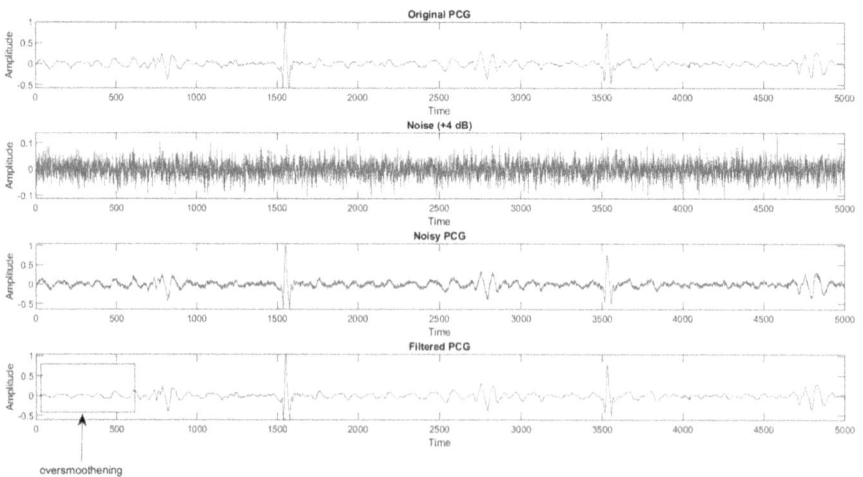

FIGURE 9.11 Over-smoothening of PCG due to small step size in LMS filter.

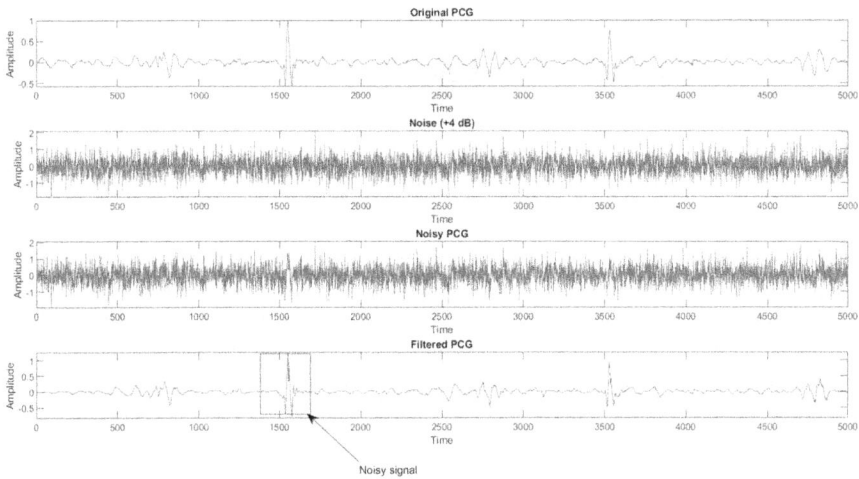

FIGURE 9.12   Under-denoising due to large step size in LMS filter.

correlation between the original PCG and the noisy PCG. Appropriate fixing of the step size may lead to under-denoising or over-denoising based on whether the step size is very large or very small. Figure 9.11 shows that a small step size results in inaccurate denoising resulting in loss of signal components and over-smoothening of the signal. Figure 9.12 shows that a large step size results in incorrect denoising, leading to the residual noisy signal at the output instead of the clean signal. Figure 9.13 shows the clean signal obtained using the proposed method with adapted step size.

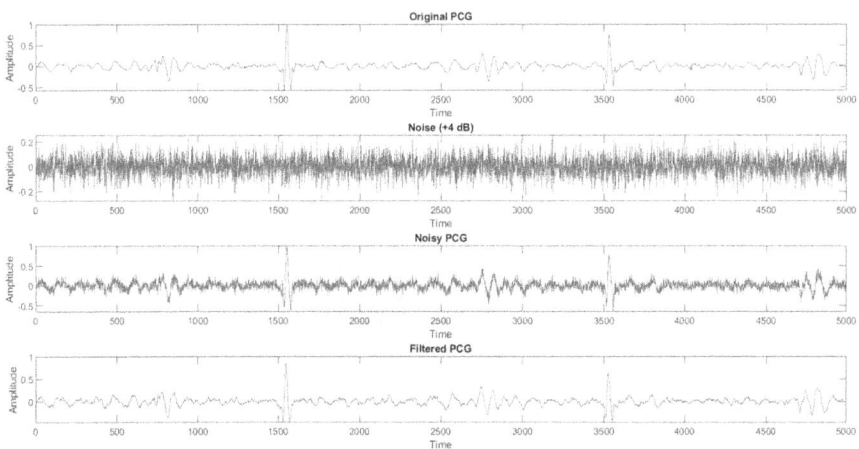

FIGURE 9.13   Accurate denoising using the Sliding Window adaptive filter

9.5 CONCLUSION

A Robust Sliding Window Adaptive Filter Model with the automatic step size adaptation is proposed in this study. The Robust Sliding Window Adaptive Filter architecture used in adaptive noise cancellation systems successfully denoises the Gaussian noise of different input signals to noise levels from normal and abnormal PCG signals by dynamically adjusting the step size. As a result, the suggested filter model offers a better solution to denoising a noisy longer-length phonocardiogram with a faster convergence time and lower MSE. According to the simulation, the suggested Robust Sliding Window Adaptive Filter outperforms conventional adaptive filter architectures, resulting in fast denoising and cost-effective noise can be tested for real-time implementation when improved denoising and fast convergence speed and accuracy are desired.

REFERENCES

1. Talbi, M. A. "A New ECG Denoising Technique Based on LWT and TVM", *Circuits, Systems, and Signal Processing* 40 (2021) 6284–6300.
2. Abbas, A. K., & Bassam, R. "Introduction to Phonocardiography Signal Processing", in *Phonocardiography Signal Processing. Synthesis Lectures on Biomedical Engineering*. Springer, Cham (2009). https://doi.org/10.1007/978-3-031-01637-0_1.
3. Alian, A., & Shelley, K. "Photoplethysmography", *Best Practice and Research Clinical Anaesthesiology* 28 (2014) 395–406.
4. Kuresan, H., Samiappan, D., & Masunda, S. "Fusion of WPT and MFCC Feature Extraction in Parkinson's Disease Diagnosis", *Technology and Health Care* 27 (2019) 1–10.
5. Kumar, D., de Carvalho, P., Antunes, M., Paiva, R. P., & Henriques, J. "Noise Detection During Heart Sound Recording Using Periodicity Signatures", *Physiological Measurement* 32 (2011) 599–618.
6. Pauline, S. H., Samiappan, D., Kumar, R., Narayanamoorthi, R., & Khin, W. L. "A Low-Cost Multistage Cascaded Adaptive Filter Configuration for Noise Reduction in Phonocardiogram Signal", *Journal of Healthcare Engineering* 2022 (2022) 24. 10.1155/2022/ 3039624.
7. Tomassini, S., Strazza, A., Sbrollini, A., Marcantoni, I., Morettini, M., Fioretti, S., & Burattini, L. "Wavelet Filtering of Fetal Phonocardiography: A Comparative Analysis", *Mathematical Biosciences and Engineering* 16 (5) (2019) 6034–6046. 10.3934/mbe.2019302.
8. Salman, A. H., Ahmadi, N., Mengko, R., Langi, A. Z. R., & Mengko, T. L. R. "Performance comparison of denoising methods for heart sound signal", in *2015 International Symposium on Intelligent Signal Processing and Communication Systems (ISPACS)* (2015) 435–440. 10.1109/ISPACS.2015.7432811.
9. Ghosh, S. K., Nagarajan, P. R., & Tripathy, R. K. "Heart Sound Data Acquisition and Preprocessing Techniques", in *Handbook of Research on Advancements of Artificial Intelligence in Healthcare Engineering,Advances in Healthcare Information Systems and Administration* (2020) 244–264. 10.4018/978-1-7998-2120-5.ch014.
10. Bai, Y. W., & Lu, C. L. "The embedded digital stethoscope uses the adaptive noise cancellation filter and the type I Chebyshev IIR bandpass filter to reduce the noise of the heart sound", in: *Proceedings of 7th International Workshop on Enterprise Networking and Computing in Healthcare Industry, 2005. HEALTHCOM 2005* (2005) 278–281. 10.1109/HEALTH.2005.1500459.

11. Kumar, A., Dhana, G. R., Albreem, M., & Le, D. "A Comprehensive Study on the Role of Advanced Technologies in 5G Based Smart Hospital", *Alexandria Engineering Journal* 2021(60) (2021) 5527–5536.
12. Ramakrishnan, B., Kumar, A., Chakravarty, S., Masud, M., & Baz, M. "Analysis of FBMC Waveform for 5G Network Based Smart Hospitals", *Applied Sciences* 11 (19) (2021) 8895. 10.3390/app11198895.
13. Song, D., Jia, L., Lu, Y., & Tao, L. "Heart sounds monitor and analysis in noisy environments", in: *2012 International Conference on Systems and Informatics (ICSAI2012)* (2012) 1677–1681. 10.1109/ICSAI.2012.6223364.
14. Tan, Z., Ma, J., Fu, B., & Dong, M. "Extract qualified heart sound in varying environment using parallel-training LMS algorithm", in: *2015 IEEE International Conference on Digital Signal Processing (DSP)* (2015) 407–411. 10.1109/ICDSP. 2015.7251903.
15. Kumar, A., & Gupta, M. "A Review on Activities of Fifth Generation Mobile Communication System", *Alexandria Engineering Journal* 57(2) (2017) 1125–1135. https://www.sciencedirect.com/science/article/pii/S1110016817300601.
16. Kumar, A., Albreem, M. A., Gupta, M., Alsharif, M. H., & Kim, S. "Future 5G Network Based Smart Hospitals: Hybrid Detection Technique for Latency Improvement", *IEEE Access* 8 (2020) 153240–153249. 10.1109/ACCESS.2020.3017625.

10 Integration of Meta Heuristic and FCM Approach for the Medical Diagnosis of an Organ Using Smart Methods

M. Jayanthi
Department of Electronics and Communication Engineering,
New Horizon College of Engineering, India

J. Joshua Daniel Raj
Department of Electric and Electronics Engineering,
New Horizon College of Engineering, India

A. B. Gurulakshmi and G. Rajesh
Department of Electronics and Communication Engineering,
New Horizon College of Engineering, India

10.1 INTRODUCTION

The pancreas is a 6-inch-long, elongated, tapered organ that is situated behind the stomach across the rear of the belly. The duodenum (the first section of the small intestine) curves at its widest point, the head, which is situated on the right side of the organ. The upper-left portion of the abdomen's left side is where the tapered left side, also known as the pancreas' body, finishes near the spleen and is referred to as the tail. Figure 10.1a shows the anatomy of the pancreas.

The pancreas performs two separate roles: digestive and hormonal functions. Pancreatic disorders can manifest in a number of different ways, diagnosing them can be challenging. Imaging is essential for the assessment of pancreatic disorders and gives clinicians vital information, that influences important management choices. Different imaging evaluations like plain radiographs, ultrasound, multi-detector computed imaging (MDCT) and magnetic resonance imaging are available to view pancreatic imaging. Each imaging technique has both benefits and

DOI: 10.1201/9781003403678-10

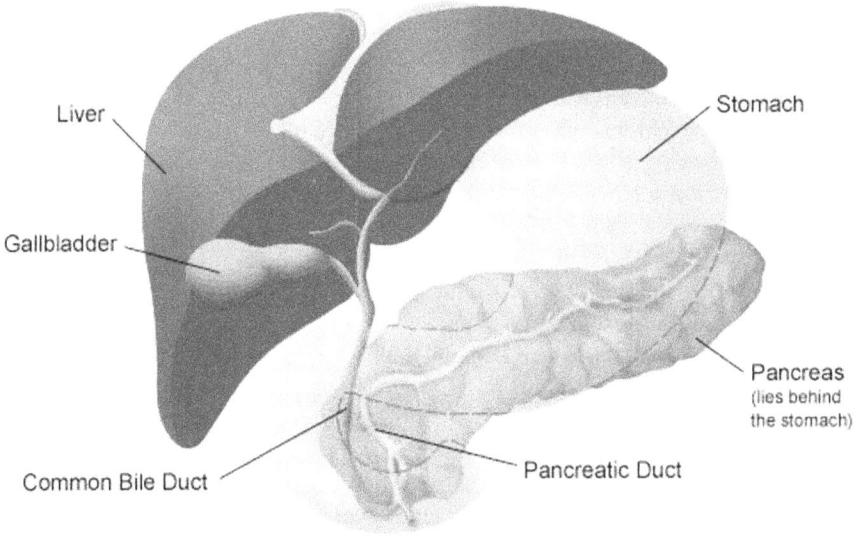

FIGURE 10.1   Anatomy of the pancreas (1).

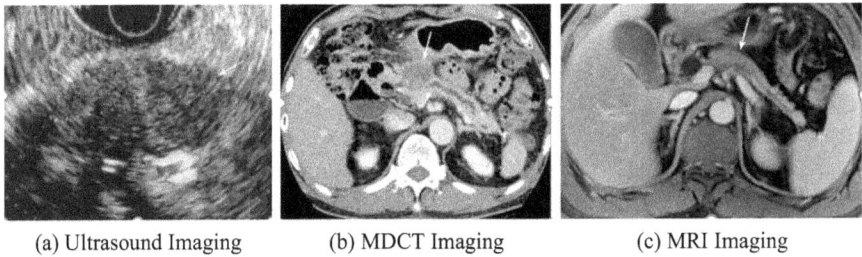

(a) Ultrasound Imaging   (b) MDCT Imaging   (c) MRI Imaging

FIGURE 10.2   Various pancreatic imaging techniques.

drawbacks. Among them, the MDCT scan is the most widely adopted non-invasive imaging modality that offers superior signal-to-noise ratio, excellent spatial resolution, patient-friendly protocols, is a relatively inexpensive, and requires minimal examination time [1]. Also, it offers more precise anatomical details about the region of interest and is more suitable for radiologists. Figure 10.2 shows different imaging of the pancreas that helps visualise the internal organs.

Due to its size, shape, and position in the abdomen on computed tomography (CT) scans, the pancreas is extremely difficult to segment. Pancreatic segmentation is an important tool for accurately diagnosing and treating pancreatic diseases as well as for advancing our understanding of this complex organ. Also, medical professionals can benefit from using pancreas segmentation to help with diagnosis, treatment, and surgery. So, there is a need for a computer-assisted system to detect the pancreas. Therefore, the proposed study combines one or more segmentation algorithms to boost segmentation accuracy and also create an optimal method to delineate the boundaries of the pancreas.

10.2 LITERATURE SURVEY

Few research studies have happened in pancreatic segmentation. Accurate segmentation of the pancreas can help researchers identify patterns and trends that may be useful for developing new therapies or improving existing one. Due to the complex and moderate structure of the pancreas very little research is done in the field of pancreatic segmentation. In this section, the survey is done in three stages consisting of pre-processing, segmentation, and optimisation.

Narain et al. [2] have published and analysed a thorough analysis of different pre-processing techniques for the suppression of noise in the medical image. The authors have also suggested an innovative technique to get rid of the tape and high rectangular label artefacts. Sonali Patil and Udupi [3] have talked about the value of pre-processing filters. The authors have provided this method to get rid of unwanted parts of the medical image as well as film artefacts. Only certain artefacts are eliminated with this technique, which has no positive impact on segmentation effectiveness. In order to reduce the noise in brain CT images, Tarandeep et al. [4] have conducted a comparative comparison of denoising filters. To choose the filter parameter for the bilateral filter in [5], the authors employed a genetic algorithm. Although the convergence rate is higher, this approach significantly improves noise suppression and edge retention.

Based on segmentation, following literature survey is made to discuss the various methods for the detection of pancreas. In [6], the authors suggest the segment and pickup (SAP) framework, which trains a neural network to segment the pancreas in the ROI using manual annotation. The authors have explained the technique [7] that is used for pancreatic segmentation with a smooth and precise output using a semantic deep learning bottom-up approach. In [8], authors present a tool for automatically segmenting the pancreas in magnetic resonance imaging and also suggest to follow the hierarchical information for pooling [9, 10], the authors have explained the revision as well as advancement of pancreatic segmentation.

Optimisation is needed to find the best possible solution to a problem within a set of constraints and objectives. The history and context related to PSO's theory are explained in [11]. The authors have examined the state of research and application in terms of algorithm structure, parameter selection, and topology. At last, the authors have analysed the issues at hand and suggestions for future research are explained. In [12], the authors have suggested combining segmentation with optimisation for better accuracy. Using a multistep pre-processing stage, a new swarm intelligence information strategy for skin lesions segmentation has been addressed in [13]. It produces the best segmentation that can be applied to a variety of images with varied possessions and deficiencies. In [14], a novel automatic segmentation method for the liver was developed and used with a smart operator for precise a 3D model.

10.3 PROPOSED METHODOLOGY

The proposed work emphasised the importance of hybrid techniques for determining pancreatic contour. We highlight the significance of bio-inspired optimisation

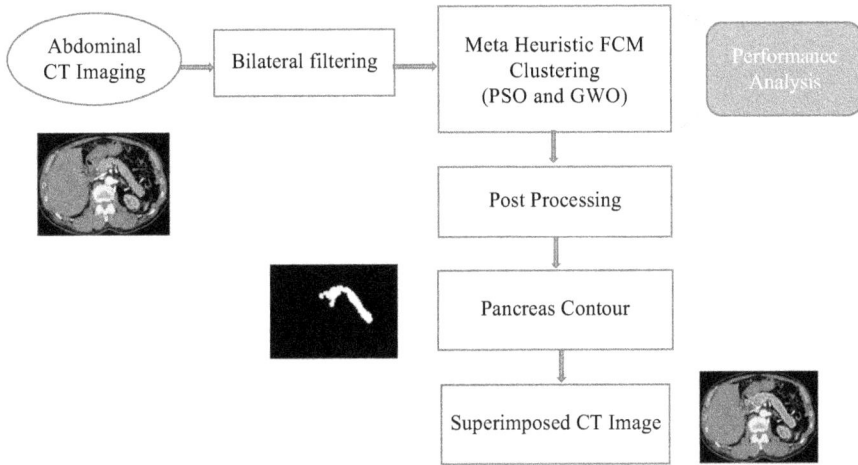

FIGURE 10.3   Framework of pancreas contour detection.

strategies to choose the optimum threshold. This recommended solution assists radiologists in detecting the pancreas' outlines.

Figure 10.3 illustrates the comprehensive framework, consisting of data acquisition, cleaning, a hybrid segmentation approach that includes a meta heuristics algorithm and morphological refinement. One of the most popular segmentation methods, Fuzzy C-Means (FCM) is used in our work because it enables each object to belong to many groups. When choosing the cluster centre, this method is prone to slipping into local minima. By integrating the FCM strategy with the optimisation technique, this issue is resolved. The FCM algorithm updates the membership values and the centroids of each cluster in each iteration until the objective function converges. The best membership values and centroids that minimise the objective function are found using optimisation techniques. Our technique provides an interactive hybrid approach to choosing the appropriate threshold by optimising cluster centre in order to visualise pancreatic contour in abdominal liver CT images.

10.3.1   DATA ACQUISITION

In this work, two types of CT image databases are used. One is a real-time database; the other is a simulation database. These images can be obtained on three different planes: the sagittal, coronal, and axial planes. These planes are used to describe the position of parts of the body. This also helps identify the extent of the disease in a patient (Figure 10.4).

10.3.2   PRE-PROCESSING

Preprocessing is a crucial step that can improve the quality of the data, reduce the complexity of the modelling task, and improve the accuracy of the final model.

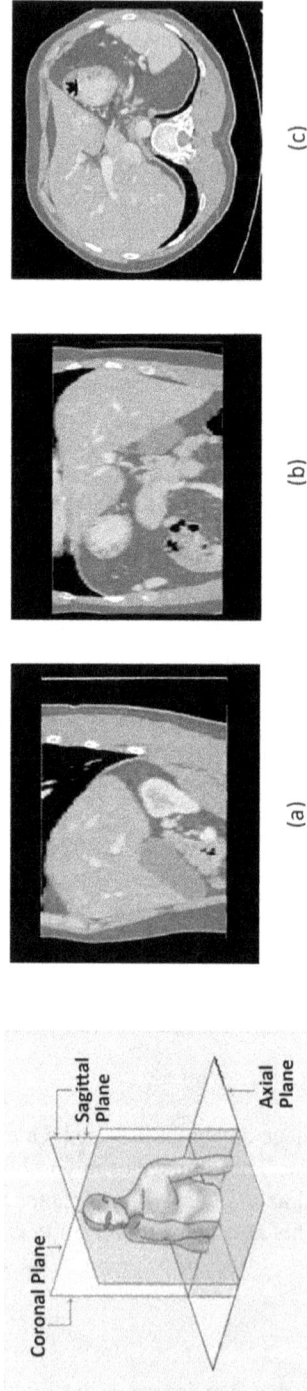

FIGURE 10.4 Image reconstruction (14). CT image view of three planes: (a) sagittal, (b) coronal, (c) axial.

Raw data often contains errors, missing values, and outliers. Pre-processing helps to identify and handle these issues to ensure the data is accurate and reliable.

10.3.2.1 Bilateral Filtering

The bilateral filter is effective in reducing noise in the image while preserving sharp edges and fine details. It is commonly used in image processing tasks such as denoising, edge detection, and tone mapping in high dynamic range (HDR) imaging. It is effective in reducing Gaussian noise, salt and pepper noise, and other types of noise.

It is a type of edge-preserving smoothing filter that applies a weighted average to each pixel in the image based on its similarity to the neighbouring pixels in both spatial distance and intensity. The weights for each pixel in the filter kernel are calculated based on these two factors, with greater weight given to pixels that are closer in both spatial and intensity domains. Figure 10.5 depicts an illustration of the bilateral filter structure. Choose an input image of 3 x 3 pixels to understand the implementation of the bilateral filter. Calculate the spatial distance and intensity difference in the input. The weighted value is multiplied by the input pixel to produce the filter's edge-preserving output. Table 10.1 shows the step-by-step process for the implementation of the bilateral filter.

10.3.3 FCM CLUSTERING

FCM (Fuzzy C-Means) clustering [15] is a well-known technique in machine learning that is used to group data points into clusters based on their similarity. It is an iterative approach to update the membership values of each data point in each cluster until the objective function converges. The convergence criterion is updating based on a maximum number of iterations or a minimum change in the objective function between iterations. The FCM algorithm can be implemented using various optimisation techniques and these optimisation techniques are used to find the

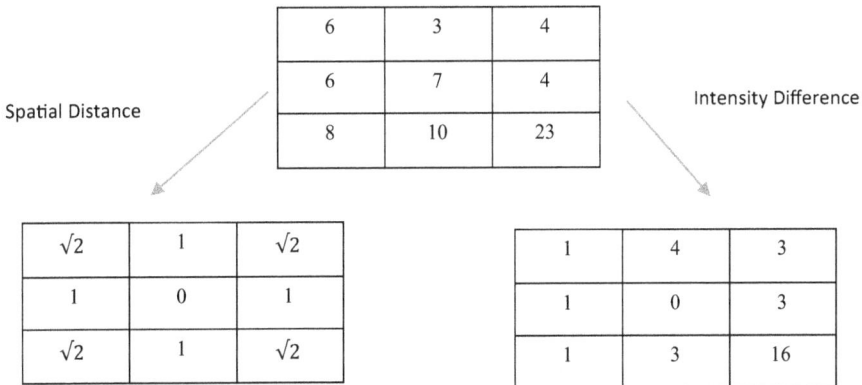

FIGURE 10.5 Example of bilateral filter.

TABLE 10.1

Pseudo Code of Bilateral Filter

Input: Abdominal CT Image

Output: Denoised Image

Step 1: Let R as the input image and Rp be the pixel value of the image at each point.

Step 2: Adjust the Window size and the tuning parameters for the bilateral filter (σ_{sd}, σ_{id}).

Step 3: Use equation 10.1 for the calculation of spatial distance noise.

$$sd\,(x,\,y) = e^{\frac{-\|x-y\|^2}{2\sigma_{sd}^2}} \qquad (10.1)$$

Step 4: Equation 10.2 is used to calculate the Gaussian intensity weight.

$$id\,(x,\,y) = e^{\frac{-|R(x)-R(y)|^2}{2\sigma_{id}^2}} \qquad (10.2)$$

Gaussian regulating kernel coefficients are σ_{sd} and σ_{id}. The spatial distance (σ_{sd}) is proportional to the size of the image and the difference in intensity σ_{id} regulates intensity differences and is inversely related to edge amplitude.

Step 5: At each pixel location, the bilateral filter output is calculated using equation 10.3.

$$\text{Bif}(x,\,y) = \frac{1}{C} \sum_{y\in\gamma(x)} Bif\,(y)sd\,(x,\,y)id\,(x,\,y) \qquad (10.3)$$

$$C = \sum_{\gamma(x)} sd\,(x,\,y)id\,(x,\,y) \qquad (10.4)$$

Where C is the normalisation factor and y(x) is the spatial neighbourhood surrounding Bif (x).

Step 6: Each individual pixel is replaced with the weighted average of the adjacent pixels in the spatial neighbourhood.

optimal values of the membership values and centroids that minimise the objective function. Implementation of FCM clustering is shown in Table 10.2. In the proposed work, optimisation-based FCM clustering is used.

10.3.4 META HEURISTIC APPROACH

A meta heuristic approach belongs to two categories: single solution-based and population-based algorithms. The first approach starts with a single solution and iteratively improves the solution's precision. The second group employs a collection of solutions and refines them over a predetermined number of iterations. A population-based algorithm is employed in the suggested work. In the proposed work, particle swarm and grey wolf optimisation method are used to detect the pancreatic contour.

TABLE 10.2

Pseudo Code of FCM Clustering

Requirement: Choose the number of cluster C, the fuzziness level m>1, and the error €

1. Initialise the $UM_{ij}(0)$ and $CV_i(0)$ matrices in the cluster's centre.

2. Set k=1

3. Calculate the centres vectors CV(k) with UM(k) for each value of K.

$$CV_j = \frac{\sum_{i=1}^{N} UM_{ij}^m \cdot DX_i}{\sum_{i=1}^{n} UM_{ij}^m} \qquad (10.5)$$

4. Revise and update the UM(k) and UM(k+1)

$$UM_{ij} = \frac{1}{\sum_{k=1}^{C} \left(\frac{\| x_i - CV_j \|}{\| x_i - CV_k \|} \right)^{\frac{2}{m-1}}} \qquad (10.6)$$

5. Stop if $UM^{(k+1)} < UM^{(k)}$. Or, go back to step 3.

10.3.4.1 Particle Swarm Optimisation (PSO)

It is a stochastic optimisation algorithm inspired by the social behaviour of fish schooling or bird flocking. In PSO [16], a population of particles moves in a multidimensional search space to find the optimal solution. Each particle in the swarm represents a potential solution to the problem and has a position and velocity in the search space. The position of each particle corresponds to a candidate solution, while the velocity represents the direction and speed of movement towards the optimal solution.

During each iteration of the PSO algorithm, each particle evaluates its fitness based on the objective function of the optimisation problem. Then, the particle updates its position and velocity based on its own best position and the best position found by its neighbours in the swarm.

The PSO algorithm has two main parameters that control its behaviour: the inertia weight and the social and cognitive parameters. The inertia weight determines the influence of the particle's previous velocity on its current velocity, while the social and cognitive parameters control the influence of the particle's best position and the best position found by its neighbours in the swarm. The search strategy of PSO is shown in Figure 10.6. The mathematical representation of PSO

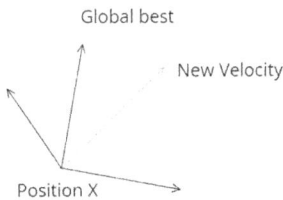

Particle best **FIGURE 10.6** PSO's search strategy

TABLE 10.3

Different Abbreviation in PSO

Ve(t)	Particle's velocity at time t
Xp(t)	Position of the particle at time t
w	Inertia weight
C1,c2	Accelerating factor
rand()	Uniformly distributed random number between 0 and 1
Xp_{pbest}, Xp_{gbest}	Particle best and global best position

implementation is presented below, and Table 10.3 gives the different abbreviations used for PSO implementation.

$$Xp(t + 1) = Xp(t) + Ve(t + 1) \tag{10.7}$$

$$Ve(t + 1) = w \times Ve(t) + c_1 \times rand() \times (Xp_{pbest} - Xp(t)) + c_2 \times rand()$$
$$\times (Xp_{gbest} - Xp(t)) \tag{10.8}$$

Table 10.3 gives the different abbreviations used for PSO implementation, and Figure 10.7 shows the optimal FCM-based PSO.

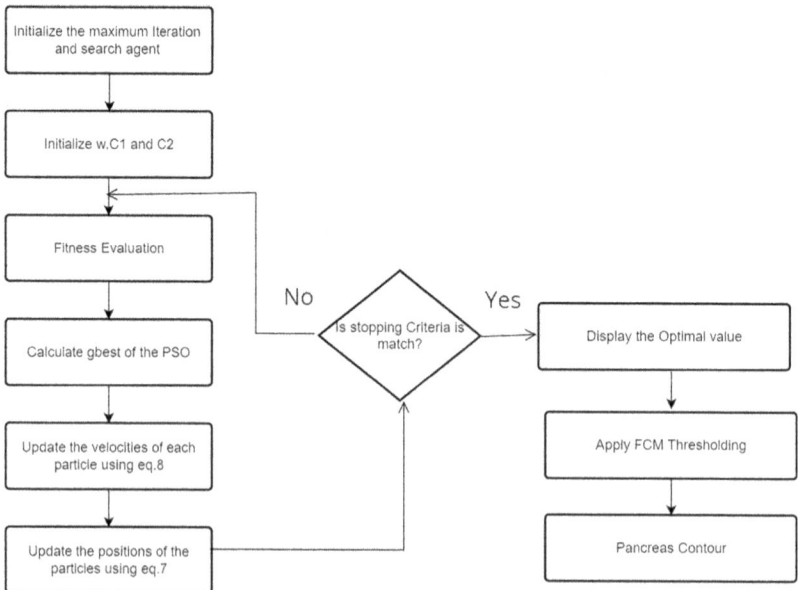

FIGURE 10.7   Optimal design implementation using PSO.

10.3.4.2 Grey Wolf Optimisation (GWO) Method

It is used as a clustering tool to provide the optimum solution. The main advantage of the grey wolf algorithm is the simple, straightforward method to implement and programme without requiring particular inputs. Grey wolves live in packs, which typically have 5 to 10 individuals each. The alpha, beta, delta, and omega breeds of grey wolves are used to imitate the leadership hierarchy. The leaders are the alpha wolves, and it is their responsibility to make choices. Second-level wolves called beta wolves aid alpha wolves in making decisions and carrying out other activities. Delta wolves obey commands from alpha and beta wolves and have the ability to lead others below them. The search strategy of GWO [17] and visualisation of the search agent are shown in Figure 10.8.

The mathematical model of grey wolves is used to create social hierarchy behaviour. The optimally fit solution is represented by the alpha. Beta and delta are the second and third most suitable solutions respectively. Before the prey is caught, the grey wolf optimisation process involves several steps. Grey wolves are randomly initialised in the search space in order to look for prey. The encirclement of prey begins after the prey is discovered. The following are the mathematical implications of encirclement:

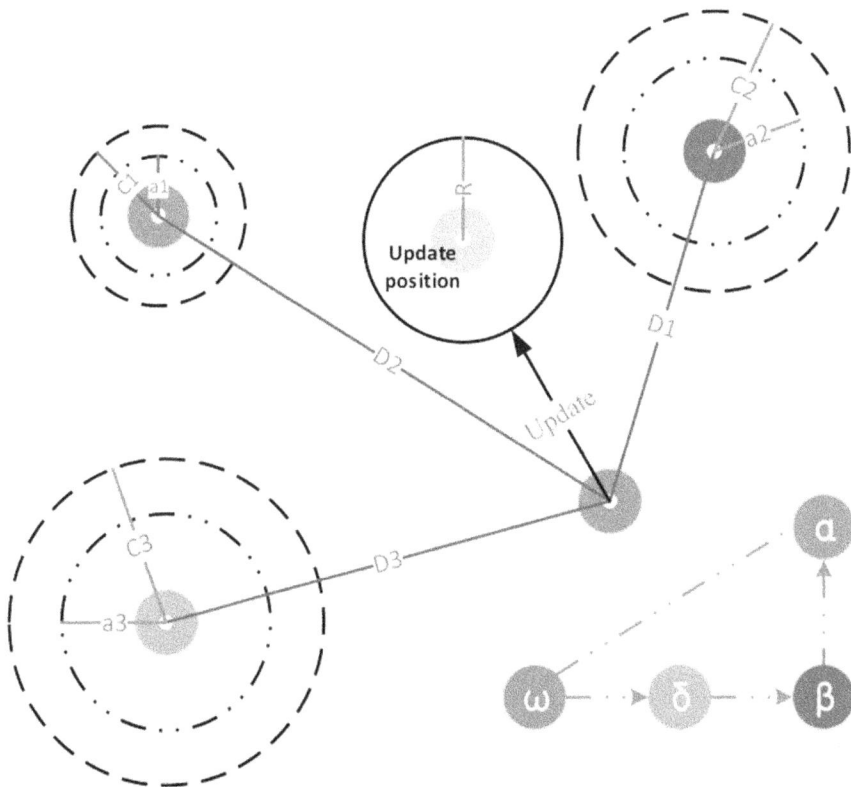

FIGURE 10.8 Visualisation of GWO [17].

$$D = C * X_{preypos}(t) - X_{greyvel\_pos}(t) \tag{10.9}$$

$$X(t + 1) = X_{prey\_pos}(t) - A. D \tag{10.10}$$

where 't' stands for the current iteration, $X_{preyposs}(t)$ is the vector of the prey's location, and $X_{greyvel\_pos}(t)$ is the vector of the position of the grey wolf.

The formulas for the coefficient vectors A and C are as follows:

$$A = 2ar_1 - a; C = 2r_2 \tag{10.11}$$

where r1 and r2 are random vectors chosen at random from the range [0, 1], and where 'a' has a linear decline value starting at 2 and increasing over the course of iteration. The finest solutions from the alpha, beta, and delta wolves are saved during the hunting process, and the omega wolf updates its positions in line with the best hunting solutions.

$$D_{alpha} = |C_1 . X_{alpha}(t) - X_{greyvel\_pos}(t)| \tag{10.12}$$

$$D_{beta} = |C_2 . X_{beta}(t) - X_{greyvel\_pos}(t)| \tag{10.13}$$

$$D_{delta} = |C_3 . X_{delta}(t) - X_{greyvel\_pos}(t)| \tag{10.14}$$

$$X_{1p} = X_{alpha}(t) - A_1 D_{alpha} \tag{10.15}$$

$$X_{2p} = X_{beta}(t) - A_2 D_{beta} \tag{10.16}$$

$$X_{3p} = X_{delta}(t) - A_3 D_{delta} \tag{10.17}$$

$$x(t + 1) = \frac{x_{1p} + x_{2p} + x_{3p}}{3} \tag{10.18}$$

where D_{alpha}, D_{beta}, and D_{delta} represent the distances between the wolves and other individuals, and $X_{greyvel\_pos}(t)$ denotes the vector location of the grey wolf. The positions of the alpha, beta, and delta wolves at the iteration of "t" are $X_{alpha}(t)$, $X_{beta}(t)$, and $X_{delta}(t)$. The optimal design of FCM-based GWO is presented in Figure 10.9.

10.3.5 POST-PROCESSING

The output of optimisation method is a binary image. Later, post-processing [18] is applied to this image to get the final segmented pancreas contour. The largest connected components are found, and the remaining gaps are filled using morphological processing. Since pancreas segmentation is difficult due to its small size and shape.

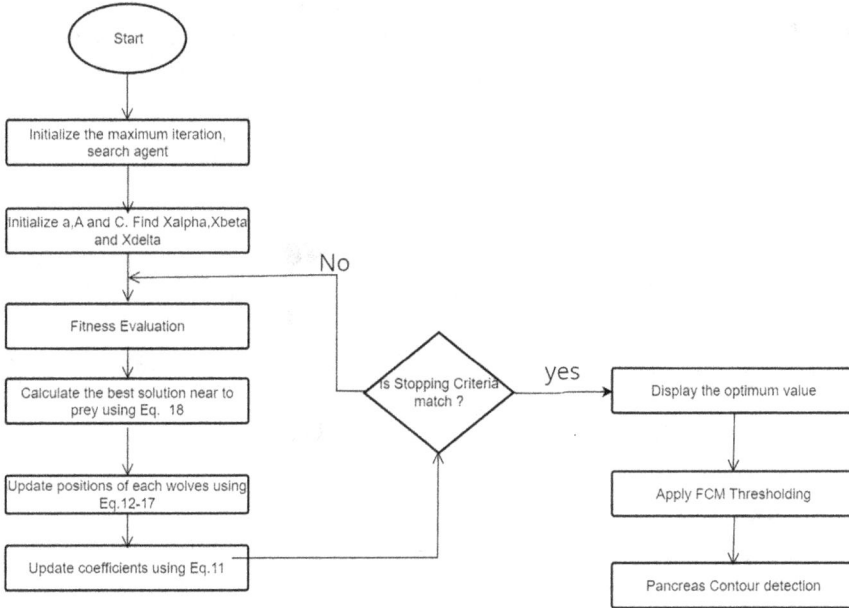

FIGURE 10.9   Optimal design implementation using GWO.

Two stages of dilation and erosion are applied in order to reach the desired region of interest. By overlaying the original image on the contour, we can determine the region of interest. By multiplying the pancreas mask with the original image, the pancreas outline is obtained.

10.4   RESULTS AND DISCUSSION

The suggested work is done using MATLAB software with a 1.8 GHz processor and 2 GB of RAM. For experimental analysis and discussion, an axial CT scan is taken. Totally, 40 data sets are used in the planned work.

Several segmentation techniques are available for the detection of the pancreas, but in this work, we proposed two optimisation methods: PSO and GWO. Both methods are used to obtain the optimal cluster centre. In PSO, few parameters need to be tuned, whereas in GWO only two parameters need to be tuned. This makes GWO implementation much easier and faster to converge. Traditional methods for pancreas segmentation often rely on manual or semi-automated segmentation, which can be time-consuming and prone to inter-observer variability. By integrating segmentation algorithms with meta heuristic approach, we can improve upon the shortcomings of the existing ones.

In the proposed work, we implemented a particle swarm optimisation (PSO) algorithm based on FCM clustering to optimise the segmentation of an abdominal data set consisting of 40 images. We incorporated PSO-based FCM clustering to obtain the cluster centre of a data set. The FCM algorithm was initialised with three randomly selected centroids and the PSO algorithm was set to run for 50 iterations

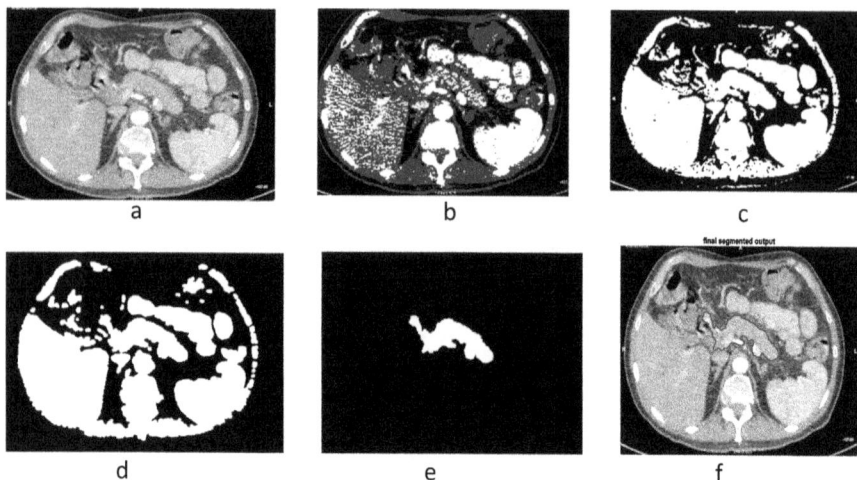

FIGURE 10.10   Results of PSO-based FCM clustering method: (a) pre-processed image, (b-c) FCM thresholding output, (d) post-processing output after morphological operation, (e) pancreas contour, (f) superimposed image.

on a dataset of 40 instances. To get the binary image of the pancreas contour, the PSO-based FCM clustering employs three classes of FCM thresholding. The numerous processing steps are used in PSO-based FCM clustering to get the pancreas contours that are shown in the aforementioned Figure 10.10. Figure 10.10a is a pre-processed image, and optimised cluster centre are shown using the PSO algorithm. Figures 10.10b and 10.10c are the outputs we obtained after FCM thresholding. In the post-processing stage, two stages of dilation and erosion are applied, and corresponding image is displayed in Figure 10.10d. Pancreas detection is depicted in Figure 10.10e and the desired region of interest is superimposed on the original image and delineated in Figure 10.10f. For implementation, we used the following parameters: number of iterations = 50, C1, C2 = 2, inertia weight of 0.9 to 0.1 linear reduction, and number of search agents = 20 for PSO-based pancreas segmentation.

In order to understand which method suits for the pancreas detection, we have used GWO-based FCM clustering to optimise the segmentation of an abdominal dataset consisting of 40 images. The GWO method was programmed to run for 50 iterations on a data set of 40 cases. The GWO-based FCM clustering makes use of three classes of FCM thresholding to obtain the binary image of the pancreatic contour. Several processing steps were used in GWO-based FCM clustering to create the pancreatic shape seen in Figure 10.11. Figure 10.11a shows a pre-processed image that utilises an optimised cluster centre. After FCM thresholding, the output is shown in Figures 10.11b and 10.11c. Two phases of dilation and erosion are applied during the post-processing stage, and the resulting image is shown in Figure 10.11d. Figure 10.11e shows the pancreas detection, and Figure 10.11f shows the delineation of the intended region of interest after superimposing it on the original image. For implementation, we used the following

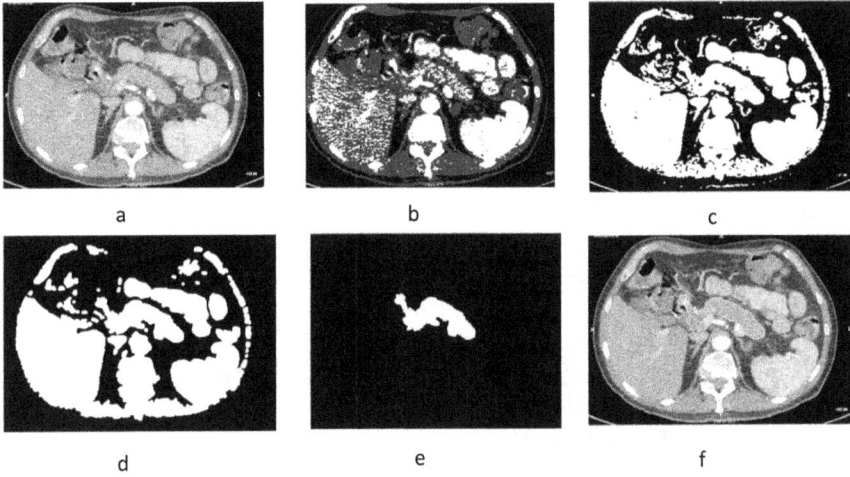

FIGURE 10.11 Results of GWO-based FCM clustering method: (a) pre-processed image, (b-c) FCM thresholding output, (d) post-processing output after morphological operation, (e) pancreas contour, (f) superimposed image.

parameters: number of iterations = 50, fuzziness = 2, cluster centres = 3, number of search agents = 20 for GWO-based pancreas segmentation.

The output of the segmentation algorithm was visually inspected to ensure accuracy and quality. Figure 10.12 is the comparative visualisation of PSO and GWO. The results showed that the algorithm was able to successfully identify and segment the regions of interest in most of the images. The segmentation results of PSO were displayed using a color-coded overlay on the original image, where the segmented regions of GWO were highlighted in green. Our results showed that

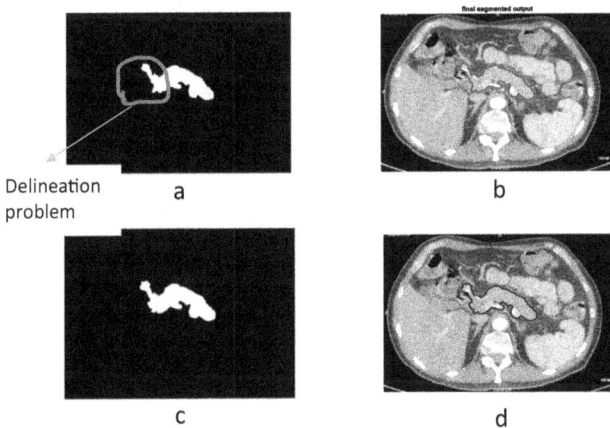

FIGURE 10.12 Comparative visualisation of PSO (a-b) and GWO (c-d) based FCM clustering.

GWO-based FCM clustering outperformed in terms of visualisation and segmentation accuracy. Figure 10.12a-b shows the results of PSO-based FCM clustering. The moderate performance of the algorithm may be attributed to a combination of factors including the complexity of the images, the limitations of the algorithm, and the inadequacy of the parameters used. In some cases, the algorithm was not able to differentiate between the region of interest and the surrounding tissue. Figure 10.12c-d shows how GWO-based FCM clustering can differentiate between the region of interest and the surrounding tissue.

In addition to visual inspection, we also quantitatively evaluated the quality of the segmentation results using the Dice Similarity Coefficient (DSC) and Jaccard metrics along with computation time. These metrics [19] are used to evaluate the performance of the clustering algorithm by comparing the output with the ground truth. The DSC measures the degree of overlap between the segmented regions and the ground truth annotations, while the Jaccard measures the intersection of two sets by the union of two sets. the ability of the algorithm to accurately identify relevant regions of interest.

$$Dice = \frac{2|Auto\_seg \cap Manual\_seg|}{|Auto\_seg + Manual\_seg|} \qquad (10.18)$$

$$Jaccard = \frac{2|Auto\_seg \cap Manual\_seg|}{|Auto\_seg \cup Manual\_seg|} \qquad (10.19)$$

We examined the performance of the proposed method in terms of segmentation metrics and computation time to assess the quality of the segmentation results. Table 10.4 displays each algorithm's top outcomes. PSO-based methods converge faster than GWO and it take less time. The average DSC score of GWO-based FCM clustering across all images was 0.913, indicating a high degree of overlap in identifying the relevant regions of interest and comparative analysis, as shown in Figure 10.13. The performance of the proposed method is verified with different abdominal image data sets taken from [20]. Both real and simulated liver data sets are taken for validation.

TABLE 10.4
Quantitative Evaluation of Proposed Method

Data Set	PSO-Based FCM Clustering			GWO-Based FCM Clustering		
	Dice	Jaccard	Computation Time	Dice	Jaccard	Computation Time
DB1	0.785	0.646	40.12	0.902	0.821	44.28
DB2	0.797	0.663	45.7	0.895	0.810	50.45
DB3	0.806	0.675	19.5	0.916	0.845	25.23
DB4	0.784	0.645	39.45	0.913	0.840	43.89
DB5	0.812	0.684	46.32	0.938	0.883	51.34
Avg	0.7968	0.662	38.21	0.913	0.839	43.03

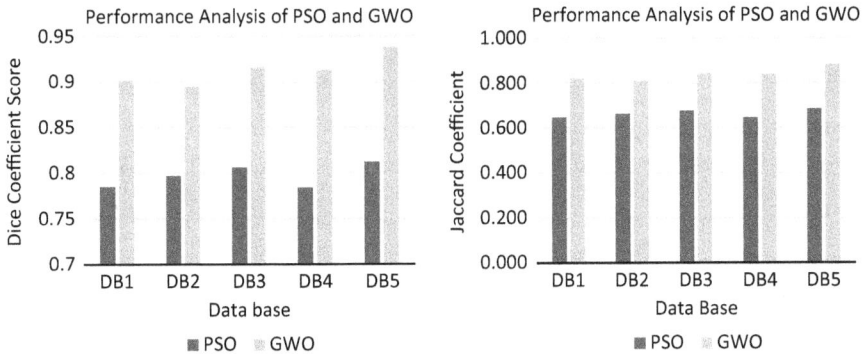

FIGURE 10.13　Comparative analysis of proposed method.

10.5　CONCLUSION

The segmentation of the pancreas is an important problem in medical image analysis with numerous clinical applications. The pancreas can be accurately segmented to improve patient care by aiding in diagnosis, planning treatments, and disease monitoring. In the proposed work, we discussed the fundamental ideas of survival of the fittest approach algorithms that draw inspiration from nature and are used for selecting optimal values. The outcomes of the experiments demonstrated how effective the two algorithms were. However, there are still several challenges in pancreas segmentation, such as the need for larger data sets, the presence of noise and intensity variations in the images, and the lack of robustness to anatomical variations across patients. In future studies, we will try to address the above challenges and provide a solution for pancreatic segmentation.

REFERENCES

1. Stanford health, 2023, March. Pancreas anatomy. Accessed date: March 12, 2023, Available: https://www.stanfordchildrens.org/en/topic/default?id=pancreas-anatomy-and-functions-85-P00682
2. Ponraj, D.N., Jenifer, M.E., Poongodi, P. and Manoharan, J.S., 2011. A survey on the preprocessing techniques of mammogram for the detection of breast cancer. *Journal of Emerging Trends in Computing and Information Sciences*, 2(12), pp.656–664.
3. Patil, S. and Udupi, V.R., 2012. Preprocessing to be considered for MR and CT images containing tumors. *IOSR Journal of Electrical and Electronics Engineering*, 1(4), pp.54–57.
4. Kumar, A., Dhanagopal, R., Albreem, A.M. and Le, D.N., 2021. A comprehensive study on the role of advanced technologies in 5G based smart hospital. *Alexandria Engineering journal*, 2021(60), pp.5527–5536.
5. Ramakrishnan, B., Kumar, A., Chakravarty, S., Masud, M., and Baz, M., 2021. Analysis of FBMC waveform for 5G network based smart hospitals. *Applied Sciences*, 11(19), p.8895. 10.3390/app11198895
6. Peng, K. and Fang, B., 2021, January. 3D segment and pickup framework for pancreas segmentation. In 2021 IEEE International Conference on Consumer Electronics and Computer Engineering (ICCECE). (pp.737–740). IEEE. 10.1109/ICCECE51280. 2021.9342350.

7. Paithane, P.M. and Kakarwal, S.N., 2022. Automatic pancreas segmentation using a novel modified semantic deep learning bottom-up approach. *International Journal of Intelligent Systems and Applications in Engineering*, 10(1), pp.98–104. 10.18201/ijisae.2022.272

8. Asaturyan, H. and Villarini, B., 2018. Hierarchical framework for automatic pancreas segmentation in MRI using continuous max-flow and min-cuts approach. In Image Analysis and Recognition: 15th International Conference, ICIAR 2018, Póvoa de Varzim, Portugal, June 27–29, 2018. Proceedings 15 (pp.562–570). 10.1007/978-3-319-93000-8_64

9. Poċė, I., Arsenjeva, J., Kielaitė-Gulla, A., Samuilis, A., Strupas, K. and Dzemyda, G., 2021. Pancreas segmentation in CT images: State of the art in clinical practice. *Baltic Journal of Modern Computing*, 9(1), pp.25–34. 10.22364/bjmc.2021.9.1.02

10. Davradou, A., 2023. Detection and segmentation of pancreas using morphological snakes and deep convolutional neural networks. *Computer Vision and Pattern Recognition*, 2023, pp.1–12. arXiv:2302.06356

11. Yao, X., Song, Y. and Liu, Z., 2020. Advances on pancreas segmentation: A review. *Multimedia Tools and Applications*, 79, pp.6799–6821. 10.1007/s11042-019-08320-7

12. Muthuswamy, J. and Kanmani, B., 2018. Optimization based liver contour extraction of abdominal CT images. *International Journal of Electrical & Computer Engineering (2088–8708)*, 8(6), pp.5061–5070. 10.11591/ijece.v8i6.pp5061-5070.

13. Abd, H.J., Abdullah, A.S. and Alkafaji, M.S., 2020. A new swarm intelligence information technique for improving information balancedness on the skin lesions segmentation. *International Journal of Electrical and Computer Engineering (IJECE)*, 10(6), pp.5703–5708. 10.11591/ijece.v10i6.pp5703-5708.

14. Radiology cafe, (2021). Anatomy of abdominal CT image. [online], Accessed date: August 8, 2022, Available: https://www.radiologycafe.com/radiology-basics/imaging-modalities/ct-overview/

15. Alomoush, W., Alrosan, A., Almomani, A., Alissa, K., Khashan, O.A. and Al-Nawasrah, A., 2021. Spatial information of fuzzy clustering based mean best artificial bee colony algorithm for phantom brain image segmentation. *International Journal of Electrical and Computer Engineering (IJECE)*, 11(5), pp.4050–4058. 10.11591/ijece.v11i5.

16. Kumar, A. and Gupta, M., 2017. A review on activities of fifth generation mobile communication system. *Alexandria Engineering Journal*, 57(2), pp.1125–1135. https://www.sciencedirect.com/science/article/pii/S1110016817300601

17. Kumar, A., Albreem, M.A., Gupta, M., Alsharif, M.H. and Kim, S., 2020. Future 5G network based smart hospitals: Hybrid detection technique for latency improvement. *IEEE Access*, 8, pp.153240–153249. 10.1109/ACCESS.2020.3017625.

18. Muthuswamy, J., 2019. Extraction and classification of liver abnormality based on neutrosophic and SVM classifier. In Progress in Advanced Computing and Intelligent Engineering: Proceedings of ICACIE 2017. Volume 1 (pp.269–279). Springer Singapore. 10.1007/978-981-13-1708-8_2.

19. Farag, A., Lu, L., Turkbey, E., Liu, J. and Summers, R.M., 2014. A bottom-up approach for automatic pancreas segmentation in abdominal CT scans. In Abdominal Imaging. Computational and Clinical Applications: 6th International Workshop, ABDI 2014, Held in Conjunction with MICCAI 2014, Cambridge, MA, USA, September 14, 2014. Proceedings 6 (pp.103–113). 10.1007/978-3-319-13692-9_10

20. Pancreas, C.T., 2023. Manual annotation and Dicom images for pancreas CT. [online], Accessed date: February 22, 2023, Available: https://wiki.cancerimagingarchive.net/display/Public/Pancreas-CT

11 A Review on Migration from 4G to 5G Network Architecture

Methods to Improve the Bandwidth, Latency, and Data Rate of a Network for Smart Hospitals

Lipsa Dash and Parag Jain
Department of Electronics and Communication Engineering,
New Horizon College of Engineering, Bengaluru, India

Mahmoud A. Albreem
Department of Electrical Engineering College of
Engineering, University of Sharjah, UAE

11.1 INTRODUCTION

Wireless mobile communication has developed by leaps and bounds in recent decades. The future communication systems also aim to provide seamless and extremely fast services to the end user with minimal latency. The need for High QoS requirements in future networks relies on newer and more adaptable technologies that have the ability to encompass complex architectures. 5G is one such booming technology that can render advanced services to users and fulfil the diverse use cases arising in today's communication scenario [1]. 5G is an open platform that will find a place in every sector, like manufacturing, automotive, agriculture, medicine, transportation, education, and intelligent communication, to name a few. There would be interoperability between a massive number of connected devices at the same time without compromising on rate and speed [2, 3]. The current 4G service would eventually upgrade to 5G, satisfying the standards laid down by 3GPP (third generation partnership project) and meeting the requirements prescribed by ITU-R (International Telecommunication Union, Radio). ITU-R releases recommendations based on the communication trends

DOI: 10.1201/9781003403678-11

prevailing worldwide, focusing on the development of emerging technologies. As we move from the "Internet of Things" era to the "Internet of Everything," 5G networks will support virtualisation of various network functions to achieve resilience accompanied by ease of deployment and configurability. The network would employ the slicing concept to handle the heterogeneous QoS requirements of individual use cases (UC). UCs focusing on critical communications would need further resources to be allocated in order to satisfy high reliability and low latency operations [4]. To empower the 5G UCs, flexibility in spectrum usage is going to play a major role in the 5G ecosystem. The different requirements of the vast network would eventually result in a more dynamic infrastructure. With the evolution of mobile systems through 2G (GSM), 3G (UMTS), and 4G (LTE/ LTEA), 5G-NR (New Radio) will now accelerate the new era of communication, building upon the established legacy [5, 6]. In contrast to the previous genera- tions, NR applies a more intelligent architecture that is no longer limited by closely located base stations (BS). With reference to 3GPP NR, the architectural requirements of both the 5G Core Network and the RAN (Radio Access Network) were reconsidered, resulting in a precise functional split between the two [7]. The intention of 3GPP in defining NR is to develop a unified air interface for faster mobile broadband experiences. NR has the capability to address UCs requiring communication at bands of 66–76 GHz and 81–86 GHz. NR categorises the 5G generic services into three broad categories: Extreme Mobile BroadBand (xMBB), Massive Machine-Type Communication (mMTC), and Ultra-reliable Machine-Type Communication (uMTC), where each category's need is met by one or more enablers. The shift from the legacy 4G LTE network to 5G NR would pose complications for service providers in terms of deployment, as it would essentially require meticulous analysis to be profitable during the changeover and later. To avoid monetary bottlenecks for the shift from the ex- isting 4G infrastructure, dual connectivity options can be exploited by market players in compliance with 3GPP regulations. The dual connectivity option originated in LTE networks with an initial focus on high individual user throughput and potent mobility by connecting to two eNBs (evolved node B) at the same time. The same strategy will enable the convenient movement to 5G with the UE's ability to establish connections with 4G and 5G base stations simultaneously. This significant embodiment will bring a great pool of ad- vantages, mainly dealing with mmWave communication, which is highly prone to signal propagation loss [8, 9]. Rapid changes in the channel would result in intermittent link failures, providing a platform for the existence of 4G/5G dual and ensuring reliable connectivity. With constraints of enhanced throughput, back compatibility during mmWave link failure, User Plane and Control Plane man- agement, RRM (radio resource management), and seamless user experience during mobility between different RATs (Radio Access Technologies), Among Options 1 to 7 laid out by 3GPP for 5G deployment, Options 3, 3a, and 3x belong to the NSA (non-standalone) scenario, differing from each other in the allocation of the data split anchor to a 4G or 5G base station [10]. Option 3x is popularly accepted for 5G network deployment by companies. NSA offers inter-system backward compatibility and is hence the top choice in the industry. During 4G deployment, due to undeveloped virtualisation technology, initial deployment was carried out on standalone physical devices, subsequently shifting to a management and orchestration (MANO)-based virtualised network function (VNF) architecture on private or public clouds. In 5G, all the network functions are virtualised and deployed in the cloud natively based on Kubernetes architecture. In contrast to 4G, 5G SBA (service-based architecture) signalling is based on REST APIs, making the system more resilient. Separation of user and control plane functionality in 5G results in system flexibility and independent scaling. The preparedness of 5G from various perspectives, such as Radio network, core network, IP transport, data centre, infrastructure, and automation, is of paramount importance [11, 12]. Either the non-disruptive approach or the green-field approach could be adopted by operators for 5G implementation. This chapter focuses on the 4G to 5G migration from an architecture standpoint, from the radio resource allocation and management point of view, and from the perspective of prominent use cases.

11.2   NETWORK ARCHITECTURE

As an enhancement in the networking domain, the 5G network meets a super speed for the future generation where technology is involved. The categories of 5G networks consist of a variety of enhancements to meet the demands of services. Therefore, the emerging technologies, based on the architectures and management schemes suggested to corelate all the challenges, comprise quality of services through data rate and traffic capacity, ensuring reliability [13]. Software-defined networking (SDN), mobile networks, and cellular networks are becoming the 5G network's most prominent technologies. Network architecture, which comprises data planes and control planes, decouples adaptability and resilience with respect to functionality for the SDN, where the scenario is very dynamic as far as support is concerned. The 5G network is also under observation and is not stable. The characteristic defined by the academician that syncs with the industry is the process that is displayed over the consultancy recommendations and is implemented [14, 15]. According to the current scenario, mobile communication is divided into two bases: outside and inside cell units, which present six issues that 4G is not able to handle in terms of data rate, latency, expenditure, and quality of service. These are some issues where 4G failed to fulfil all promises in comparison to the new design, which can handle the same to some extent effectively by overcoming all the loopholes present in the existing system [16]. On contrast, the major objective focuses on all the aspects relevant to the emerging technologies based on free apparition, where extensive labour has been done reciting about 5G mobile communications.

11.2.1   SOFTWARE-DEFINED NETWORKING (SDN) FOR 5G

Network services involve data forwarding, programmability, and application infrastructure and are the main parameters that are directly associated with the control. Such emerging architecture falls under this category and is manageable, flexible, familiar, and less expensive with respect to other network architecture [17, 18].

11.2.1.1 SDN (Software-Defined Networking) and NFV (Network Function Virtualisation)

The next-generation internet and data networks are the key components present in the SDN architecture. The description of SDN is very wide and can be defined in a few ways. The Open Networking Foundation (ONF) elaborated on an explicit and stable definition in terms of commercialisation, standardisation, and dealing with the public where development is associated [19]. It is observed that NFV is the key component in the design of SDN. NFV is not entirely dependent on SDN, but somehow both terms are advantageous together (Figure 11.1).

11.2.1.2 SDN Functionalities

Multiple functions can be supported by the functionalities present in SDN as architecture comprises of a control plane, centralised controller, and data plane. From Figure 11.2, the mechanism of planes and layer(s) can be easily understood [20].

11.2.1.3 SDN Architecture for 5G

The model proposed by ONF is quite easy as its architecture is very superior with respect to SDN. From Figure 11.3, it is clearly depicted that the model is categorised in three different layers [21].

11.2.2 Design of 5G Mobile Network Architecture

As per the next-generation network, the 5G system was deployed after considering all the suggestions driven by the real-time scenario, where all the components of the architecture have been covered, namely IP structure, interoperability of the cellular network, and software-based networking. From the below-mentioned Figure 11.4, we can easily draw an inference about the technical flow with respect to OSI layers, radio access techniques, different server configurations, and intermediate networking devices [22, 23].

11.2.2.1 Interoperability of Heterogeneous Wireless Networks

To adapt the improvements along with the legacy system is very challenging, as heterogeneity in networking is increasing in terms of spectrum efficiency, networking architecture, and resource allocation [24, 25]. The main concern is how to make the wide variety of different networks into one cluster so that we can overcome the issue of interoperability.

11.2.2.2 Functional Entities and Functionalities Proposed in Architecture

The function of the network layer has its own advantages because of its basic features, which are directly related to connectivity and security. The modules are separated based on client operability and the quality characteristics of the server. All the different modules are aligned together to employ a virtual scenario in terms of the network layer [26].

(a)

(b)

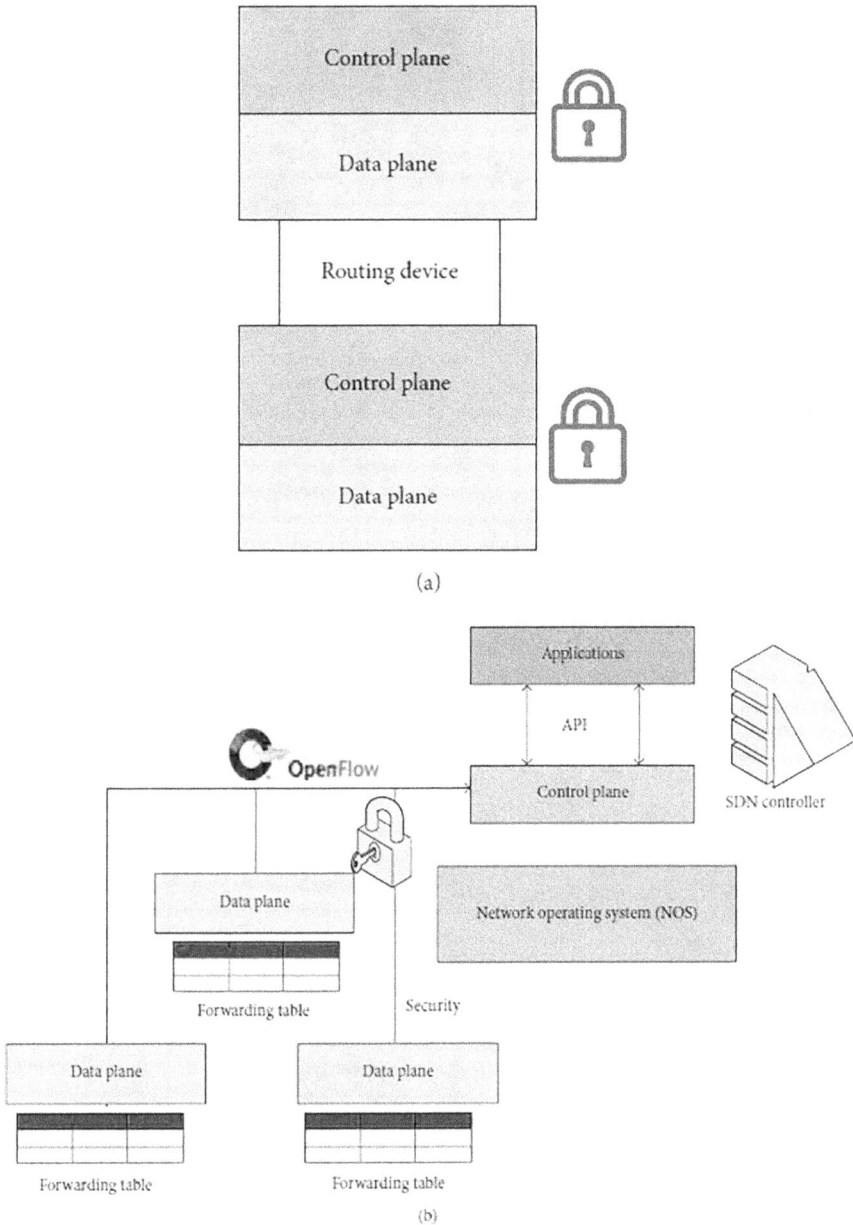

FIGURE 11.1 Comparison between (a) traditional hardware-based network and (b) SDN.

11.2.3 5G Cellular Network Architecture

As per the growing demand and to fulfill huge requirements, the existing system will not sustain itself for a longer duration. The technology needs to be updated in such a way that it can satisfy the user's growing day-to-day needs [27]. The current

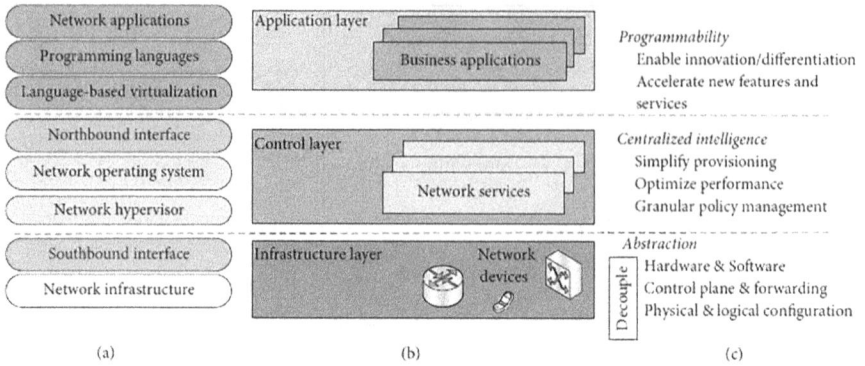

Network applications	Application layer		Programmability

FIGURE 11.2   SDN (a) layers, (b) planes, and (c) functionalities.

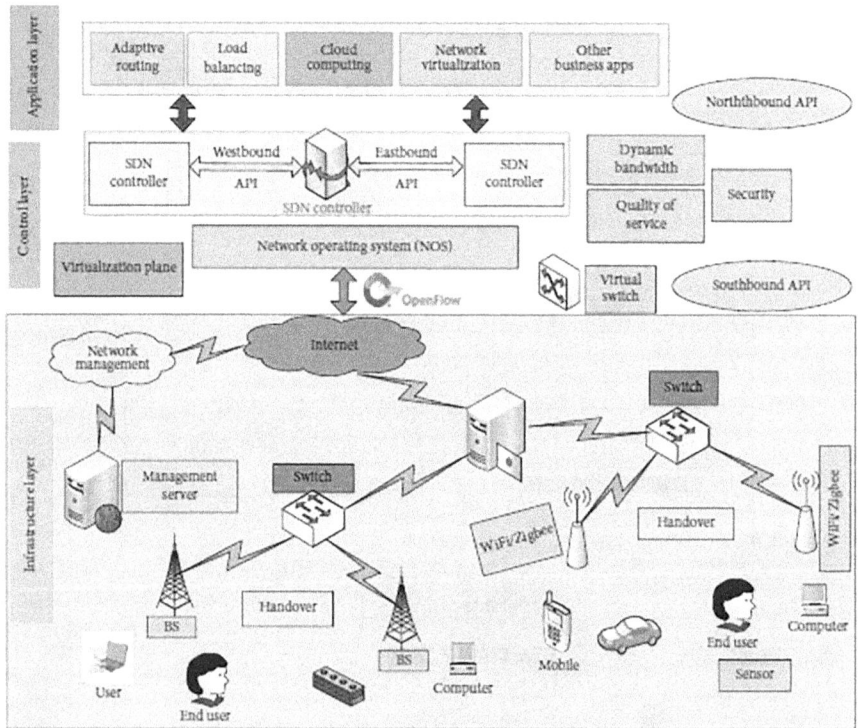

FIGURE 11.3   SDN architecture for 5G.

mobile architecture is broadly categorised based on inside and outside location in terms of base station. Because of these setup issues, the transmitted signal faces various kinds of losses, which result in reductions in spectral utility, energy efficiency, and data capacity [28]. Keeping these issues in mind, it is worthwhile to develop new ideas that bring a number of solutions to the problems faced by the

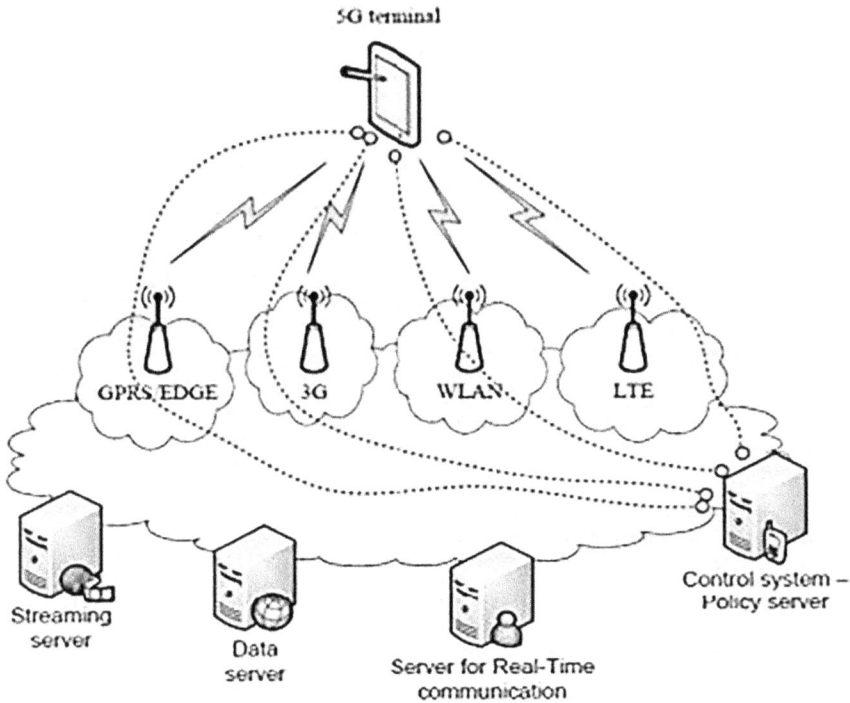

FIGURE 11.4   Practical architecture for 5G mobile networks.

current mobile communication technology. As an outcome of deep studies and tireless research, the evolution of 5G came into the picture. Initially, this idea was implemented through MIMO technology; later, it was modified by massive MIMO systems. All the major components of 5G mobile networking are explicitly depicted in Figure 11.5.

11.3   LATENCY REDUCTION IN 5G-BASED SMART HOSPITAL

Reducing latency in a 5G-based smart hospital involves optimising various aspects of the network infrastructure and implementing technologies designed to minimise delays in data transmission. Here are some approaches to reducing latency in a 5G-based smart hospital [28, 29, 30]:

- Leveraging edge computing technologies can significantly reduce latency by processing data closer to the source. By deploying computing resources at the network edge, near the medical devices or sensors, data can be processed and analysed locally, minimising the need for data to travel back and forth to centralised servers.
- Network Slicing: 5G allows for network slicing, which involves dividing the network into multiple virtual networks optimised for specific use cases. By allocating a dedicated slice of the network for critical medical

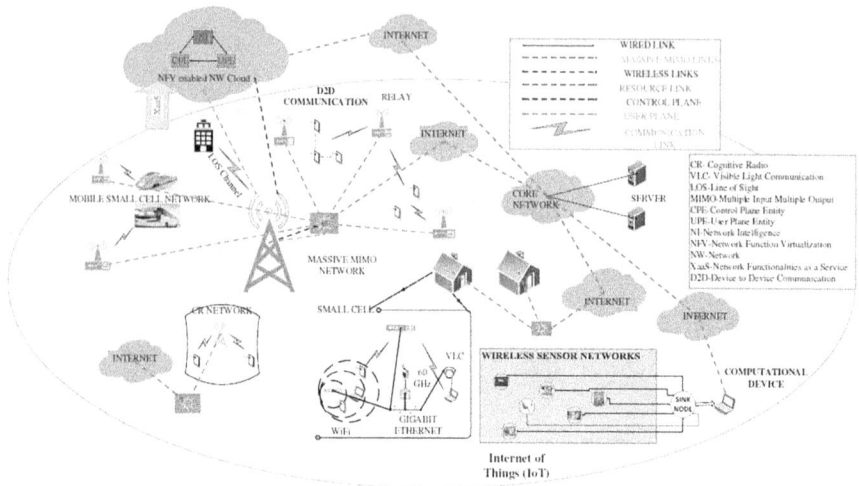

FIGURE 11.5 A general 5G cellular network architecture.

applications, healthcare providers can ensure low-latency connectivity and prioritise the transmission of real-time data.

- Small Cell Deployment: Smart hospitals can deploy a dense network of small cells throughout their facilities. Small cells are low-power, short-range base stations that improve coverage and capacity in localised areas. By strategically placing small cells, hospitals can enhance signal strength and reduce latency, particularly in high-traffic areas.

- Quality of Service (QoS) Prioritisation: Implementing QoS mechanisms allows healthcare applications to be given priority over non-critical traffic. By assigning higher priority to medical data traffic, hospitals can ensure low-latency transmission of vital information.

- Device-to-Device (D2D) Communication: 5G supports direct communication between devices without routing data through a central network. Leveraging D2D communication can reduce latency by enabling devices to exchange information directly, minimising the need for data to traverse the network infrastructure.

- Network Optimisation: Optimising the network infrastructure, including reducing interference, improving signal strength, and minimising packet loss, can help reduce latency. This involves ensuring proper network planning, optimising antenna placement, and using advanced technologies such as beamforming.

- Caching and Content Delivery Networks (CDNs): By implementing local caching mechanisms and CDNs within the hospital premises, frequently accessed content, such as medical records and imaging data, can be stored closer to the end users. This reduces the latency associated with retrieving data from distant servers.

- Real-Time Analytics: Employing real-time analytics and machine learning algorithms at the edge can enable quicker processing and decision making.

By analysing data locally and generating insights in real time, healthcare providers can respond faster to critical situations, reducing latency in the decision-making process.

- Redundancy and Failover Mechanisms: Implementing redundant network links and failover mechanisms can help ensure continuous connectivity and minimise downtime. By quickly switching to alternative network paths in the case of network failures, hospitals can reduce the impact of latency due to network disruptions.

It's important to note that reducing latency in a 5G-based smart hospital requires careful planning, optimisation, and collaboration between healthcare providers and network operators. Additionally, the specific implementation strategies may vary depending on the hospital's infrastructure, size, and requirements.

11.3.1 Spectral Access in 5G-Based Smart Healthcare

Spectral efficiency plays a crucial role in enhancing the capabilities and performance of 5G-based smart healthcare systems. Spectral efficiency refers to the amount of data that can be transmitted over a given bandwidth. By improving spectral efficiency, 5G networks can accommodate a higher volume of data traffic. In smart healthcare, this translates to the ability to handle a larger number of connected devices, such as medical sensors, wearables, and monitoring equipment, without compromising performance. The increased data capacity enables real-time monitoring, remote consultations, and seamless transmission of medical data. Spectral efficiency improvements in 5G networks enable the delivery of high-quality video and imaging applications [31]. This is particularly valuable in smart healthcare, where high-resolution videoconferencing, telemedicine consultations, and remote surgeries require low-latency and high-bandwidth connections. Efficient spectrum utilisation allows for the transmission of high-definition video streams, enabling healthcare professionals to assess patient conditions accurately and make informed decisions. Spectral efficiency enhancements in 5G help ensure reliable and real-time communication between healthcare providers, medical devices, and patients. By optimising the utilisation of available spectrum resources, 5G networks can maintain a stable connection even in high-density environments like hospitals. This reliability is critical for transmitting vital patient data, alerts, and emergency notifications without delays or interruptions, enabling prompt actions and timely interventions [32]. The IoMT ecosystem in smart healthcare relies on seamless connectivity between various medical devices, wearables, and infrastructure components. Spectral efficiency improvements in 5G facilitate the simultaneous connection of numerous IoT devices, allowing them to exchange data efficiently. This connectivity is vital for collecting real-time health data, managing patient information, and supporting advanced applications such as remote patient monitoring, medication adherence tracking, and preventive care. Spectral efficiency improvements in 5G can also contribute to energy savings. By optimising the use of spectrum resources, 5G networks can transmit data more efficiently, reducing the energy consumption of network components. This energy efficiency is beneficial in smart healthcare, where numerous devices and systems are interconnected and power management is crucial for extended battery life in wearable devices, IoT sensors, and medical equipment. Spectral efficiency advancements in 5G networks enable seamless mobility, allowing healthcare providers and patients to maintain uninterrupted connectivity while moving within the hospital premises or even between different healthcare facilities. Continuous and reliable connectivity enhances the effectiveness of mobile healthcare applications, location-based services, and real-time tracking of patients and medical assets. Overall, spectral efficiency improvements in 5G-based smart healthcare systems ensure reliable, high-capacity, low-latency, and energy-efficient communication, facilitating enhanced patient care, remote diagnostics, telemedicine, and efficient healthcare management [33].

11.3.2 Power Optimisation for 5G-Based Hospital

Optimising power consumption in 5G radio for a smart hospital is crucial to ensuring efficient operations and minimising energy costs. Here are some strategies to optimise power in 5G radio for a smart hospital [34, 35, 36]:

I. Power Management Techniques: Implement power management techniques at various levels, including base stations, small cells, and IoT devices. This involves optimising power amplifier efficiency, reducing power consumption during low-traffic periods through sleep mode activation, and dynamically adjusting transmit power based on the signal quality and distance.

II. Network Planning and Optimisation: Conduct thorough network planning and optimisation to minimise unnecessary power consumption. This includes optimising the placement and coverage of base stations and small cells to minimise signal interference and reduce the overall transmit power required.

III. Smart Antenna Systems: Utilise advanced antenna technologies such as beamforming and beam steering to improve signal strength and coverage. Smart antenna systems can dynamically adapt their radiation patterns to focus the signal on the intended recipients, reducing the need for excessive transmit power.

IV. Spectrum Efficiency: Enhance spectrum efficiency to minimise power consumption. Techniques such as carrier aggregation, which allows for the aggregation of multiple frequency bands, help maximise data throughput while utilising the spectrum efficiently. Efficient spectrum usage reduces the need for high-power transmissions.

V. Device-to-Device Communication: Leverage device-to-device (D2D) communication capabilities within 5G to enable direct communication between nearby devices without routing through base stations. This approach reduces the need for transmitting data over long distances, resulting in lower power consumption.

VI. Energy-Efficient Hardware: Deploy energy-efficient radio equipment, base stations, and IoT devices that adhere to industry standards for power consumption. Utilise hardware components with low-power modes and advanced power management features to minimise energy usage during idle periods or low-demand scenarios.

VII. Sleep Mode Activation: Enable sleep mode or power-saving mode in IoT devices and network equipment during periods of inactivity or when the devices are not in use. This allows for significant power savings without compromising the functionality or responsiveness of the smart hospital system.

VIII. Energy Harvesting: Explore opportunities for energy harvesting techniques, such as solar panels or energy harvesting from ambient sources to power low-power devices or recharge batteries. This can help reduce reliance on external power sources and lower overall energy consumption.

IX. Data Compression and Offloading: Implement data compression techniques to reduce the size of data transmitted over the network. Offload non-critical data or computing tasks to edge servers or cloud infrastructure, reducing the processing and transmission workload on devices and minimising power consumption.

X. Continuous Monitoring and Optimisation: Regularly monitor and optimise power consumption in the 5G radio network by analysing power usage patterns, network performance, and energy efficiency metrics. This allows for ongoing improvements and adjustments to optimise power utilisation based on the specific requirements and dynamics of the smart hospital environment.

Implementing these power optimisation strategies can contribute to a more sustainable and energy-efficient 5G radio network in a smart hospital, reducing operational costs and minimising the environmental impact.

11.3.3 CHALLENGES OF IMPLEMENTING 5G SMART HOSPITALS IN RURAL AREAS

Implementing a 5G smart hospital in villages poses several challenges due to the unique characteristics and infrastructure limitations of rural areas. Rural areas often lack the necessary infrastructure required for 5G deployment, such as high-speed internet connectivity, fibre-optic networks, and a robust power supply. Upgrading the existing infrastructure to support 5G technology can be costly and time-consuming. Providing reliable and widespread 5G coverage in rural areas can be challenging due to the scattered population and geographical obstacles [37]. Rural areas may have remote or hilly terrain that hinders signal propagation, requiring additional infrastructure investments to ensure comprehensive coverage. Deploying and maintaining 5G infrastructure in rural areas may have high costs, considering the lower population density and potential lack of financial resources in those regions. Balancing the cost-effectiveness of the deployment while ensuring affordability for healthcare providers and residents is a significant challenge. Building and operating a 5G smart hospital requires a skilled workforce capable of managing and maintaining the complex infrastructure. In rural areas, there may be a shortage of trained professionals with expertise in 5G technologies, necessitating training and capacity-building initiatives. Integrating various healthcare systems, medical devices, and IoT technologies within the 5G smart hospital architecture can be challenging, particularly if the systems and devices come from different vendors. Ensuring seamless interoperability and data exchange requires standardised protocols and robust integration frameworks. Protecting patient data and ensuring privacy are critical concerns in healthcare [38]. Establishing robust security measures in a 5G smart hospital in villages may pose challenges, as the infrastructure and networks may be more susceptible to cybersecurity threats due to limited resources and technical capabilities. Adhering to regulatory requirements and aligning with government policies can be complex when implementing a 5G smart hospital in rural areas. Navigating the legal and regulatory landscape, obtaining necessary permissions, and complying with healthcare regulations are important considerations. Promoting awareness and fostering acceptance of 5G technology and its benefits among rural communities, healthcare providers, and local authorities is crucial. Overcoming resistance to change and addressing concerns related to the impact of advanced technologies on traditional healthcare practises can be a challenge. Addressing these challenges requires collaboration between government bodies, telecommunication providers, healthcare organisations, and local communities. It involves careful planning, investment in infrastructure, capacity building, and tailored solutions that consider the specific needs and limitations of rural areas. Additionally, public-private partnerships and innovative financing models may be required to overcome the financial barriers associated with implementing 5G smart hospitals in villages [39].

11.4 CONCLUSION

The upcoming mobile technology is intended to deliver data at super-speed, irrespective of time and location. Because of this trend, the current networking architecture needs to work on several aspects of communication, like low latency, maximum throughput, more security, fewer losses, and minimum error rates. This chapter justifies the significance of the transition from the current 4G network to the future 5G network in terms of its networking architecture, use cases, and resource allocation. All the migration components are compared and elaborated well with the help of the respective figures. This chapter discussed all the possible aspects of 5G network architecture, which helps fulfill the needs expected in 2023. This literature has gone through a deeper analysis of the 5G mobile technology by covering all the practical aspects in terms of its architecture, use cases, and resource allocation. This chapter can also provide good intuition to other researchers for solving more complicated issues that may be encountered in future generation networks.

REFERENCES

1. A. Kumar, M. A. Albreem, M. Gupta, M. H. Alsharif and S. Kim, "Future 5G Network Based Smart Hospitals: Hybrid Detection Technique for Latency Improvement," *IEEE Access*, vol. 8, pp. 153240–153249, 2020, 10.1109/ACCESS. 2020.3017625.

2. K. Kour and K. Ali, "A Review Paper on 5G Wireless Networks," *International Journal of Engineering Research & Technology (IJERT) V-IMPACT – 2016*, vol. 4, no. 32, pp. 24–32, 2016.

3. A. Kumar and M. Gupta, "A Review on Activities of Fifth Generation Mobile Communication System," *Alexandria Engineering Journal*, vol. 57, no. 2, pp. 1125–1135, 2018, 10.1016/j.aej.2017.01.043.

4. J. Moysen and L. Giupponi, "From 4G to 5G: Self-Organized Network Management Meets Machine Learning," *Computer Communications*, vol. 129, pp. 248–268, 2018, ISSN 0140-3664, 10.1016/j.comcom.2018.07.015.

5. A. Kumar and S. Chakravarty, "Dynamic Power Allocation to Improve an Existing SWIPT Cooperative NOMA Network," *National Academy Science Letters*, vol. 45, pp. 507–510, 2022, 10.1007/s40009-022-01141-7.

6. M. Shariat, Ö. Bulakci, A. De Domenico, C. Mannweiler, M. Gramaglia, Q. Wei, A. Gopalasingham, E. Pateromichelakis, F. Moggio, D. Tsolkas, B. Gajic, M. Rates Crippa and S. Khatibi, "A Flexible Network Architecture for 5G Systems," *Wireless Communications and Mobile Computing*, vol. 2019, Article ID 5264012, p. 19, 2019, 10.1155/2019/5264012.

7. M. R. Noohani and K. U. Magsi, "A Review of 5G Technology: Architecture, Security, and Wide Applications," *International Research Journal of Engineering and Technology (IRJET)*, vol. 07, pp. 3440–3471, 2020, 10.5281/zenodo.3842353.

8. P. Suthar, V. Agarwal, R. S. Shetty and A. Jangam, "Migration and Interworking between 4G and 5G," 2020 IEEE 3rd 5G World Forum (5GWF), Bangalore, India, 2020, pp. 401–406, doi:10.1109/5GWF49715.2020.9221021.

9. M. Agiwal, H. Kwon, S. Park and H. Jin, "A Survey on 4G-5G Dual Connectivity: Road to 5G Implementation," *IEEE Access*, vol. 9, pp. 16193–16210, 2021, 10.1109/ACCESS.2021.3052462.

10. Y. Hao, "Investigation and Technological Comparison of 4G and 5G Networks," *Journal of Computer and Communications*, vol. 9, pp. 36–43, 2021, 10.4236/jcc.2021.91004.

11. A. Kumar, K. Rajagopal, G. Gugapriya, H. Sharma, N. Gour, M. Masud, M.A. AlZain and S. H. Alajmani, "Reducing PAPR with Low Complexity Filtered NOMA Using Novel Algorithm," *Sustainability*, vol. 14, p. 9631, 2022a, 10.3390/su14159631.

12. V. Pana, V. Balyan and B. Groenewald, "Fair Allocation of Resources on Modulation and Coding Scheme in LTE Networks with Carrier Aggregation," 2018 International Conference on Advances in Computing, Communication Control and Networking (ICACCCN), Greater Noida, India, 2018, pp. 467–470, 10.1109/ICACCCN.2018.8748355.

13. N. Singh, S. Agrawal, T. Agarwal and P. K. Mishra, "RBF-SVM Based Resource Allocation Scheme for 5G CRAN Networks," 2018 3rd International Conference and Workshops on Recent Advances and Innovations in Engineering (ICRAIE), Jaipur, India, 2018, pp. 1–6, 10.1109/ICRAIE.2018.8710423.

14. M. Y. Ramadhan and M. I. Nashiruddin, "Performance Evaluation of Radio Resource Allocation Algorithm for 5G Device-to-Device Communication Underlying on 4G LTE Networks," 2020 International Conference on Radar, Antenna, Microwave, Electronics, and Telecommunications (ICRAMET), Tangerang, Indonesia, 2020, pp. 91–96, 10.1109/ICRAMET51080.2020.9298685.

15. L. N. Degambur, A. Mungur, S. Armoogum and S. Pudaruth, "Resource Allocation in 4G and 5G Networks: A Review," *International Journal of Communication Networks and Information Security (IJCNIS)*, vol. 13, p. 3, April 2022, 10.17762/ijcnis.v13i3.5116.

16. M. A. Kamal, H. W. Raza, M. M. Alam, M. M. Su'ud and A. B. A. B. Sajak, "Resource Allocation Schemes for 5G Network: A Systematic Review," *Sensors (Basel)*, vol. 21, no. 19, p. 6588, October 2, 2021, 10.3390/s21196588. PMID: 34640908; PMCID: PMC8512213.

17. A. Kumar and N. Kumar, "OFDM System with Cyclo-Stationary Feature Detection Spectrum Sensing," *ICT Express*, vol. 5, pp. 21–25, 2018.

18. O. O. Erunkulu, A. M. Zungeru, C. K. Lebekwe, M. Mosalaosi and J. M. Chuma, "5G Mobile Communication Applications: A Survey and Comparison of Use Cases," *IEEE Access*, vol. 9, pp. 97251–97295, 2021, 10.1109/ACCESS.2021.3093213.

19. J. Mendoza, I. de-la-Bandera, C. S. Álvarez-Merino, E. Jatib Khatib, J. Alonso, S. Casalderrey-Díaz and R. Barco, "5G for Construction: Use Cases and Solutions," *Electronics*, vol. 10, no. 14, p. 1713, 2021, 10.3390/electronics10141713

20. P. G. Kuppusamy, "A Comparative Study on 4G and 5G Technology for Wireless Applications," *IOSR Journal of Electronics and Communication Engineering (IOSR-JECE)*, vol. 2015, pp. 1–32, 2015.

21. A. Kumar and M. Gupta, "Design of 4:8 MIMO OFDM with MSE Equalizer for Different Modulation Techniques," *Wireless Personal Communications*, vol. 95, pp. 4535–4560, 2017.

22. B. Keogh and A. Zhu, "Wideband Self-Interference Cancellation for 5G Full-Duplex Radio Using a Near-Field Sensor Array," 2018 IEEE MTT-S International Microwave Workshop Series on 5G Hardware and System Technologies (IMWS-5G), Dublin, Ireland, 2018, pp. 1–3, 10.1109/IMWS-5G.2018.8484398.

23. X. Wang et al., "Holistic Service-Based Architecture for Space-Air-Ground Integrated Network for 5G-Advanced and Beyond," *China Communications*, vol. 19, no. 1, pp. 14–28, January 2022, 10.23919/JCC.2022.01.002.

24. V. Agarwal, C. Sharma, R. Shetty, A. Jangam and R. Asati, "A Journey Towards a Converged 5G Architecture & Beyond," 2021 IEEE 4th 5G World Forum (5GWF), Montreal, QC, Canada, 2021, pp. 18–23, 10.1109/5GWF52925.2021.00011.

25. A. Kumar and M. Gupta, "A Comprehensive Study of PAPR Reduction Techniques: Design of DSLM-CT Joint Reduction Technique for Advanced Waveform," Soft Computing, vol. 24, pp. 11893–11907, 2020.

26. X. Liang and X. Qiu, "A Software Defined Security Architecture for SDN-Based 5G Network," 2016 IEEE International Conference on Network Infrastructure and Digital Content (IC-NIDC), Beijing, China, 2016, pp. 17–21, 10.1109/ICNIDC.2016.7974528.

27. A. Kumar, "PAPR Minimization in FBMC Multi-Carrier Waveform by Particle Transmission Sequence-Particle Swarm Optimization Algorithm," *Journal of Communications Technology and Electronics*, vol. 66, pp. 155–163, 2021, 10.1134/S106422692102008X.

28. E. M. Oproiu, M. Iordache, C. Patachia, C. Costea and I. Marghescu, "Development and Implementation of a Smart City Use Case in a 5G Mobile Network's Operator," 2017 25th Telecommunication Forum (TELFOR), Belgrade, Serbia, 2017, pp. 1–4, 10.1109/TELFOR.2017.8249292.

29. S. Chakravarty and A. Kumar, "PAPR Reduction of GFDM Signals Using Encoder-Decoder Neural Network (Autoencoder)," *National Academy Science Letters*, vol. 46, pp. 213–217, 2023, 10.1007/s40009-023-01230-1.

30. W. S. H. M. W. Ahmad et al., "5G Technology: Towards Dynamic Spectrum Sharing Using Cognitive Radio Networks," *IEEE Access*, vol. 8, pp. 14460–14488, 2020, 10.1109/ACCESS.2020.2966271.

31. A. Kumar, "PAPR Reduction in beyond 5G Waveforms Using a Novel SLM Algorithm", *National Academy Science Letters*, 2023, 10.1007/s40009-023-01289-w.

32. M. Parvini et al., "Spectrum Sharing Schemes from 4G to 5G and Beyond: Protocol Flow, Regulation, Ecosystem, Economic," *IEEE Open Journal of the Communications Society*, vol. 4, pp. 464–517, 2023, 10.1109/OJCOMS.2023.3238569.

33. M. Agiwal, A. Roy and N. Saxena, "Next Generation 5G Wireless Networks: A Comprehensive Survey," *IEEE Communications Surveys & Tutorials*, vol. 18, no. 3, pp. 1617–1655, 3rd Quart. 2016.

34. A. Kumar, H. Sharma, N. Gour and R. Pareek, "A Hybrid Technique for the PAPR Reduction of NOMA Waveform," *International Journal of Communication Systems*, vol. 36, no. 4–10, 2022b, 10.1002/dac.5412.

35. E. Sisinni, A. Saifullah, S. Han, U. Jennehag and M. Gidlund, "Industrial Internet of Things: Challenges Opportunities and Directions," *IEEE Transactions on Industrial Informatics*, vol. 14, no. 11, pp. 4724–4734, November 2018.

36. A. Kumar and H. Sharma, "Intelligent Cognitive Radio Spectrum Sensing Based on Energy Detection for Advanced Waveforms," *Radio Electronics and Communication Systems*, vol. 65, no. 3, pp. 175–181, 2022.

37. M. K. Sharma and A. Kumar, "NOMA Waveform Technique Using Orthogonal Supplementary Signal for Advanced 5G Networks Security," *Journal of Discrete Mathematical Sciences and Cryptography*, vol. 25, pp. 1125–1136, 2022, 10.1080/09720529.2022.2075088.

38. S. Alraih et al., "Revolution or Evolution? Technical Requirements and Considerations Towards 6G Mobile Communications," *Sensors*, vol. 22, no. 3, p. 762, January 2022.

39. M. A. Albreem et al., "Low Complexity Linear Detectors for Massive MIMO: A Comparative Study," *IEEE Access*, vol. 9, pp. 45740–45753, 2021, 10.1109/ACCESS.2021.3065923.

12 Analysis of Routing Protocols for Wireless Sensor Network for Remote Healthcare System

Amit Kumar Jain
Research Scholar, Poornima University, India

Garima Mathur
Department of Electronics & Communication Engineering,
Poornima College of Engineering, India

Prashant Jamwal
Department of Electrical and Computer Engineering, School
of Engineering and Digital Sciences, Republic of Kazakhstan

12.1 INTRODUCTION

The data aggregation protocol aims to exclude redundant data transmissions, thus reducing resources and extending the life of wireless sensor networks. The above solution is not energy efficient as the same data can be collected from nodes in close proximity. An improvement over the above method is a cluster where each node sends data to the cluster head (CH), which aggregates the raw data received and sends it to the sink [1] (Figure 12.1).

12.1.1 OVERVIEW OF ROUTING PROTOCOL

Comparison of routing in WSNs is extra attractive due to the inherent characteristics of ad-hoc networks. First, transmission resource availability, processing power, and bandwidth are very low. Second, a global approach to Internet Protocol (IP) is difficult to design. This is because updating addresses in large or complex WSNs can have high overhead. Third, resource scarcity makes it difficult to deal with frequent changes in evolving topologies, especially in

DOI: 10.1201/9781003403678-12

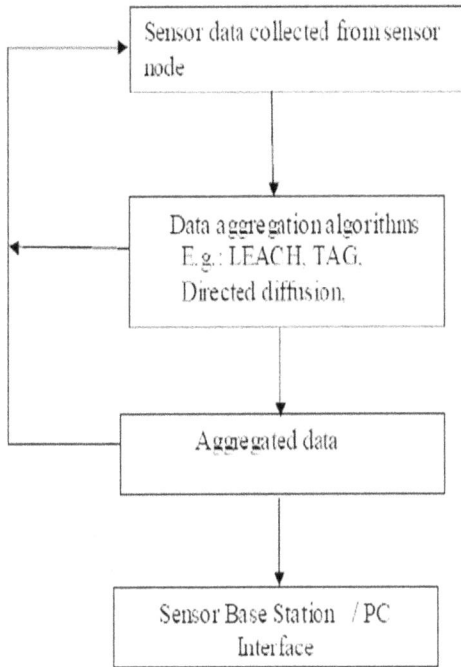

FIGURE 12.1   Basic architecture for data aggregation.

mobile environments. Fourth, the processing of data by multiple sensor nodes creates a high degree of consistency in the data computed by routing protocols. Most WSN applications do not allow a single communicating device from multiple sources to be a multicast or pair-to-peer application. Finally, transmission of WSN application data should be limited to a certain period of time. Therefore, these types of applications should consider minimum latency for data transfer. However, in many applications, power security is more important than quality of service (QoS), as power is limited by all sensor nodes that are directly related to the life of the network [2].

12.2   LITERATURE SURVEY

In this text, the purpose of this chapter is to ensure reliability and a coherent data supply and limitless network life for a query-driven energy neutral guided diffusion (ENDD) protocol. Traffic flow input controls are performed on the basis of their own energy collection status on any sensor, preventing sensors from shutting down due to excessive energy use. In order to increase the reliability of the admitted control mechanism, we suggest a practical energy consumption estimation model in real time. In addition, we demonstrate analytically that the ENDD protocol is extremely scalable since the total number of communications control messages exchanged for road setup can provide a linear upper boundary. In order to determine and compare performance of our proposed ENDD protocol to other query-based routing protocols, detailed simulations are also performed [3].

This chapter proposed a new algorithm for goal tracking for RDPSO (random drift swarm optimization algorithm). RDPSO increases regional integration and is more effective in contrast with PSO and QPSO. A sequential RDPSO tracking algorithm was suggested based on a conventional PSO-based tracking system. We adjust the initialization process, using the Gaussian mixture model to determine the fitness value to further increase the efficiency of the proposed tracking algorithm. The efficiency and performance of our algorithm are shown in numerous experimental findings, particularly in cases of major changes in the context, deformities or rapid movements and camera waves [4].

This chapter reviews the variants proposed in LEACH routing protocols so far and addresses their development and functioning. This survey classifies all of the protocols in two parts, i.e., single-hop and multi-hop communication based on cluster head to base station data transfer. A comparative study was performed in sequential fashion using nine different criteria, including energy consumption, overhead, scalability complexity, etc. The article also addresses the strengths and limitations of any LEACH type. Finally, the chapter ends with recommendations for potential fields of study in the WSN area [5, 6].

The distance between the transmitter and the recipient can be deduced on the basis of the signal intensity (RSS) that was received by implementing a radio diffusion model. This approach is generally used in the positioning systems of wireless sensor networks (WSNs). Owing to slow and quick decay, the scope precision of such a system is extremely small. While the first has been examined extensively, the second is seldom debated. This is based on the premise that averages compensate for fast decline, but how much a certain degree of precision can be calculated by RSS remains uncertain. Furthermore, positioning errors are related to the sensor distribution, rendering them both unstable and inaccurate. This chapter deals extensively with the range error and positioning error to better understand the system's poor performance [7, 8].

12.3   PROPOSED METHODOLOGY

To begin the simulation, we used a set of predefined parameters in this study. After the necessary number of cycles has been completed, the data are gathered and analyzed. The results are used to show the diagrams, while the diagrams themselves are used to explain the results. Finally, we compared our findings to similar studies in the literature.

LEACH is the first mesh networking protocol that uses hierarchical routing to increase network lifetime. In Figure 12.2, all nodes in the network are grouped into local cluster groups, with a single node as the cluster head. Although all non-cluster head nodes transmit their data to the cluster head, the cluster head node collects data from all cluster members, performs data signal processing functions (e.g., data

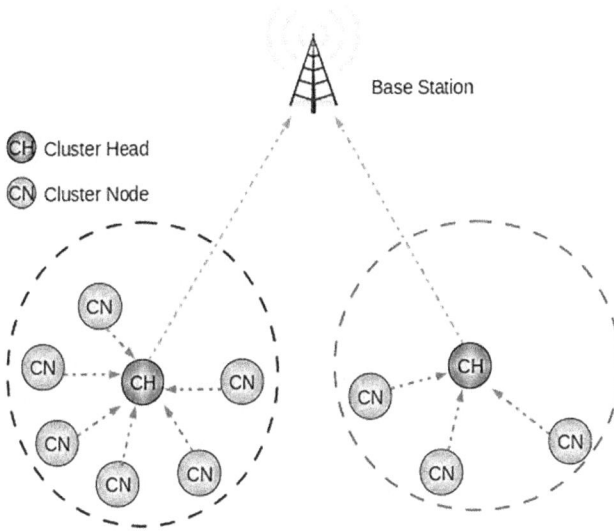

FIGURE 12.2 Illustration of LEACH protocol [7].

aggregation), and transmits data to the remote baseline. Thus, as a cluster head node, it needs much more resources than a non-cluster head node.

LEACH combines random rotation of cluster head positions with high-energy effects to rotate between sensors so that no single sensor in the network drains the battery. The cluster head energy load is evenly distributed across the nodes. Because the cluster head node is aware of all cluster members, it can create time division multiple access (TDMA) schedules that specify when each node should send information. In addition, using a TDMA data transmission schedule avoids collisions within the cluster. The LAUSCH process is divided into several parts. A cluster round begins with a buildup process, followed by a continuation phase, followed by several data frames from the nodes to the cluster head and base stations, which are then sent to the cluster head.

12.4 RESULT ANALYSIS

According to Figures 12.3 to 12.14, both LEACH and EAMMH improvements over time lose energy as rounds increase. When a node reaches zero, it is often unusable and is called a dead node. Figures 12.5–12.7 show that his EAMMH curve of average power of each node gets slightly better as the number of nodes increases. The number of dead nodes is also less in compared to LEACH, increasing the total number of nodes. Therefore, EAMMH outperforms LEACH with a probability of 0.01 as the number of nodes increases. In Figures 12.3 to 12.14, we can see that the number of EAMMH nodes increases in relation to the average energy of each node and the total number of dead nodes at each probability level. However, LEACH improved overall performance on a small number of nodes.

12.4.1 Simulation of Protocols at 0.01 Probabilities

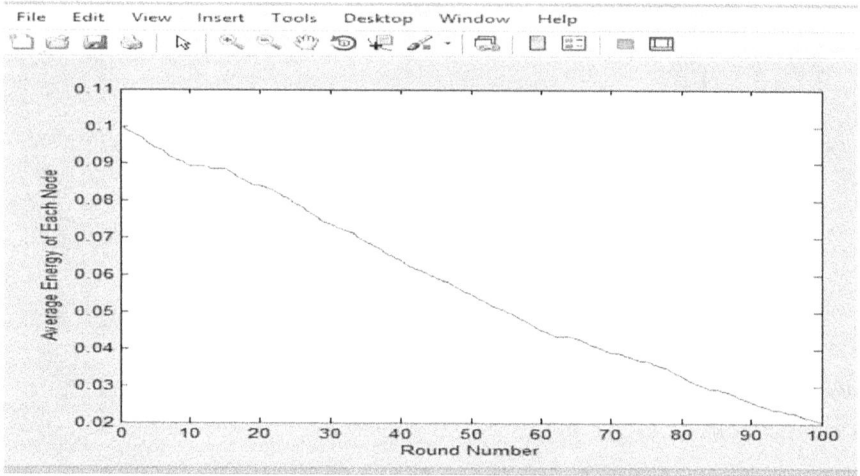

FIGURE 12.3   Average energy v/s round no. (EAMMH).

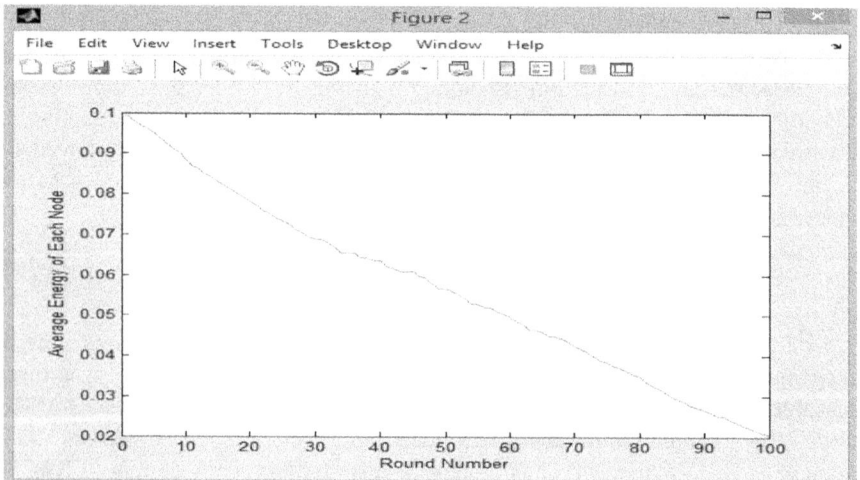

FIGURE 12.4   Average energy v/s round no. (LEACH).

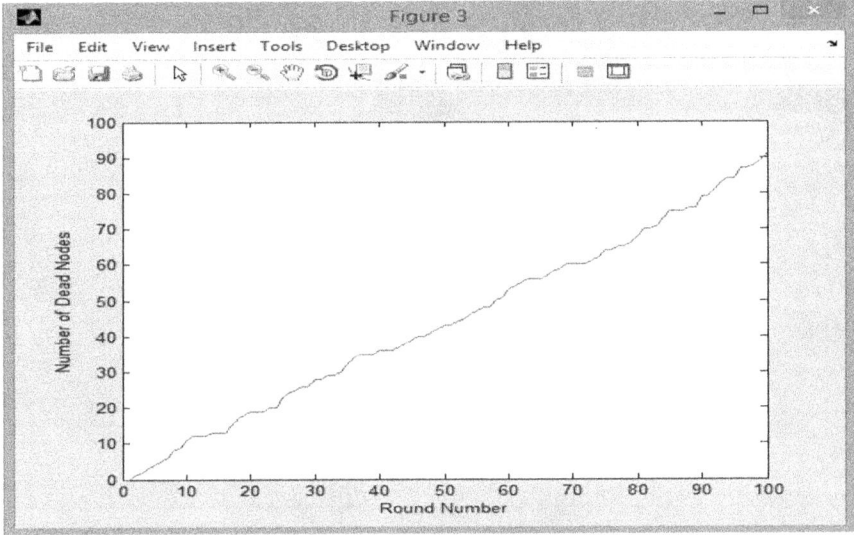

FIGURE 12.5 No. of dead nodes v/s round no. (EAMMH).

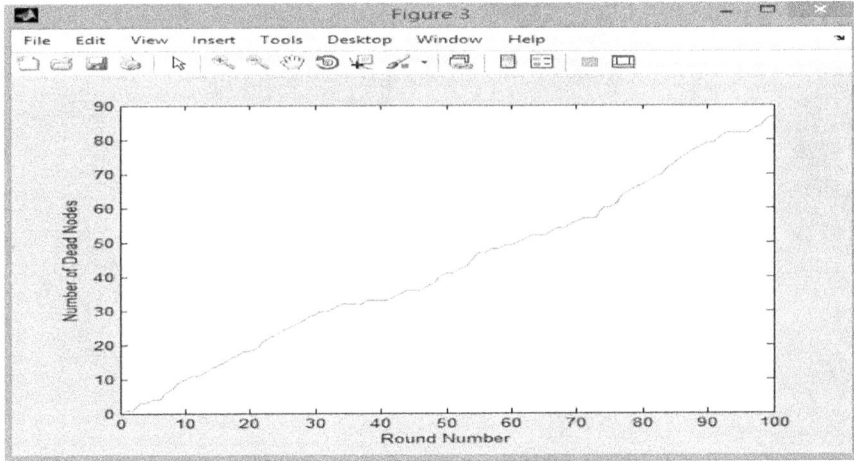

FIGURE 12.6 No. of dead nodes v/s round no. (LEACH).

12.4.2 SIMULATION OF PROTOCOLS AT 0.50 PROBABILITY

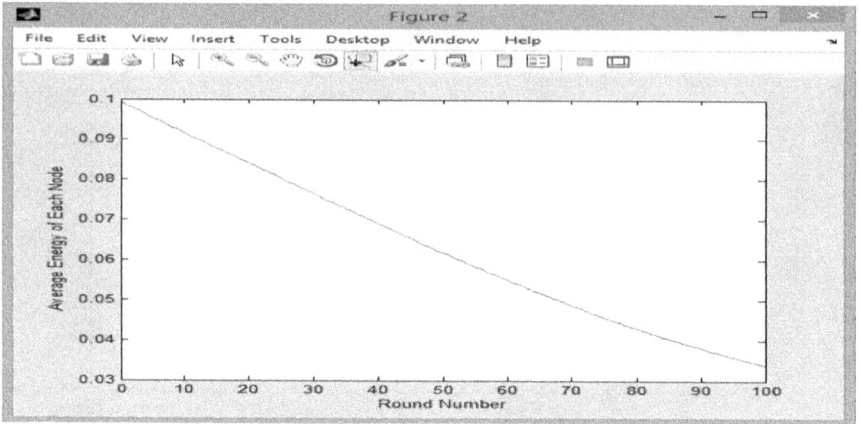

FIGURE 12.7 Average energy v/s round no. (EAMMH).

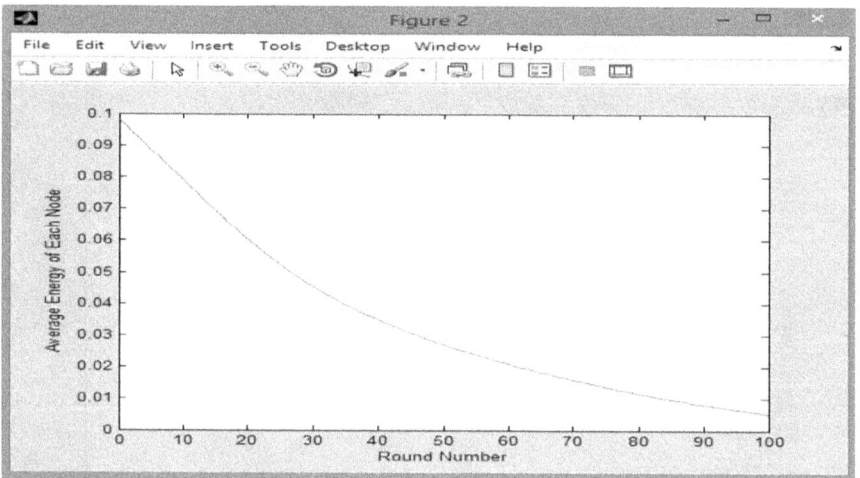

FIGURE 12.8 Average energy v/s round no. (LEACH).

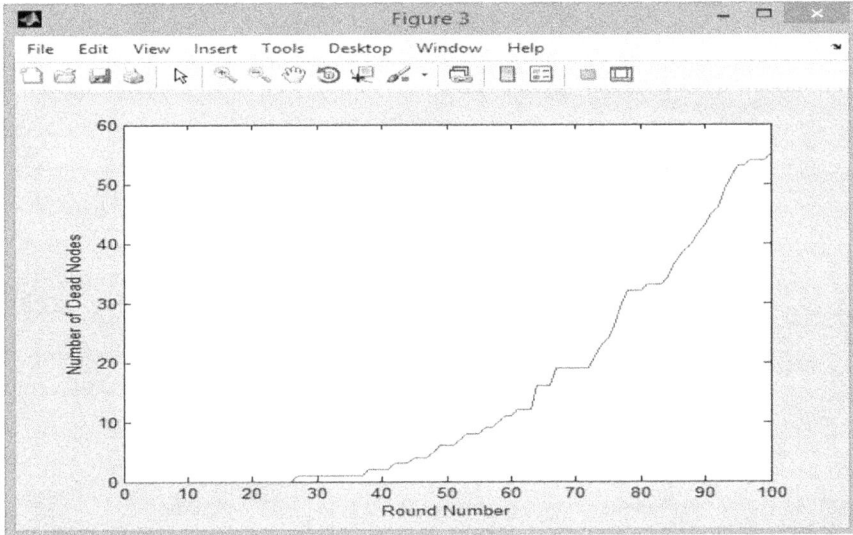

FIGURE 12.9   No. of dead nodes v/s round no. (EAMMH).

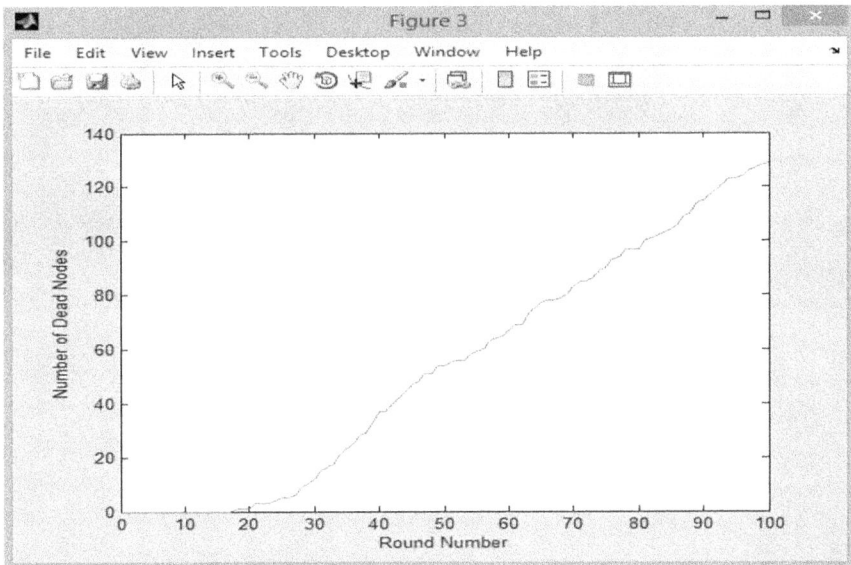

FIGURE 12.10   No. of dead nodes v/s round no. (LEACH).

12.4.3   SIMULATION OF PROTOCOLS AT 0.20 PROBABILITIES

Tables comparing the performance of LEACH and EAMMH based on different parameters are provided below. Based on the number of dead nodes, we compare the performance of the three protocols (Tables 12.1 and 12.2).

TABLE 12.1

Comparison of Number of Dead Nodes for 100 Rounds

	Total Dead Nodes	
Probability	LEACH	EAMMH
.01	85	**90**
.50	140	**55**
.20	130	**98**

TABLE 12.2

Comparison of Average Energy for 100 Rounds

	Average Energy (J)	
Probability	LEACH	EAMMH
.01	.02	**.02**
.50	.005	**.032**
.20	.0013	**.012**

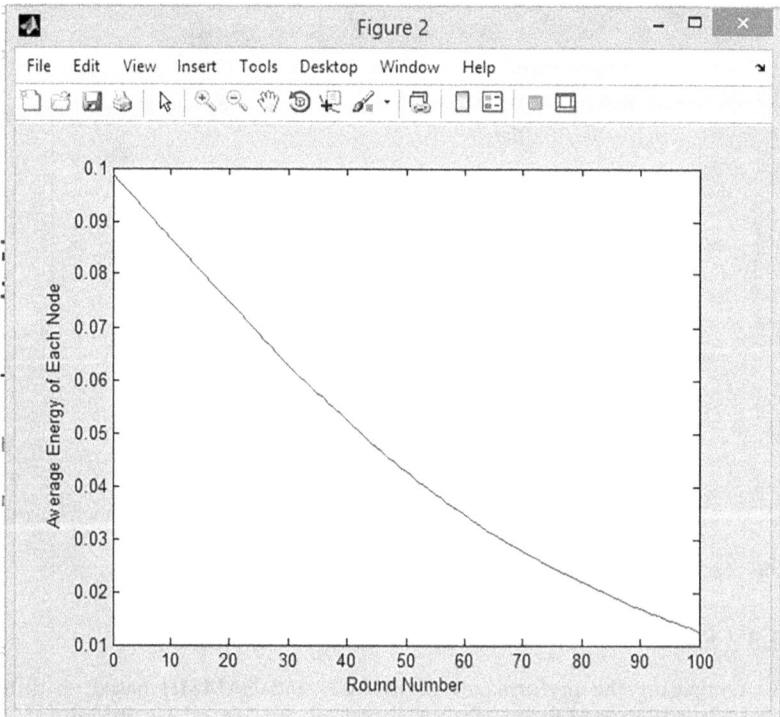

FIGURE 12.11   Average energy v/s round no. (EAMMH).

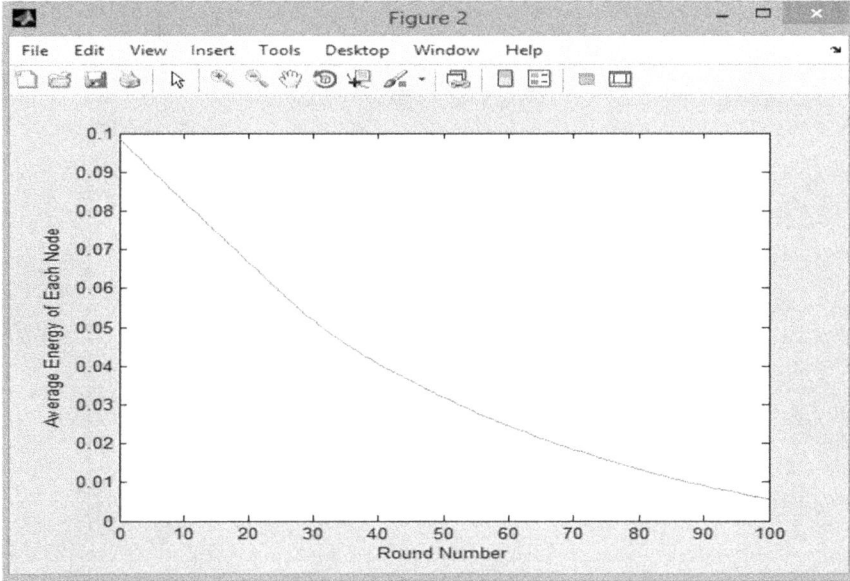

FIGURE 12.12   Average energy v/s round no. (LEACH).

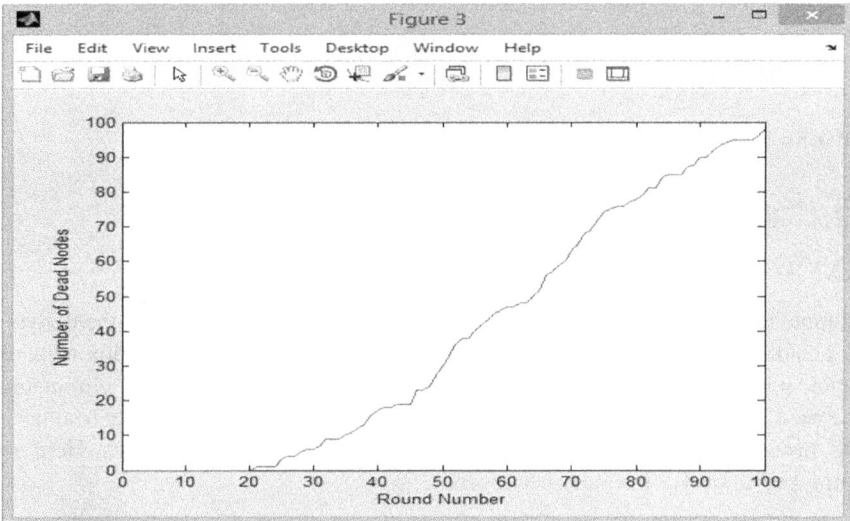

FIGURE 12.13   No. of dead nodes v/s round no. (EAMMH).

In Tables 12.1 and 12.2, a comparison of LEACH and EAMMH performance is presented depending on various factors. The number of dead nodes is used to compare the output of the three methods. The efficiency of the two protocols is compared using their average energy.

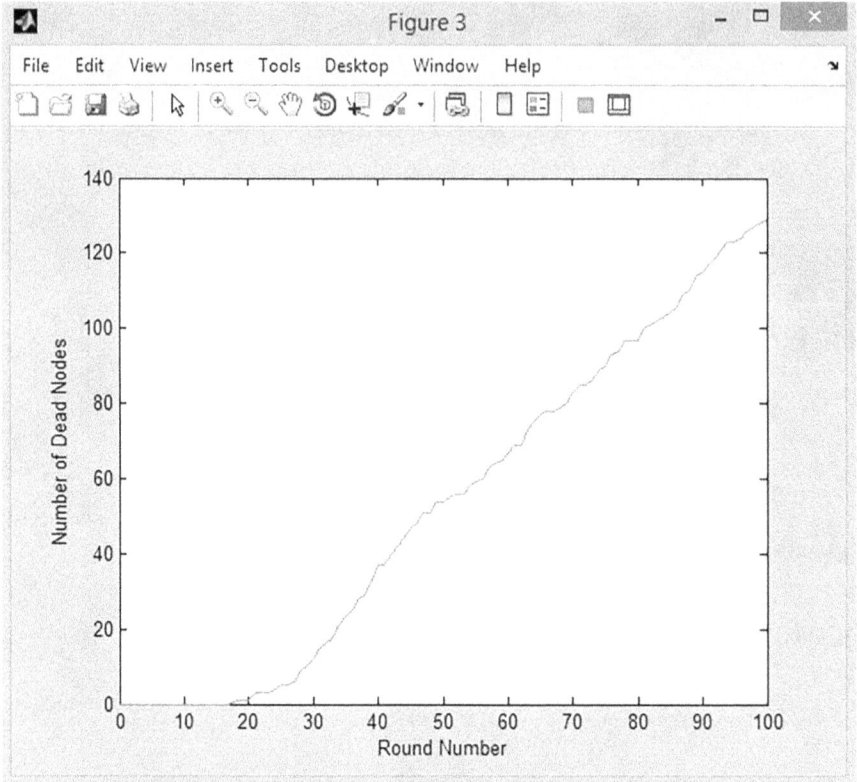

FIGURE 12.14   No. of dead nodes v/s round no. (LEACH).

12.5   REMOTE HEALTHCARE

12.5.1   REMOTE HEALTHCARE AND ITS IMPACT

Remote healthcare, also known as telehealth or telemedicine, refers to the delivery of healthcare services and information through electronic communication technologies. It enables patients and healthcare providers to interact remotely, eliminating the need for in-person visits to healthcare facilities. The impact of remote healthcare has been significant and continues to grow, especially in recent times. Here are some key impacts of remote healthcare:

- Improved Access to Healthcare: Remote healthcare has addressed barriers to access by bringing healthcare services to patients, regardless of their geographical location. It is particularly beneficial for individuals living in rural or underserved areas who may have limited access to healthcare facilities. Through telehealth, patients can consult with healthcare professionals, receive diagnoses, and access treatment without the need for travel.

- Increased Convenience: Remote healthcare provides patients with convenient access to healthcare services. They can schedule appointments and consultations at their preferred time without the need to take time off work or arrange transportation. It reduces waiting times, as patients can connect with healthcare providers virtually and receive prompt attention.
- Cost Savings: Telehealth has the potential to reduce healthcare costs for both patients and providers. Patients can save on transportation expenses and avoid the costs associated with in-person visits, such as parking fees. Remote healthcare also reduces healthcare facility overhead costs and enables providers to reach a larger patient population efficiently, potentially leading to cost savings in the long run.
- Efficient Healthcare Delivery: Remote healthcare improves the efficiency of healthcare delivery. It enables healthcare providers to manage and monitor patients' conditions remotely, reducing the need for frequent hospital visits. Remote monitoring of vital signs, wearable devices, and electronic health records facilitate real-time data collection, analysis, and proactive intervention when necessary.
- Continuity of Care: Telehealth promotes continuity of care by allowing patients to maintain regular contact with their healthcare providers. Follow-up appointments, medication management, and routine check-ups can be conducted remotely, ensuring ongoing care for chronic conditions or post-treatment monitoring.
- Emergency and Disaster Management: Remote healthcare plays a crucial role in emergency and disaster management situations. It allows healthcare providers to triage and provide initial assessments remotely, enabling rapid response and potentially saving lives. Telehealth also helps manage surges in patient volume during public health emergencies by reducing the strain on physical healthcare facilities.
- Patient Engagement and Empowerment: Telehealth promotes patient engagement and empowerment by involving patients in their own healthcare. It encourages active participation, education, and self-management of health conditions. Patients can access educational resources, track their progress, and communicate with healthcare providers, fostering a collaborative approach to healthcare.

It's important to note that while remote healthcare offers numerous benefits, certain limitations exist. Not all medical conditions can be addressed through telehealth, and in-person visits may still be necessary for some situations. Additionally, reliable internet access and technological literacy are essential for effective remote healthcare implementation.

12.5.2 REMOTE HEALTHCARE: GROWING POPULATIONS

Remote healthcare has the potential to tackle the challenges posed by growing populations in several ways:

- Efficient Resource Utilization: As populations grow, healthcare systems face increased pressure on their resources. Remote healthcare helps optimize resource allocation by reducing the burden on physical infrastructure, such as hospitals and clinics. It allows for more efficient use of healthcare personnel, as they can attend to patients remotely, reducing wait times and improving overall efficiency.
- Enhanced Patient Convenience: Remote healthcare offers patients the convenience of accessing medical care from their homes or workplaces. It eliminates the need for traveling long distances, waiting in crowded waiting rooms, or taking time off work. This convenience encourages more individuals to seek timely medical advice, leading to better overall health outcomes.
- Continuous Monitoring and Chronic Disease Management: With remote healthcare technologies, patients can be remotely monitored, allowing for continuous tracking of vital signs, symptoms, and disease progression. This is particularly valuable for managing chronic conditions, where regular check-ups and monitoring are crucial. Remote monitoring helps detect early warning signs, enables timely interventions, and reduces the risk of complications.
- Health Education and Preventive Care: Remote healthcare facilitates the dissemination of health education and preventive care information to a larger population. Through teleconferencing, video consultations, or online platforms, healthcare providers can educate individuals on healthy lifestyles, disease prevention, and self-care strategies. This proactive approach can help reduce the burden on healthcare systems by preventing the onset of avoidable diseases.
- Support for Specialized Consultations: Remote healthcare allows patients to access specialized consultations that may be limited in their local areas. Virtual visits enable patients to connect with experts and specialists remotely, gaining access to specialized knowledge and opinions. This helps ensure that patients receive appropriate care, even if the required expertise is not available locally.

It's important to note that while remote healthcare offers many benefits, it is not a substitute for in-person care in all situations. Certain medical conditions and emergencies may still require physical examinations and interventions. However, when appropriately integrated into healthcare systems, remote healthcare can play a vital role in tackling the challenges posed by growing populations and enhancing healthcare access and delivery.

12.5.3 REMOTE HEALTHCARE: APPLICATIONS

- Remote Consultations: Patients can connect with healthcare professionals remotely, through video calls or phone calls, to discuss their symptoms, receive medical advice, and obtain prescriptions or referrals. This approach is particularly useful for patients in rural or underserved areas who may have limited access to healthcare facilities.

- Monitoring and Management of Chronic Conditions: Remote healthcare enables healthcare providers to remotely monitor patients with chronic conditions such as diabetes, hypertension, or heart disease. Patients can use wearable devices or self-reporting tools to collect and transmit vital signs, medication adherence data, or other relevant information to healthcare professionals. This allows for timely intervention, adjustment of treatment plans, and early detection of potential complications.

- Mental Health Support: Remote healthcare has become increasingly important in the field of mental health. It allows individuals to access counseling, therapy, or psychiatric consultations from the comfort of their homes, removing barriers such as transportation or stigma. Videoconferencing platforms and secure messaging applications facilitate ongoing communication between mental health professionals and their patients.

- Remote Monitoring of Postoperative Patients: After surgical procedures, patients often need close monitoring and follow-up care. Remote healthcare technologies enable healthcare providers to remotely assess patients' recovery progress, review postoperative instructions, and address any concerns. This approach reduces the need for unnecessary hospital visits and minimizes the risk of postoperative complications.

- Remote Education and Training: Remote healthcare extends beyond patient care and can be used for education and training purposes. Healthcare professionals can participate in webinars, online courses, or virtual conferences to enhance their skills and knowledge. Additionally, remote healthcare platforms can facilitate remote supervision and mentoring for medical students, residents, or healthcare professionals in training.

- Health Information Exchange and Collaboration: Remote healthcare technologies allow healthcare providers to securely exchange patient information, medical records, and test results, facilitating collaboration and coordination among different healthcare professionals. This improves the continuity of care, particularly in complex cases or when involving multiple specialists.

- Health and Wellness Monitoring: Remote healthcare applications can be used to monitor individuals' overall health and wellness. For example, wearable devices or smartphone applications can track physical activity, sleep patterns, heart rate, or stress levels. These data can be shared with healthcare providers, who can provide personalized recommendations and interventions to improve health outcomes.

- Remote healthcare has the potential to enhance access to healthcare services, improve patient outcomes, and reduce healthcare costs. However, it is important to note that certain medical conditions or emergencies may still require in-person care. Remote healthcare should be used as a complement to traditional healthcare and tailored to the specific needs of each patient [9].

12.5.4 REMOTE HEALTHCARE: MONITORING SYSTEM

A remote health monitoring system refers to a technology-enabled platform that allows healthcare providers to monitor and track the health status of patients remotely, without the need for in-person visits. This system typically involves the use of various devices, sensors, and communication technologies to collect and transmit patient data to healthcare professionals for analysis and intervention [10].

Here are some key components and features commonly found in a remote health monitoring system:

- Monitoring Devices: These can include wearable devices such as fitness trackers, smart watches, or medical-grade sensors that can measure vital signs like heart rate, blood pressure, blood glucose levels, oxygen saturation, or even activity levels.
- Data Transmission: Patient data collected from monitoring devices is transmitted securely through wireless technologies like Bluetooth, Wi-Fi, or cellular networks to a centralized platform or healthcare provider's system.
- Cloud-Based Platform: The collected data is stored and processed in a secure cloud-based platform accessible to healthcare providers. This platform allows real-time monitoring, analysis, and interpretation of the patient's health status.
- Alerts and Notifications: The system can generate alerts and notifications based on predefined thresholds or abnormal data patterns. This enables healthcare providers to receive timely information about changes in a patient's condition that may require immediate attention or intervention.
- Electronic Health Records Integration: Remote health monitoring systems can integrate with electronic health record (EHR) systems, ensuring seamless integration of patient data with the existing healthcare infrastructure. This facilitates a comprehensive view of the patient's health history and enhances clinical decision making.
- Patient Engagement: Remote monitoring systems often include patient-facing applications or portals that allow individuals to actively participate in their own care. They can view their health data, set personal goals, receive educational materials, and communicate with healthcare providers through secure messaging [11].
- Analytics and Insights: Advanced analytics tools enable healthcare professionals to derive meaningful insights from the collected data. These insights can help identify trends, predict potential health issues, and personalize treatment plans based on individual patient needs.

12.5.5 REMOTE HEALTHCARE: BENEFITS

- Improved access to healthcare, especially for individuals in remote areas or with limited mobility.
- Early detection of health problems and proactive intervention, potentially reducing hospital admissions and emergency room visits.

- Enhanced patient engagement and self-management, empowering individuals to actively participate in their care.
- Continuous monitoring of chronic conditions, allowing healthcare providers to make data-driven decisions and adjust treatment plans as needed.
- Cost savings for patients and healthcare systems, as remote monitoring can reduce the need for frequent in-person visits and hospital stays.
- It's important to note that while remote health monitoring systems can provide valuable insights and support, they should not replace face-to-face medical care entirely. They are most effective when used in conjunction with traditional healthcare services and under the guidance of healthcare professionals [12].

12.5.6 Remote Healthcare: Features

- Virtual Consultations: Remote healthcare allows patients to consult with healthcare providers through video or audio calls, eliminating the need for in-person visits. Patients can discuss their symptoms, receive medical advice, and get prescriptions remotely.
- Real-Time Communication: Remote healthcare platforms facilitate real-time communication between patients and healthcare professionals. This enables patients to ask questions, seek clarifications, and receive immediate guidance, ensuring timely access to medical advice.
- Electronic Health Records (EHRs): Remote healthcare systems often integrate electronic health records, allowing healthcare providers to access patients' medical history, test results, and treatment plans remotely. This promotes continuity of care and assists in making informed decisions.
- Remote Monitoring: Advanced remote healthcare solutions enable the monitoring of patients' health parameters from a distance. This may involve wearable devices, sensors, or home monitoring kits that collect and transmit data, such as heart rate, blood pressure, glucose levels, or sleep patterns. Healthcare providers can remotely analyze this data and intervene when necessary.
- Prescription and Refill Management: Remote healthcare platforms enable healthcare professionals to issue electronic prescriptions and manage prescription refills. Patients can receive their prescribed medications through online pharmacies, saving time and effort.
- Online Health Portals and Apps: Many remote healthcare services offer dedicated online portals or mobile apps that allow patients to schedule appointments, access medical records, communicate with healthcare providers, and receive educational resources or preventive care guidance.
- Remote Diagnostic Support: Remote healthcare can leverage technologies like high-quality imaging, remote pathology, and diagnostic tools that enable healthcare providers to remotely assess and diagnose certain

conditions. This can be particularly useful in situations where in-person consultations are not readily available.

- Behavioral Health Support: Remote healthcare extends to mental health services as well. Patients can receive counseling, therapy sessions, and support for mental health conditions through video or audio calls, providing accessibility and privacy.

- Remote Second Opinions: Remote healthcare facilitates obtaining second opinions from specialists located anywhere in the world. Patients can share their medical reports and diagnostic images securely for remote review, enabling them to benefit from diverse medical expertise.

- Education and Training: Remote healthcare platforms can be utilized for educational purposes, such as conducting virtual medical conferences, training programs, and continuing medical education (CME) sessions. This allows healthcare professionals to stay updated with the latest advancements and enhance their skills.

12.6   CONCLUSION AND FUTURE RESEARCH

Wireless sensor networks are often largely distributed over a wide area. In this regard, we need a way to better manage our WSNs. Limited battery capacity is used for wireless sensor networks. A major challenge in developing protocols for wireless sensor networks is energy efficiency due to the limited capacity of sensor nodes. The ultimate motivation behind any routing protocol is to keep the network running as energy efficiently as possible for the long term. In this work, we introduced clustering as a means to overcome this energy efficiency problem. A detailed description of the process of the two protocols, LEACH and EAMMH, is available. From a brief analysis of simulations, we conclude that LEACH can be used on small grids with a total of less than 50 nodes when LEACH slightly outperforms EAMMH and LEACH, and when the heuristic probability of cluster head selection is high.

Remote healthcare collectively enhances healthcare accessibility, enables early intervention, reduces geographical barriers, and improves patient outcomes by offering remote medical services. However, it's important to note that not all medical conditions can be effectively addressed through remote healthcare, and in certain cases, in-person consultations may still be required.

REFERENCES

1. O. Younis and S. Fahmy, "HEED: A Hybrid, Energy Efficient, Distributed Clustering Approach for Ad Hoc Sensor Networks," *IEEE Transaction on Mobile Computing*, vol. 3, no. 4, pp. 366–379, 2004.
2. V. Mhatre and C. Rosenberg, "Homogeneous vs Heterogeneous Clustered Sensor Networks: A Comparative Study," Communications, 2004 IEEE International Conference on, vol. 6, pp. 3646–3651. IEEE, 2004. 10.1109/ICC.2004.1313223
3. S. Peng, "Energy Neutral Directed Diffusion for Energy Harvesting Wireless Sensor Networks," *Computer Communication*, vol. 63, pp. 40–52, 2015. 10.1016/j.comcom.2015.02.017

4. A. Kumar, R. Dhanagopal, M. A. Albreem and D. Le, "A Comprehensive Study on the Role of Advanced Technologies in 5G Based Smart Hospital," *Alexandria Engineering Journal*, vol. 60, pp. 5527–5536, 2021.
5. B. Ramakrishnan, A. Kumar, S. Chakravarty, M. Masud and M. Baz, "Analysis of FBMC Waveform for 5G Network Based Smart Hospitals," *Applied Sciences*, vol. 11, no. 19, pp. 8895, 2021. 10.3390/app11198895
6. S. K. Singh, P. Kumar and J. P. Singh, "A Survey on Successors of LEACH Protocol," *IEEE Access*, vol. 5, pp. 4298–4328, 2017. 10.1109/access.2017.2666082
7. S. Han, Z. Gong and W. Meng, "Automatic Precision Control Positioning for Wireless Sensor Network," *IEEE Sensors Journal*, vol. 16, no. 7, pp. 2140–2150, 2016. 10.1109/JSEN.2015.2506166
8. A. Kashaf et al., "TSEP: Threshold-Sensitive Stable Election Protocol for WSNs," 10th International Conference on Frontiers of Information Technology (FIT), pp. 164–168, 2012. 10.1109/FIT.2012.37
9. S. Jiang, "LEACH Protocol Analysis and Optimization of Wireless Sensor Networks Based on PSO and AC," 2018 10th International Conference on Intelligent Human-Machine Systems and Cybernetics (IHMSC), pp. 246–250, 2018. 10.1109/IHMSC.2018.10163.
10. G. S. Kumar, M. Paul and K. Jacob, "Mobility Metric Based LEACH Mobile Protocol," Proceedings of 16th International Conference on Advanced Computing and Communications, 2008. 10.1109/ADCOM.2008.4760456.
11. A. Kumar, M. A. Albreem, M. Gupta, M. H. Alsharif and S. Kim, "Future 5G Network Based Smart Hospitals: Hybrid Detection Technique for Latency Improvement," *IEEE Access*, vol. 8, pp. 153240–153249, 2020. 10.1109/ACCESS.2020.3017625.
12. A. Kumar and M. Gupta, "A Review on Activities of Fifth Generation Mobile Communication System," *Alexandria Engineering Journal*, vol. 57, no. 2, pp. 1125–1135, 2017.

13 Smart Wearable Devices for Healthcare Applications Using 5G Network

Murthy Muniyappa, Mahesh Shastri, S Rohith, and K N Nagesh
Department of Electronics and Communication,
Nagarjuna College of Engineering and Technology, India

K Aravinda
Department of Electronics and Communication,
New Horizon College of Engineering, India

Dinesh Rangappa
Department of Applied Science (Nanotechnology),
Visvesvaraya Technological University, India

13.1 INTRODUCTION

By delivering vital signs in real time, smart wearables improve the quality of healthcare and allow improved diagnostic tools to treat patients with advanced treatments. The purpose of smart wearable technology is to provide information about medical problems and associated solutions [1]. To monitor patient health status continually medical equipment's based on IoT connections play a major role. Even applications of wearable devices are commonly found in IoT for 5G connectivity, fog computing to monitor health, sports, and fitness [2]. Recent research surveys indicate that the IoT-based healthcare sector attracted investments worth $330 billion. Telemedicine services gained popularity after the COVID-19 outbreak. Systems are coupled to wearable technology that allows for constant patient monitoring. Many healthcare practitioners were able to offer their services remotely and on demand because of technology [3]. For the patients with chronic illnesses, such as cardiovascular diseases, neurological disorders, and diabetes, real-time and continuous monitoring highly recommended.

DOI: 10.1201/9781003403678-13

The World Health Organization (WHO) estimates that chronic diseases cause three-quarters (75%) of global mortality and have significant economic costs. Therefore, many approaches are needed for the monitoring and diagnosis of such disorders, and in this regard, wearable health monitoring wearable devices (HWDs) are a successful approach.

Wearable devices are the devices worn on the human body or on cloth. Wearable devices are designed using a transducer and a target receptor. When a receptor detects the target analyte, it reacts appropriately. The response from the receptor is subsequently transformed into a meaningful signal by the transducer. Wearable technology has been used in numerous studies across a variety of industries, and thanks to their flexibility and compliance, these gadgets have demonstrated promising outcomes in the healthcare sector. These HWDs aid in avoiding and treating diseases by giving a clearer understanding of the alterations that occur within the human body.

It allows remote health diagnosis facility that in turn helps in reduction of travel time treatment costs and aids in expanding their services beyond geographical region. Smart devices for healthcare are necessary to ensure that people receive health services as smart cities grow in number. In addition to improving well-being, prompt diagnosis can significantly lower healthcare costs. For instance, it is projected that the market for smart healthcare that makes use of the IoT will reach $158.1 billion in 2022 [2].

The 5G networks will be important for facilitating the broad adoption of IoT [3]. Also, smart healthcare services are important applications for the 5G network [4]. Figure 13.1 shows the general architecture of the 5G-based smart healthcare network and its main entities.

IoT can enhance a number of applications in smart healthcare, such as quality management in hospitals, remote monitoring, smarter medication, and telemedicine [2]. In the near future, these applications will be crucial to the medical industry.

Smart antennas are crucial for 5G network connectivity [5]. To increase 5G coverage and capacity, smart antennas make use of numerous significant advancements [6]. One such breakthrough is beam forming, which concentrates RF energy into a small beam where it is needed rather than diffusing it over a wide area [7]. The higher frequency millimeter wave RF is susceptible to fading due to authentication loss and distance caused by objects striking it (such as cars, buildings, etc.). Hence, beam forming is especially helpful for 5GNR [8]. A more well-coordinated RF energy beam makes it more likely that the transmission capacity and signal quality will be optimal. But it's crucial to remember that the line of location without any interference [9].

The 5G networks are projected to offer a higher data rate for many IoT devices, even though it is very dense. It must be versatile and adaptable to support new applications. Along with large data rates, these applications must also offer massive connection, compact distribution, dependability, excellent efficiency in energy, and long-distance coverage.

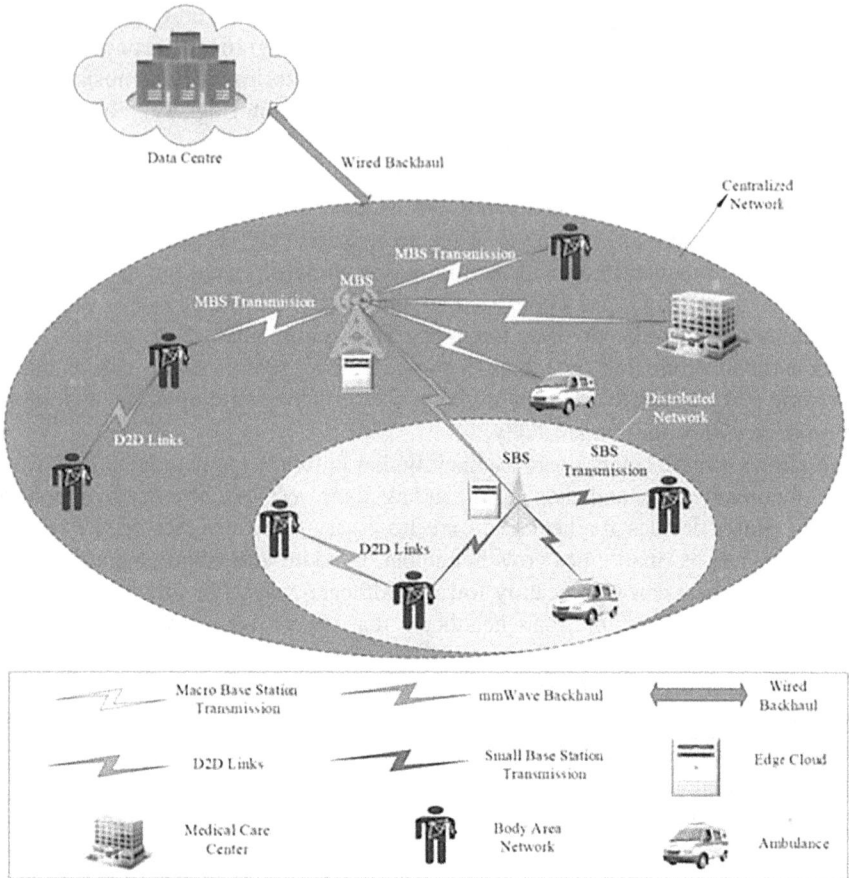

FIGURE 13.1   A general architecture of smart healthcare network based on 5G [4].

13.2   SMART DEVICES

For various medical applications, several distinct non-intrusive sensor types have been developed, making them appropriate for wireless sensor network-dependent medical healthcare services [10]. They are also adequate for the IoT to provide the same services. In addition to network densification and assistance for many IoT-based devices, 5G is projected to offer a higher data rate. Also, 5G must be versatile and adaptable to support new applications. Along with large data rates, these applications must also offer massive connection, dense deployment, dependability, low latency, excellent energy efficiency, and long-distance communication [11].

13.2.1   WEARABLE DEVICE ACCESS (WDA)

The 5G networks must be versatile and adaptable to support new applications (4). Along with large data rates, these applications must also offer massive connection and long-distance coverage. Semantic-oriented systems should be able to handle natural language execution techniques in order to enhance user experience, generate identifiable specimens based on previously obtained knowledge, and have impressive computing capabilities [12].

13.2.2 Applications of Wearable Devices

There are many applications of wearable devices such as the following.

Glucose Sensing: Diabetes is a group of metabolic disorders characterized by elevated blood glucose levels (sugar). A diet, exercise routine, and medication schedule can all be planned with the use of blood glucose monitoring, which also detects variations in blood glucose levels [13]. The strategy described in this article involves connecting patient-related sensors to leading healthcare organizations using an IPv6 network.

Electrocardiogram (ECG) Monitoring: The examination of the human heart's electrical activity record, or an ECG, includes estimating the simple pulse and identifying the vital rhythm in addition to identifying complicated late QT intervals, arrhythmias, and myocardial ischemias [14].

Blood Pressure (BP) Monitoring: It uses sensors to detect the signal of pulse and pressure and then shows the result in digital format. These sensors include electronic pressure and pulsating sensors. In this article, a gadget that collects data and sends it over the network is demonstrated [4]. A mechanical assembly for measuring blood pressure and a communication component make up the gadget. The authors [15] present a location-aware intelligent terminal for IoT network-supported continuous blood pressure monitoring.

Body Temperature Supervising: A key component of intelligent healthcare is the control of body temperature. Consequently, a critical indicator in the body is temperature, which maintains stability of the body. A sensor that measures body temperature that is implanted in the TelosB is used to realize the m-IoT idea. The constructed m-IoT system's functionality is then demonstrated by checking the mill trail for actual body temperature data [16].

Checking Saturation of Oxygen: Monitoring blood oxygen saturation secretly with heartbeat oximetry is possible. Applications for smart healthcare that are driven by change can benefit from the integration of heartbeat oximetry and IoT [17]. The system makes use of sensors and Bluetooth health device profiles that are directly connected to the secure platform.

13.3 CIRCUMSTANCES OF 5G NETWORK AND ITS PREREQUISITES

Four possible 5G network circumstances shown below can be categorized. The specifications and technology advancements needed are shown in Figure 13.2.

13.3.1 Enhanced Mobile Broadband (EMB)

The specifications, for instance, are as follows: The maximum data rate and capacity is 20 Gbps and 10 Mbps, respectively. The important objectives are to boost the network's data throughput and traffic capacity [18].

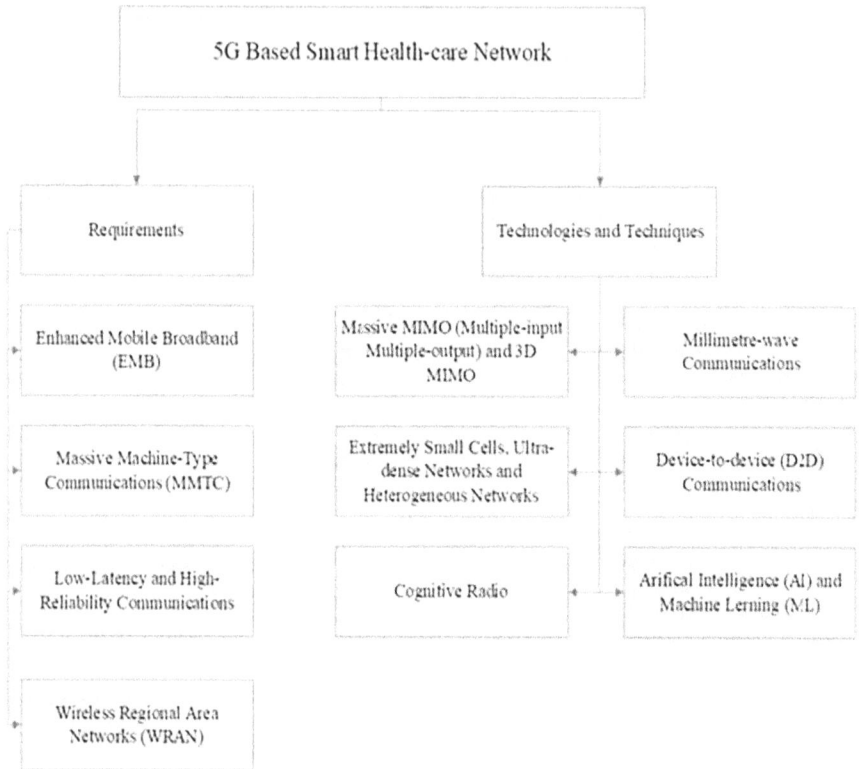

FIGURE 13.2 Technologies and prerequisite trend of smart healthcare powered by 5G [4].

13.3.2 MASSIVE MACHINE-TYPE COMMUNICATIONS (MMTC)

The machine-to-machine (M2M), wireless sensor networks (WSNs) and Internet of Things are all referenced in the scenario. In this scenario, density of connectivity and power efficiency are the main objectives. For instance, the connectivity density is 106 devices/m^2. The network's devices must have ten-year usable life span [19].

13.3.3 LOW-LATENCY AND HIGH-RELIABILITY COMMUNICATIONS

The issue is related to tactile internet applications and extremely trustworthy connectivity, such as autonomous car communications with ambulances and remote surgery. Excellent reliability and low latency are crucial in this situation [20].

13.4 TECHNOLOGIES REQUIREMENTS IN THE 5G NETWORK

The key requirements are extremely high connection density, traffic capacity, and high data rates. These criteria can be realized through a variety of technology advancements, which can also be leveraged to help realize the stated 5G network needs [21].

13.4.1 MULTIPLE-INPUT MULTIPLE-OUTPUT (MIMO)

The MIMO system can address the initial trend for the fifth-generation (5G) network by achieving a high data rate [22].

A massive MIMO uses multiple antennas that support numerous terminals simultaneously [23]. The 3D MIMO controls the horizontal and vertical directions and cell partitioning. However, SNR can be enhanced to manage antenna coverage, which results in a reduction in transmission power or an increase in link capacity. Figure 13.3 depicts the MIMO and 3D MIMO concepts [24].

13.4.2 MILLIMETER WAVE COMMUNICATIONS

An increased data rate is the effect of the high bandwidth channel. However, millimeter wave communications have a lot of drawbacks. The millimeter wave free-space propagation causes increased signal attenuation [26]. Second, reasonable observers of this band include rain, atmospheric gases, and structures [27].

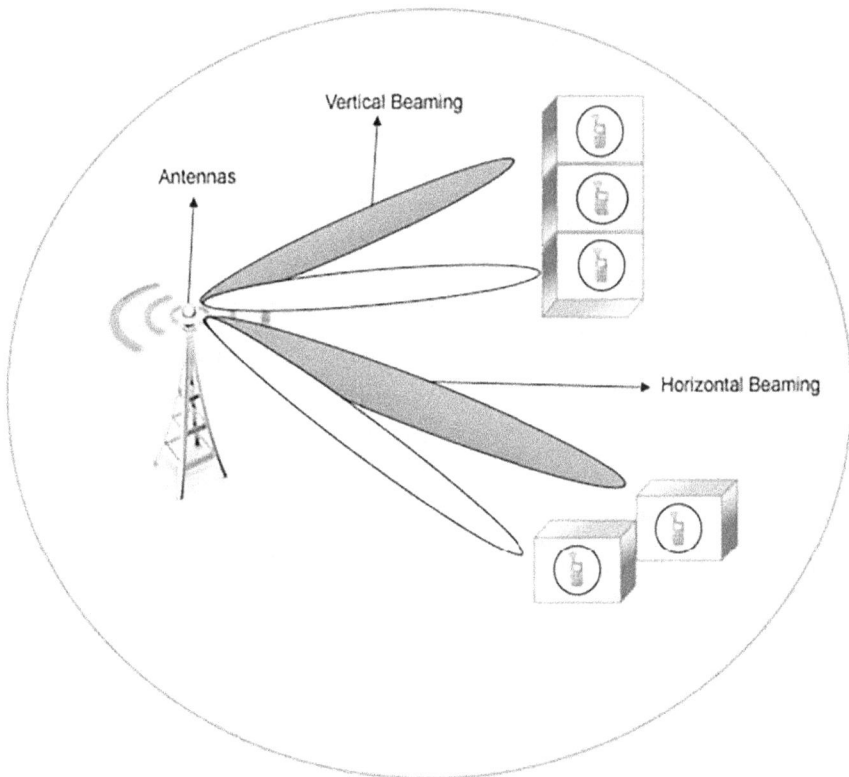

FIGURE 13.3 Massive MIMO and 3D MIMO [25].

There are several potential solutions to the problem, as was previously mentioned: smaller cells will reduce attenuations; for larger attenuations, directed antennas or inside base stations should be utilized to minimize the problem of building absorption.

13.4.3 SMALL CELLS AND HETEROGENEOUS NETWORKS

In 5G, the employment of small cells in the context of an extremely dense network is the key feature in addition to cell sectoring and frequency reutilisation. Additionally, the usage of tiny cells maximizes SNR while minimizing transmission power; this lowers communication power, increases link capacity, and increases energy savings. Another trend for 5G is a heterogeneous network made up of tiny cells, macro cells, pico cells, and femto cells. In this scenario, the macro cells help the control panel by providing connectivity and mobility [27]. Figure 13.4 depicts this concept. However, it is crucial to remember that tiny cells are not appropriate.

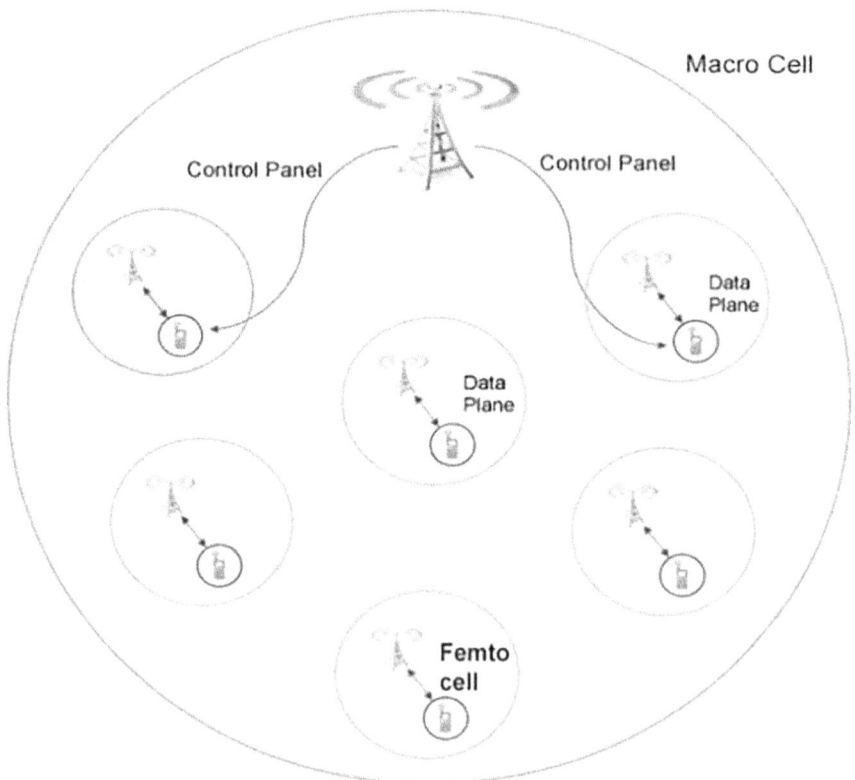

FIGURE 13.4   Heterogeneous network [25].

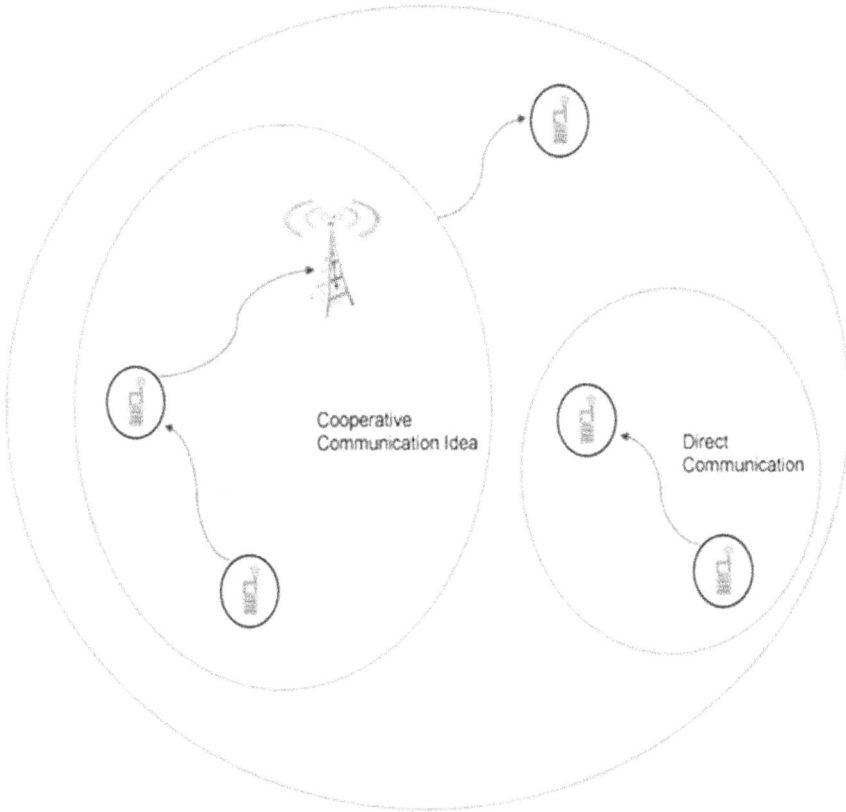

FIGURE 13.5 D2D approaches [25].

13.4.4 DEVICE-TO-DEVICE (D2D) COMMUNICATIONS

In direct terminal-to-terminal communication, the base station is excluded. It can increase system throughput, channel dependability, and operating costs. Figure 13.5 depicts both base stations working and D2D strategies. It enables several D2D lines to share the common bandwidth simultaneously, resulting in an increase in cell traffic capacity. Finally, D2D direct communication provides the reduction in radio link latency in the network [28].

13.4.5 COGNITIVE RADIO

The cognitive radio (CR) technology is considered as an important future for 5G. The WRAN scenario may only be enabled through the use of cognitive radio technology [29]. In CR, users are sub-divided into two groups. In the first group, the primary users are allocated and in the second group, secondary users are allocated. The CR system uses the concept of spectrum overlay and spectrum underlay. In the spectrum overlay, both primary and secondary users can transmit the data at the same time.

13.4.6 ARTIFICIAL INTELLIGENCE (AI) AND MACHINE LEARNING (ML) IN SMART HEALTHCARE

Artificial intelligence and machine learning are still being used in the early stages of developing smart healthcare apps for wireless networks. The 5G network's topology, propagation models, mobility of nodes, and network design can all be intricate. In order to help and manage various network resources, AI and ML can therefore play crucial roles [30]. Three methods can be used to implement AI and ML in a network. The network's edge devices can each use AI and ML algorithms for speedy operations requirements [31]. These algorithms can be implemented on a per-device basis in edge devices to enable rapid calculation and decision making for low latency IoT services [32].

13.5 FUTURE PERSPECTIVES

In addition to the above-mentioned developments, implementing 5G for smart healthcare comes with a number of difficulties and open research challenges.

13.5.1 INTEROPERABILITY

The IoT devices in a smart healthcare network come in a variety of shapes and interoperability is essential because it provides a foundation for connecting to many devices using various communication techniques. Yet, because there aren't any widely established standards for communications technology, the interoperability between different sectors is a significant obstacle to the adoption of the IoT [33]. In order to ensure interoperability at various levels and enable millions of devices in the network to connect with one another, a vital intelligent strategy is needed. Multiple organizations, including FIWARE and oneM2M, are collaborating with various standardizations, including 3GPP, OMA, and ETSI [34].

13.5.2 BIG DATA ANALYSIS

Big data analysis is a critical field of study in a smart healthcare network. The future smart healthcare network's millions of gadgets will produce vast volumes of data that can be analyzed [35]. Private user information about the patient (also known as patient data) and details about the patient's surrounding environment are among these data (i.e., heartbeat rate, ECG, etc.). As a result, data analysis requires innovative algorithms and approaches.

13.5.3 IoT CONNECTIVITY

The IoT devices have the ability to offer information after sensing. Any contemporary communication technology, including Bluetooth, Wi-Fi, and cellular networks, can be used by IoT devices to connect to this network (5G and LTE) [36]. The smart healthcare network faces numerous difficulties in ensuring connectivity to every device, including ensuring connectivity to the network's high mobility devices (such as moving patients and high-speed ambulances).

13.5.4 ATTAINING SECURITY, TRUST, AND PRIVACY

Security is a major problem because many IoT devices are connected to one another. IoT devices have limited battery life and computing capacity make it difficult to integrate complex security algorithms and protocols. The majority of IoT devices will be vulnerable to assault in the future. This could lead to a range of risks and assaults with regard to privacy and security [37].

13.6 CONCLUSIONS

It will be vital to deploy fifth-generation (5G) networks in applications for wearable and IoT technology in the healthcare sector. From the perspectives of functional and financial, applications of IoT are essential to the 5G network. This study compared the range, frequency, power consumption, and data rate of short- and long-range communication technologies for smart healthcare from various perspectives. Four distinct scenarios were also taken into consideration in accordance with various 5G network requirements and various technology trends were presented and thoroughly discussed in order to meet these requirements.

REFERENCES

1. P. Sundaravadivel, E. Kougianos, S. Mohanty, and M. Ganapathiraju, "Everything You Wanted to Know about Smart Health Care: Evaluating the Different Technologies and Components of the Internet of Things for Better Health," *IEEE Consumer Electronics Magazine*, vol. 7, pp. 18–28, January 2018, 10.1109/MCE.2017.2755378.
2. J. M. C. Brito, "Technological Trends for 5G Networks Influence of E-Health and IoT Applications," *International Journal of E-Health and Medical Communications*, vol. 9, no. 1, pp. 1–22, January 2018, 10.4018/IJEHMC.2018010101.
3. J. J. P. C. Rodrigues, L. M. C. C. Pedro, T. Vardasca, I. de la Torre-Díez, and H. M. G. Martins, "Mobile Health Platform for Pressure Ulcer Monitoring with Electronic Health Record Integration," *Health Informatics Journal*, vol. 19, no. 4, pp. 300–311, December 2013, 10.1177/1460458212474909.
4. A. Kumar, M. A. Albreem, M. Gupta, M. H. Alsharif, and S. Kim, "Future 5G Network Based Smart Hospitals: Hybrid Detection Technique for Latency Improvement," *IEEE Access*, vol. 8, pp. 153240–153249, 2020, 10.1109/access.2020.3017625.
5. N. O. Parchin, H. J. Basherlou, Y. I. A. Al-Yasir, R. A. Abd-Alhameed, A. M. Abdulkhaleq, and J. M. Noras, "Recent Developments of Reconfigurable Antennas for Current and Future Wireless Communication Systems," *Electronics*, vol. 8, no. 2, pp. 1–17, 2019a, 10.3390/electronics8020128.
6. N. O. Parchin, "Low-Profile Air-Filled Antenna for Next Generation Wireless Systems," *Wireless Personal Communications*, vol. 97, no. 3, pp. 3293–3300, December 2017, 10.1007/s11277-017-4519-2.
7. N. O. Parchin, M. Alibakhshikenari, H. J. Basherlou, R. A. Abd-Alhameed, J. Rodriguez, and E. Limiti, "MM-Wave Phased Array Quasi-Yagi Antenna for the Upcoming 5G Cellular Communications," *Applied Sciences*, vol. 9, no. 5, 2019b, 10.3390/app9050978.

8. H. Saeidi-Manesh and G. Zhang, "Low Cross-Polarization, High-Isolation Microstrip Patch Antenna Array for Multi-Mission Applications," *IEEE Access*, vol. 7, pp. 5026–5033, January 2019, 10.1109/ACCESS.2018.2889599.

9. M. Alibakhshi-Kenari, M. Naser-Moghadasi, R. A. Sadeghzadeh, B. S. Virdee, and E. Limiti, "Periodic Array of Complementary Artificial Magnetic Conductor Metamaterials-Based Multiband Antennas for Broadband Wireless Transceivers," *IET Microwaves, Antennas & Propagation*, vol. 10, no. 15, pp. 1682–1691, 2016, 10.1049/iet-map.2016.0069.

10. A. Haleem, M. Javaid, R. P. Singh, R. Suman, and S. Rab, "Biosensors Applications in Medical Field: A Brief Review," *Sensors International*, vol. 2, p. 100100, 2021, 10.1016/j.sintl.2021.100100.

11. M. Attaran, "The Impact of 5G on the Evolution of Intelligent Automation and Industry Digitization," *Journal of Ambient Intelligence and Humanized Computing*, vol. 14, pp. 5977–5993, 2021, 10.1007/s12652-020-02521-x.

12. B. Manaris, "Natural Language Processing: A Human-Computer Interaction Perspective," *Advances in Computers*, vol. 47, pp. 1–66, December 1998, 10.1016/S0065-2458(08)60665-8.

13. R. S. H. Istepanian, S. Hu, N. Philip, and A. Sungoor, "The Potential of Internet of M-Health Things M-IoT for Non-invasive Glucose Level Sensing," *Annual International Conference of the IEEE Engineering in Medicine and Biology Society*, vol. 2011, pp. 5264–5266, August 2011, 10.1109/IEMBS.2011.6091302.

14. S. H. Liu, C. B. Lin, Y. Chen, W. Chen, T. S. Huang, and C. Y. Hsu, "An EMG Patch for the Real-Time Monitoring of Muscle-Fatigue Conditions During Exercise," *Sensors (Basel)*, vol. 19, no. 14, July 2019, 10.3390/s19143108.

15. A. Al-Qatatsheh et al., "Blood Pressure Sensors: Materials, Fabrication Methods, Performance Evaluations and Future Perspectives," *Sensors*, vol. 20, no. 16, pp. 1–75, 2020, 10.3390/s20164484.

16. J. Hill and D. Culler, "A Wireless Embedded Sensor Architecture for System-Level Optimization," November 2002.

17. H. A. Khattak, M. Ruta, and E. Di Sciascio, "CoAP-Based Healthcare Sensor Networks: A Survey," *Proceedings of 2014 11th International Bhurban Conference on Applied Sciences & Technology (IBCAST) Islamabad, Pakistan, 14th–18th January, 2014*, Islamabad, Pakistan, 2014, pp. 499–503, 10.1109/IBCAST.2014.6778196.

18. H. Yu, H. Lee, and H. Jeon, "What is 5G? Emerging 5G Mobile Services and Network Requirements," *Sustainability*, vol. 9, no. 10, 2017, 10.3390/su9101848.

19. N. Al-Falahy and O. Y. Alani, "Technologies for 5G Networks: Challenges and Opportunities," *IT Professional*, vol. 19, no. 1, pp. 12–20, 2017, 10.1109/MITP.2017.9.

20. S. Tanwar, S. Tyagi, I. Budhiraja, and N. Kumar, "Tactile Internet for Autonomous Vehicles: Latency and Reliability Analysis," *IEEE Wireless Communications*, vol. 26, no. 4, pp. 66–72, April 2019, 10.1109/MWC.2019.1800553.

21. Z. Ma, Y. Xiao, H. V. Poor, B. Vucetic, and M. Xiao, "High-Reliability and Low-Latency Wireless Communication for Internet of Things: Challenges, Fundamentals and Enabling Technologies," *IEEE Internet Things J.*, vol. 6, pp. 7946–7970, October 2020, 10.1109/JIOT.2019.2907245.

22. A. Kartun-Giles, S. Jayaprakasam, and S. Kim, "Euclidean Matchings in Ultra-Dense Networks," *IEEE Communications Letters*, vol. 22, no. 6, pp. 1216–1219, 2018, 10.1109/LCOMM.2018.2799207.

23. M. Usama and M. Erol-Kantarci, "A Survey on Recent Trends and Open Issues in Energy Efficiency of 5G," *Sensors*, vol. 19, no. 14. 2019, 10.3390/s19143126.

24. R. Chataut and R. Akl, "Massive MIMO Systems for 5G and beyond Networks-Overview, Recent Trends, Challenges, and Future Research Direction," *Sensors (Basel)*, vol. 20, no. 10, May 2020, 10.3390/s20102753.

25. K. N. R. S. V. Prasad, E. Hossain, and V. K. Bhargava, "Energy Efficiency in Massive MIMO-Based 5G Networks: Opportunities and Challenges," *IEEE Wireless Communications*, vol. 24, no. 3, pp. 1–8, 2020.
26. Federal Communications Commission Office of Engineering and Technology New Technology Development Division, "Federal Communications Commission Office of Engineering and Millimeter Wave Propagation: Spectrum Management Implications Mail Stop Code 1300-E," no. 70, 1997.
27. L. Wei, R. Q. Hu, Y. Qian, and G. Wu, "Key Elements to Enable Millimeter Wave Communications for 5G Wireless Systems," *IEEE Wireless Communications*, vol. 21, no. 6, pp. 136–143, 2014, 10.1109/MWC.2014.7000981.
28. M. Kazeminia, M. Mehrjoo, and S. Tomasin, "Delay-Aware Spectrum Sharing Solutions for Mixed Cellular and D2D Links," *Computer Communications*, vol. 139, pp. 58–66, 2019, 10.1016/j.comcom.2019.03.011.
29. G. P. Joshi, S. Y. Nam, and S. W. Kim, "Cognitive Radio Wireless Sensor Networks: Applications, Challenges and Research Trends," *Sensors (Basel)*, vol. 13, no. 9, pp. 11196–11228, August 2013, 10.3390/s130911196.
30. Y. Fu, S. Wang, C. X. Wang, X. Hong, and M. Stephen, "Artificial Intelligence to Manage Network Traffic of 5G Wireless Networks," *IEEE Network*, vol. 32, pp. 58–64, November 2018, 10.1109/MNET.2018.1800115.
31. A. Kumar and H. Sharma, "Intelligent Cognitive Radio Spectrum Sensing Based on Energy Detection for Advanced Waveforms," *Radio Electronics and Communication Systems*, vol. 65, no. 3, pp. 175–181, 2022.
32. D. K. Kumar, "IoT-Edge Communication Protocol Based on Low Latency for Effective Data Flow and Distributed Neural Network in a Big Data Environment," *Microprocessors and Microsystems*, vol. 81, p. 103642, 2021, 10.1016/j.micpro.2020.103642.
33. S. Cheruvu, A. Kumar, N. Smith, and D. M. Wheeler (Eds.), "IoT Frameworks and Complexity BT - Demystifying Internet of Things Security: Successful IoT Device/Edge and Platform Security Deployment," in *Demystifying Internet of Things Security: Successful IoT Device/Edge and Platform Security Deployment Paperback*, Berkeley, CA: Apress, 2020, pp. 23–148.
34. AIOTI WG Standardisation, "Edge Computing Standard Framework Concepts," *Alliance for Internet of Things Innovation (AIOTI)*, pp. 1–95, 2021, https://aioti.eu/wp-content/uploads/2021/09/AIOTI-SDOs_alliance_landscape_edge_computing_standard_framework_R1-Published.pdf
35. S. Dash, S. K. Shakyawar, M. Sharma, and S. Kaushik, "Big Data in Healthcare: Management, Analysis and Future Prospects," *Journal of Big Data*, vol. 6, no. 1, p. 54, 2019, 10.1186/s40537-019-0217-0.
36. P. Sethi and S. R. Sarangi, "Internet of Things: Architectures, Protocols, and Applications," *Journal of Electrical and Computer Engineering*, vol. 2017, p. 9324035, 2017, 10.1155/2017/9324035.
37. K. T. Nguyen, M. Laurent, and N. Oualha, "Survey on Secure Communication Protocols for the Internet of Things," *Ad Hoc Networks*, vol. 32, pp. 17–31, 2015, https://doi.org/10.1016/j.adhoc.2015.01.006.

14 Semantic Separation-Based Kinematic Tracking with IoT and AI
Implementation and Challenges

Sumit Chakravarty
Electrical and Computer Engineering, Kennesaw State University, USA

Imtiaz Ahmed
Department of Electrical Engineering and Computer Science, Howard University, USA

Arun Kumar
Department of Electronics and Communication, New Horizon College of Engineering, India

14.1 INTRODUCTION

With the developing advantages of applied machine learning in regard to image processing applications, the efficacy of automating complex data collection schemes in the field is becoming more and more feasible. The aim of this project is to construct a modular and adaptive framework of image processing technologies, in order to efficiently generate kinematic models of a batter's motion in swing [1]. This framework is devised with the intent for use in the field, capable of functioning with real-world footage of the batter's box. In the following sections, each aspect of such a framework will be discussed in order of importance. Written primarily within the MATLAB interface and supplemented by several excursions into C++ and Python, Scap-Trac (the program) has been designed to accomplish outlined goals. As outlined in the Program Block Diagram (Figure 14.1) in the appendix, the primary script follows a loosely guided order of execution. To maintain robustness, as well as to facilitate modified and/or new method injection, each block denotes class-specific structures and their purpose, arguments, and data types. Called from the primary script class, these class executions can be rearranged within the primary

DOI: 10.1201/9781003403678-14

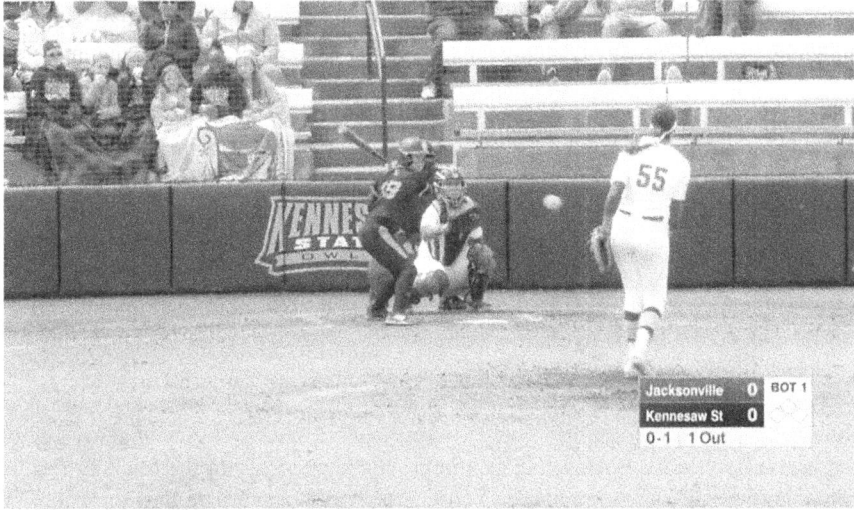

FIGURE 14.1   Example source frame.

chain execution, and are designed to preserve parsing accessibility to adjacent classes. All classes can be categorized with such adjacency into five distinct stages of computation [2]:

- Initialization
- Pre-Processing and Segmentation
- Neural Network Manipulation
- Environment Construction
- Data Packaging

In the following sections, each stage will be further expanded upon, accompanied by several satellite scripts/solutions that serve to prepare relevant workspaces. At the start of runtime, housekeeping and import directives are evaluated from configuration parameters. It is at this stage that the rebuilding of MEX structures can be ordered and performed, should changes to other implementation require such action. The source video data is allocated to the workspace in frames, a set of which is stored as an index four-dimensional matrix. These matrices will traverse the length of the program, allowing each clip to be processed by frame, while retaining the ability to interpolate data over time when needed. Once all preliminary workspace objects are built, a call is made to the present blockchain, and a frame matrix is passed into pre-processing. Semantic separation–based kinematic tracking (SSKT) is a technique used in computer vision and motion tracking to accurately estimate the 3D pose and movements of objects or body parts in a video sequence [2]. It aims to separate the semantic information of different objects or body parts and track their movements independently. Traditional motion tracking methods often face challenges when multiple objects or body parts occlude or overlap each other in a video. This makes it difficult to accurately track individual objects or body parts and estimate their movements. SSKT addresses this issue by utilizing semantic information and applying it to the tracking process. The first step in SSKT is to perform semantic segmentation, which involves segmenting the video frames into different regions based on their semantic content. For example, in the context of tracking body parts, semantic segmentation can identify and separate the regions corresponding to different body parts such as the head, torso, arms, and legs. Once the semantic segmentation is obtained, SSKT utilizes the semantic information to track the individual body parts independently. This is achieved by associating the segmented regions across consecutive frames using various techniques such as feature matching or optical flow. By leveraging the semantic information, SSKT can handle occlusion or overlap situations more effectively, as it can distinguish between different body parts and track their movements separately [3]. SSKT also benefits from the knowledge of the kinematic constraints of the tracked objects or body parts. By incorporating prior knowledge about the expected range of motion and anatomical constraints, SSKT can improve the accuracy of the tracking results. For example, when tracking human body parts, SSKT can utilize the constraints on joint angles and limb lengths to refine the estimated poses and improve the overall tracking performance. The application of SSKT extends beyond tracking human body parts. It can be used in various scenarios where there is a need to track and analyze the movements of objects with semantic significance. For instance, it can be employed in sports analysis to track the movements of players, in robotics to track the motions of robotic limbs, or in augmented reality applications to accurately overlay virtual objects on real-world scenes. Overall, SSKT is a technique that utilizes semantic segmentation and kinematic constraints to accurately track and estimate the movements of objects or body parts in videos. By separating the semantic information and leveraging prior knowledge, SSKT addresses the challenges of occlusion and overlap, enabling more precise and reliable motion tracking in various applications [4].

14.1.1 MOTIVATION

The motivation for research in SSKT is from the need to address the limitations of traditional motion tracking techniques and improve the accuracy and robustness of pose estimation and object tracking in complex and dynamic scenarios. Traditional motion tracking methods often struggle with occlusion and overlap, leading to inaccurate tracking results. SSKT aims to overcome these challenges by leveraging semantic information and separating the tracked objects or body parts based on their semantic content. This semantic separation enables more accurate and reliable tracking, as it allows for individual parts to be tracked independently, reducing the ambiguity and errors caused by occlusion or overlap [5]. Real-world scenarios often involve complex scenes with multiple objects or body parts moving simultaneously. Conventional tracking techniques may fail to accurately estimate the poses and movements in such dynamic environments. SSKT addresses this challenge by incorporating semantic segmentation to identify and track individual parts separately, even in complex and crowded scenes. This capability is particularly beneficial in applications such as sports analysis, robotics, and augmented reality, where tracking accuracy is critical for meaningful interpretation and interaction. Occlusion occurs when objects or body parts are partially or completely blocked from view. It poses a significant challenge for accurate motion tracking since the information required for tracking is missing or corrupted. By utilizing semantic separation, SSKT can better handle occlusion scenarios [6]. By tracking each part independently, SSKT can maintain the tracking of visible parts even when occlusion occurs, providing more robust and continuous tracking results. SSKT has significant implications for human-computer interaction (HCI) applications, such as gesture recognition, motion-based interfaces, and augmented reality. Accurate and real-time tracking of human body parts is crucial for these applications to interpret user actions and provide appropriate responses. SSKT can improve the accuracy and responsiveness of such systems by accurately tracking individual body parts and capturing their movements in real time. This enhances the user experience and opens up new possibilities for natural and intuitive interactions with digital environments. Understanding human movement patterns and biomechanics is essential in various fields, including sports science, rehabilitation, and ergonomics. SSKT can play a significant role in analyzing human motion and assessing biomechanical parameters. By accurately tracking body parts and estimating their movements, SSKT enables researchers and practitioners to analyze motion patterns, identify anomalies, and provide feedback for rehabilitation exercises or ergonomic adjustments [7]. This can lead to improved injury prevention strategies, personalized rehabilitation programs, and enhanced ergonomic design. SSKT is at the intersection of computer vision and machine learning, and its research contributes to the advancement of these fields. Developing robust and efficient algorithms for semantic segmentation, object tracking, and pose estimation requires innovations in computer vision techniques and the application of deep learning models. The research in SSKT not only improves motion tracking but also pushes the boundaries of computer vision and machine learning, contributing to the development of more sophisticated algorithms and methodologies in these domains [8]. SSKT has practical applications in various domains, including healthcare, sports analysis, robotics, augmented reality, and entertainment. In healthcare, SSKT can aid in the analysis of human motion for diagnosis, treatment planning, and monitoring the progress of rehabilitation programs. In sports analysis, SSKT can provide valuable insights into athletes' movements, enhancing performance analysis and training strategies [9]. In robotics, SSKT can enable more precise and natural interaction between humans and robots. In augmented reality and entertainment, SSKT can create immersive and interactive experiences by accurately overlaying virtual objects on real-world scenes. These practical applications highlight the importance of researching and advancing SSKT for real-world impact [10].

The motivation for research in SSKT arises from the need to overcome the limitations of traditional motion tracking techniques and improve accuracy, robustness, and applicability in complex scenarios. By leveraging semantic information, handling occlusion, enhancing human-computer interaction, enabling biomechanical analysis, advancing computer vision and machine learning, and facilitating practical applications, SSKT research contributes to the progress of multiple domains and has the potential to revolutionize motion tracking and pose estimation [11].

14.2   INTEGRATION OF SSKT WITH IoT AND AI

SSKT can be significantly improved by leveraging the capabilities of artificial intelligence (AI) and the Internet of Things (IoT). The combination of AI and IoT technologies can enhance the accuracy, efficiency, and applicability of SSKT in various domains. Here are some ways in which AI and IoT devices can play a crucial role in collecting data for SSKT. By integrating sensors into wearable devices, smart clothing, or even environment-based sensors, a wealth of data can be captured in real time. These sensors can provide precise measurements of body movements, joint angles, or limb positions, allowing for accurate tracking and pose estimation. Additionally, IoT-enabled cameras or depth sensors can capture detailed visual information to supplement the tracking process. AI algorithms can then analyze this collected data to extract relevant features and information, enabling more robust and accurate tracking [12]. AI algorithms can be applied to process and analyze the data collected by IoT devices in real time. By utilizing deep learning and computer vision techniques, AI can identify and track individual body parts, segment them semantically, and estimate their poses and movements. Real-time processing enables immediate feedback and intervention, making SSKT suitable for applications such as interactive rehabilitation, sports analysis, or real-time motion-based interfaces [13]. AI-powered algorithms can also adapt and learn from incoming data, improving tracking performance over time. The combination of AI and IoT can benefit from edge computing, where data processing and analysis occur closer to the data source. Edge devices, such as local servers or edge computing nodes, can execute AI algorithms directly on the IoT devices or within the local network, reducing the latency and bandwidth requirements. This is particularly relevant for SSKT applications that demand real-time tracking, where low latency is critical. By processing data at the edge, AI algorithms can provide faster and more efficient pose estimation, enabling immediate responses and feedback. AI algorithms can enable adaptive tracking in SSKT by incorporating contextual information. By integrating contextual cues, such as environmental conditions, user-specific characteristics, or activity patterns, AI algorithms can enhance tracking accuracy and robustness. For example, by considering contextual information, AI algorithms can differentiate between normal and abnormal movements, adapt tracking parameters based on user capabilities or limitations, or adjust tracking strategies to handle challenging scenarios [14]. Context-aware tracking improves the reliability and versatility of SSKT in various real-world situations. AI techniques can enable predictive analysis and anomaly detection in SSKT. By training AI models on a large data set of tracked movements and poses, algorithms can learn patterns, predict future movements, and detect anomalies or deviations from expected behaviors. This capability is valuable in rehabilitation settings, where AI algorithms can analyze and predict the progress of rehabilitation exercises, detect incorrect movements, and provide real-time feedback to patients. Predictive analysis and anomaly detection enhance the effectiveness and safety of SSKT-based interventions [15]. AI algorithms can facilitate data fusion and multi-modal integration in SSKT. By combining information from different sensors, such as inertial sensors, cameras, or depth sensors, AI algorithms can integrate the strengths of each modality to improve tracking accuracy and robustness. For example, sensor fusion techniques can combine visual information with motion data to overcome occlusion or partial visibility challenges. AI algorithms can fuse data from multiple sources and extract meaningful features, enabling a comprehensive understanding of body movements and poses. AI and IoT enable continuous learning and improvement in SSKT. By leveraging AI techniques such as online learning or reinforcement learning, SSKT algorithms can adapt and improve over time. Continuous learning allows the algorithms to adapt to individual users, accommodate changes in body dynamics or sensor characteristics, and refine the tracking performance based on real-time feedback. IoT connectivity facilitates the collection of data from a large user base, enabling the algorithms to learn from diverse movement patterns and improve their generalization capabilities. The combination of AI and IoT technologies provides significant potential for improving SSKT. Through enhanced data collection, real-time processing, edge computing, adaptive tracking, predictive analysis, data fusion, and continuous learning, AI and IoT can enhance the accuracy, efficiency, and applicability of SSKT in various domains, including healthcare, sports analysis, rehabilitation, and motion-based interfaces. The integration of AI and IoT in SSKT opens up new possibilities for precise, real-time tracking and analysis of body movements, leading to improved outcomes in multiple fields [16].

14.2.1 Requirement for SSKT with IoT and AI

SSKT combined with the IoT and AI brings numerous advantages and fulfills specific requirements that are essential for accurate and robust motion tracking. This combination addresses the limitations of traditional tracking techniques and opens up new possibilities for various applications. Let's delve into the requirements and benefits of SSKT with IoT and AI [17; 18; 19]:

- Real-time Tracking and Analysis: SSKT integrated with IoT and AI enables real-time tracking and analysis of body movements. The data captured by IoT devices, such as wearable sensors or cameras, is processed in real time using AI algorithms. This real-time capability is crucial for applications like interactive rehabilitation or sports analysis, where immediate feedback and intervention are necessary. SSKT with IoT and AI ensures that tracking results are updated in real time, providing accurate and timely information.
- High Accuracy and Precision: Accurate and precise motion tracking is a fundamental requirement for numerous applications. SSKT, combined with AI algorithms, leverages advanced computer vision techniques to accurately track and estimate the poses of body parts. By incorporating semantic information and context-awareness, SSKT ensures precise tracking even in challenging scenarios like occlusion or complex movements. The integration of IoT enables the collection of high-quality sensor data, enhancing the accuracy and reliability of SSKT.

- Adaptability and Customization: SSKT with IoT and AI allows for adaptability and customization to cater to individual needs and preferences. AI algorithms can learn and adapt to different users' movement patterns, body characteristics, and abilities. By continuously analyzing and processing data, SSKT can personalize tracking algorithms to provide customized feedback, adjust tracking parameters, and accommodate changes in movement patterns or environmental conditions. This adaptability enhances the user experience and improves the effectiveness of applications like personalized rehabilitation or motion-based interfaces.
- Robustness to Challenging Environments: SSKT with IoT and AI addresses the challenges posed by complex and dynamic environments. IoT devices provide a diverse range of sensors, such as accelerometers, gyroscopes, or depth cameras, which capture rich contextual information. AI algorithms process this information to enhance tracking robustness. By leveraging contextual cues, SSKT can differentiate between normal and abnormal movements, handle occlusion or partial visibility, and adapt tracking strategies to challenging environments. The combination of IoT and AI ensures robust tracking performance even in complex real-world scenarios.
- Data Fusion and Multi-modal Integration: SSKT with IoT and AI facilitates data fusion and multi-modal integration. IoT devices can capture data from various sources, including sensors, cameras, or depth cameras. AI algorithms can fuse and integrate data from these sources to obtain a comprehensive understanding of body movements. By combining different modalities, SSKT achieves a more holistic view of motion, enhancing tracking accuracy and robustness. For example, depth information from cameras can complement the measurements from wearable sensors, improving the tracking of body parts even in challenging scenarios.
- Scalability and Connectivity: The integration of IoT in SSKT enables scalability and connectivity. IoT devices can be easily deployed and interconnected, allowing for the seamless collection and sharing of data. This scalability is particularly important for applications that involve multiple users or distributed environments. SSKT with IoT ensures that tracking algorithms can handle the simultaneous tracking of multiple individuals or objects, enabling applications like group-based rehabilitation or sports team analysis. The connectivity provided by IoT ensures that data can be efficiently transmitted and shared among different devices or systems, supporting collaborative tracking scenarios.
- Privacy and Security: SSKT with IoT and AI requires careful consideration of privacy and security aspects. As IoT devices collect and transmit sensitive motion data, privacy safeguards and secure data transmission protocols are crucial. The implementation of privacy-preserving techniques, encryption, and authentication mechanisms ensures the confidentiality and integrity of collected data. Additionally, AI algorithms should comply with privacy regulations and follow ethical guidelines to protect the privacy rights of individuals.

SSKT integrated with IoT and AI fulfills several crucial requirements for accurate and robust motion tracking. Real-time tracking and analysis, high accuracy and precision, adaptability and customization, robustness to challenging environments, data fusion and multi-modal integration, scalability and connectivity, as well as privacy and security considerations, are all addressed by combining SSKT with IoT and AI. These advancements open up new possibilities for applications in areas such as healthcare, sports analysis, rehabilitation, virtual reality, and human-computer interaction, enhancing the overall performance and impact of motion tracking systems.

14.2.2 Procedure for Semantic Separation-Based Kinematic Tracking

Pre-processing and segmentation play a crucial role in SSKT by improving the accuracy and robustness of the tracking process. Pre-processing techniques are applied to the input data, such as sensor readings or image frames, to reduce noise and artifacts that can affect tracking accuracy. Noise can arise from various sources, including sensor inaccuracies, environmental factors, or imperfect data acquisition. By applying filters and noise reduction algorithms, pre-processing helps to smooth the data and remove unwanted fluctuations, ensuring that the subsequent tracking algorithms operate on clean and reliable input signals. Pre-processing involves calibrating and aligning the data to ensure consistency and accuracy across different sensors or modalities. This step is particularly important when using multiple sensors or cameras for tracking [20]. Data calibration involves mapping the sensor readings to physical measurements or coordinates, correcting for any sensor biases or misalignments. Alignment ensures that data from different sensors are synchronized in time and spatial reference frames, enabling accurate fusion and integration during the tracking process. Pre-processing includes extracting relevant features from the input data that capture distinctive characteristics of the tracked objects or body parts. These features can include shape descriptors, motion characteristics, color information, or texture patterns, depending on the modality and application [21]. Pre-processing algorithms are used to extract these features and select the most informative ones, reducing the dimensionality of the data and focusing on the relevant aspects for tracking. Feature extraction and selection enable more efficient and accurate tracking by providing discriminative information for subsequent analysis. Segmentation is the process of dividing the input data into meaningful regions or segments corresponding to individual objects or body parts. In SSKT, segmentation is crucial for separating different body parts and distinguishing them from the background or other objects. By segmenting the input data, such as images or point clouds, into distinct regions corresponding to body parts, the subsequent tracking algorithms can focus on each part separately, enabling more accurate and reliable pose estimation. Segmentation algorithms can utilize various techniques, such as thresholding, edge detection, region growing, or machine learning–based approaches, to identify and extract relevant regions of interest. Pre-processing includes the selection of the region of interest (ROI) within the input data that contains the relevant body parts or objects to be tracked [22]. This step helps to narrow down the focus of the tracking algorithms, reducing computational complexity and improving efficiency. ROI selection can involve manually or automatically identifying the regions that encompass the body parts of interest or the objects to be tracked. By restricting the analysis to the selected ROI, the tracking algorithms can concentrate their efforts on the critical regions, improving tracking accuracy and performance [23]. Overall, pre-processing and segmentation play a vital role in SSKT by preparing the input data, reducing noise, calibrating and aligning sensor readings, extracting informative features, and segmenting the data into relevant regions. These steps enhance the accuracy, efficiency, and robustness of the tracking process, enabling more precise and reliable pose estimation and motion tracking in applications such as human motion analysis, rehabilitation, sports performance monitoring, and virtual reality interactions [24].

14.3   PRE-PROCESSING AND SEGMENTATION

Before complex processing procedures can be applied to the frame set of each play, hereafter denoted *Case*, each frame must be prepared in order to improve data collection efficacy in subsequent steps. *Pre-processing* techniques applied include spatial filtering, lighting compensation, and otherwise HSV marginalization, as shown in Figure 14.2. A relevant class operates by frame, and as such remains indifferent of changes over time [3]. To perform single pass processing for each *Case*, the *Sequencer* class matches argument specific pointers to a given *Case*, from which each frame can be processed and packaged for return to the chain. For most non-transient procedures, the *Sequencer* orchestrates operations performed by frame, thus simplifying the procedure solutions themselves. At this point, processed matrices are normalized prior to segmentation [4].

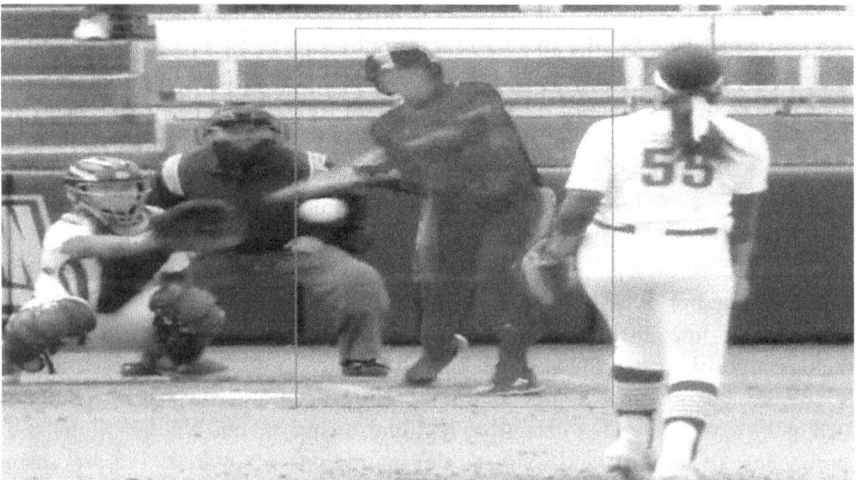

FIGURE 14.2   ROI, filtered frame.

14.3.1 Neural Network Manipulation

To segment each frame, Scap-Trac utilizes a K-means algorithm, supplemented by a set of gabor filters created for the *Case*, indicated in Figure 14.3. These filters can be configured to carry some magnitude of mask equivalent between frames, to interpolate missing information during movement or extrinsic obscurity [5]. This second pass is once again performed by the *Sequencer*, returning segmented *Cases* to the chain.

The third pass of segmentation imposes a combination surface feature track and foreground manipulation. This procedure serves to isolate moving objects of interest, generating a frame indexed structure containing all tracked regions of interest, or ROIs. Frame matrices are not altered with this pass, but *Cases* are packaged into cell arrays with resulting ROI indices. This pass can be toggled at Initialization to generate heat maps for entire regions as needed. Once all segmentation has been performed by the *Sequencer*, the *Case* cell array can be returned to the chain. To evaluate configured *Case* ROIs, Scap-Trac utilizes the OpenPose [6] library, a convolutional neural network (CNN) designed to generate heat maps of estimated joint positions within a given image. Trained with the COCO data set [7], OpenPose estimates this data with great efficacy. For use within this program, the network has been repackaged with Caffe [8], utilizing compatible MEX functions built by the framework. Handler methods within this stage parse frame ROIs through the network, returning evaluated heat maps and key-point link matrices. With the appropriate pointer ordered, full *Case* sets are parsed via the *Sequencer*. Using original frame dimensions, the processed ROIs are placed within a null matrix, effectively returning the isolated model to the full scene [8]. In Figure 14.4, heat maps generated represent joint position confidence with magnitude, and joint orientations with labeled color. Linked key-point matrix sets are exported to output folders here, as beyond generation they are not utilized.

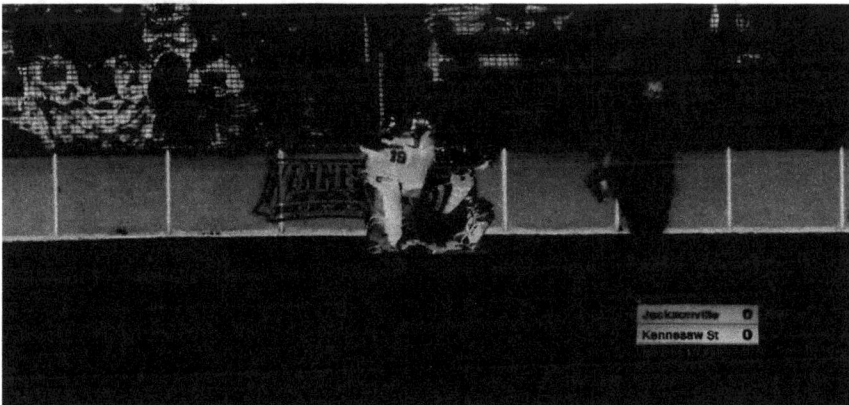

FIGURE 14.3   Segmented applied filter, second pass.

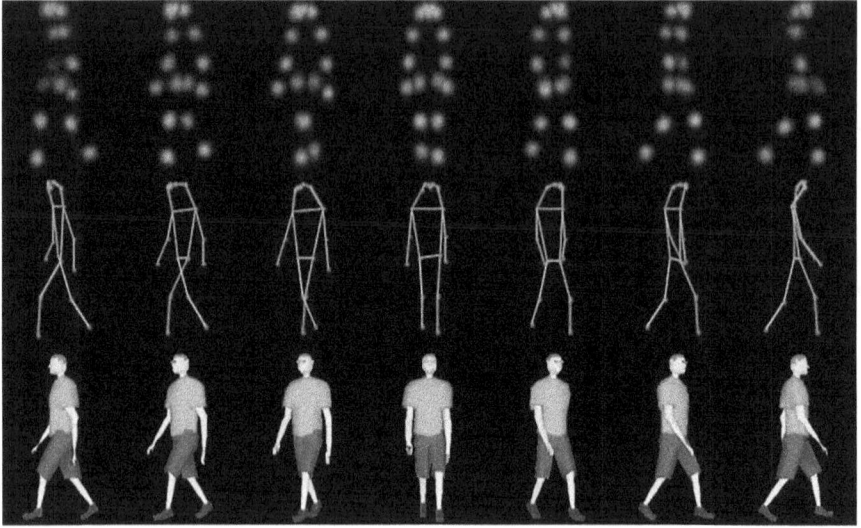

FIGURE 14.4 *OpenPose* heat maps and key-points, rotational test.

For an individual event, a cell array containing heat-map data from each source covering the event is created and shown in Figure 14.5. Each source set is indexed likely, hereby matching each perspective per unit time. With the x and y dimensions restored to each frame, the data is primed for geometric interpretation.

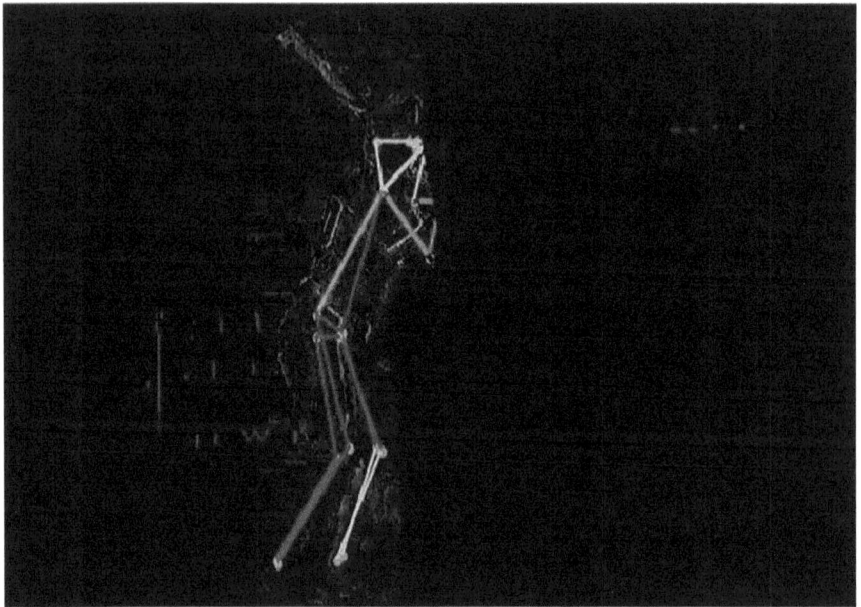

FIGURE 14.5 Key-points paired to split frame.

14.3.2   ENVIRONMENT CONSTRUCTION

Scene geometry estimation classes operate with two distinct strategies, deter-mined at *Initialization* by the number of different sources available for any given *Case*: For single-source *Cases*, estimation tends towards speculative results; to compensate, linked joint maps are delivered in tandem with frame indexed heat maps. In this scenario, the *CNN* pass bears most of the computational workload for geometric estimation. However, without known extrinsic parame-ters, desired *Case* characteristics such as joint velocity and target distance lack any substantial frame of reference [9]. This caveat can be remedied after completion by introducing known geometry into the system, albeit a somewhat non-ideal solution. For multiple-source *Cases*, a more pragmatic approach is performed. With multiple heat maps gathered for any given frame of the *Case*, feature tracking can be performed, relating each source by transformation links [10]. These links exist as orthographic projections of shift and rotation matrices from each available perspective. Furthermore, by isolating possible extrinsic source parameters, the links can be computed into such matrices, and therefore source positions within the scene. Assuming that no source can exist outside of [11]:

$$0 \leq \theta \leq 180^o, 0 \leq \phi \leq 30^o,$$

The inter-source transformations can be calculated. To achieve this goal, Scap-Trac utilizes *surface feature tracking* to generate the links, and passes the resulting array indexed by source to the *camera parameter estimator*, both con-structed from tools contained within the *Computer Vision Toolbox* shown in Figure 14.6.

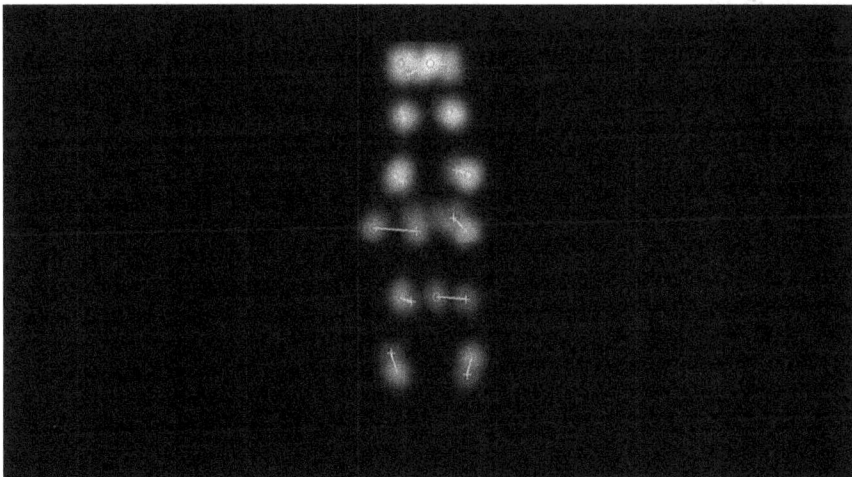

FIGURE 14.6   Multi-source transformation vectors.

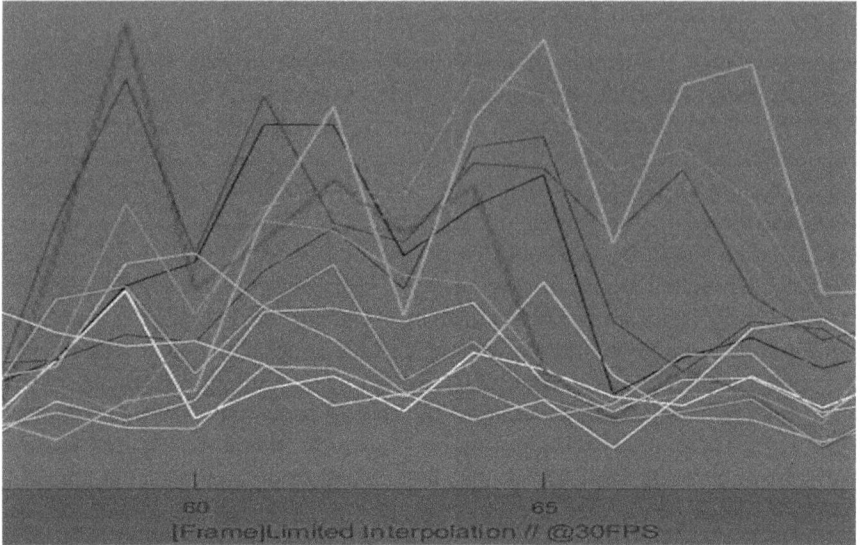

FIGURE 14.7   Skeletal velocities.

14.3.3 DATA PACKAGING

To make use of estimated joint positions, a separate workspace is used. The gui_master.m script serves as the primary controller for this final stage of computation. Saved positional data is imported to the workspace, and separate consecutive methods return estimated joint velocities and musculature action. As before, source count determines both the form in which joint positions are imported, and which procedures can be performed at this stage [12]. For single-source cases, joint velocities relative to the structural center are derived by measuring changes with respect to each joint's parent structure. While this method is capable of producing testable results, the algorithm is currently limited in its ability to detect movement along the perspective vector to the subject. This can be seen as a "ringing" of joint velocity functions as the subject's movement leaves the orthogonal plane, as shown in Figure 14.7.

For multi-source cases, this procedure would be much more refined. As the joint position data would be already contained as a four-dimensional matrix, the skeletal velocities would be carried from the environment. Utilizing the interpolated skeletal velocities, musculature action over the sequence can also be derived. A single-source example of this calculated action is shown in Figure 14.8, derived from joint respective velocities for each muscle group.

14.4   PROCEDURAL CONCERNS

Each source processed for each *Case* of Events must be clipped and synchronized within a global frame count, to be indexed upon case-by-case initialization. Currently, a manual initialization triggering will be required, and should the

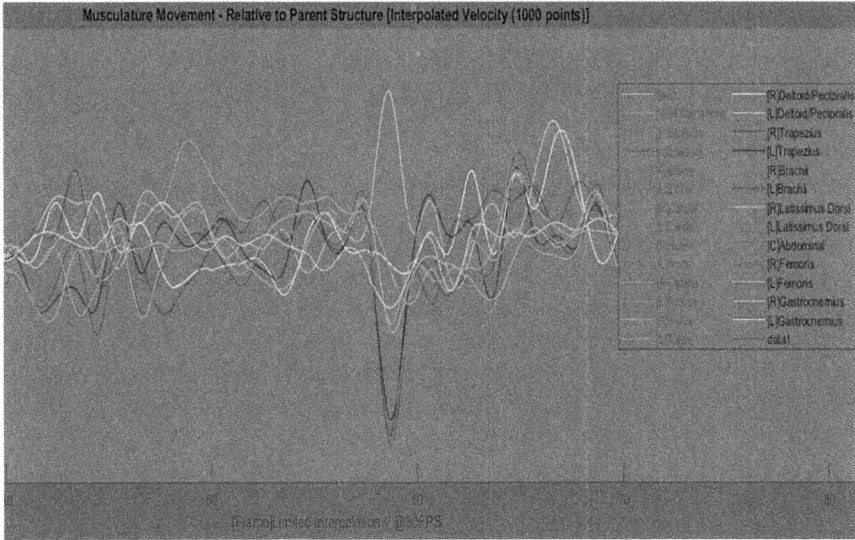

FIGURE 14.8 Musculature action.

framework prove effective, an automatic solution will be pursued. In order to accurately map the frame-wise position of the batter, a collaborative recognition effort will occur with the set of sources for each case. The first pass of recognition will occur for each source and frame, drawing from both the edge detection frame and learned positions by frame index. Base unit position values will occur in terms of actor joints; the actor object itself being connected in amalgamation of known links between said joints. Positions will be compared with known limits per frame index, scaled by both margin and aforementioned scene scale. Because of frame-wise occlusion, these links cannot be assigned directly; rather, visible joint vectors will be assigned "confidence magnitudes," in order to assess the most probable identity of the joint. These values, together with those of the other sources for the given frame, can be used to estimate the most probable joint identity above a certain threshold of total confidence. Ideally, every frame would contain every joint from at least one of the sources; however, it should be expected that for any one *Case* at least 35–40% of all source joint data will be unobtainable simply because of occlusion. All identified joints existing as vectors within the virtual space, some extent of interpolation will be required to complete the model. This process can be augmented by the geometry of the links themselves, as known limits can be applied to their lengths.

14.4.1 NEURAL NETWORKS

Neural networks play a significant role in SSKT by enabling accurate and robust pose estimation and motion tracking. Neural networks are a class of machine learning algorithms inspired by the structure and function of the human brain [9]. They excel at learning complex patterns and relationships from data, making them well-suited for tasks like image analysis, object recognition, and pose estimation. Neural networks excel at learning high-level feature representations from raw sensor data. In SSKT, neural networks can be used to extract informative features from input data, such as images or sensor readings. By learning feature representations directly from the data, neural networks can capture relevant patterns and discriminative information that aids in accurate pose estimation and motion tracking. For example, convolutional neural networks (CNNs) are commonly used to extract spatial features from images, while recurrent neural networks (RNNs) are effective at capturing temporal dependencies in time-series data. The neural networks are used to estimate the poses of body parts or objects in SSKT. Given the extracted features, neural networks can learn to map the input data to the corresponding pose parameters, such as joint angles or 3D coordinates. Various neural network architectures, such as convolutional pose machines (CPMs) or recurrent neural network–based pose estimation models (e.g., LSTM-based models), have been developed specifically for accurate pose estimation. These models learn to associate visual or sensor information with specific poses, enabling precise tracking of body movements [9]. It also facilitates the semantic separation of body parts or objects in SSKT. By leveraging semantic segmentation techniques, neural networks can assign distinct labels or masks to different body parts or objects in the input data. This semantic separation is essential for accurately tracking individual body parts or objects and distinguishing them from the background or other entities. Neural network–based semantic segmentation models, such as fully convolutional networks (FCNs) or U-Net architectures, can learn to identify and segment relevant regions of interest, aiding in precise pose estimation and tracking. It is capable of incorporating contextual information into the tracking process. By considering the contextual cues in the input data, neural networks can improve the understanding of body movements and enhance tracking accuracy. For example, recurrent neural networks can capture temporal dependencies and long-term context, enabling smoother and more coherent tracking. Additionally, attention mechanisms can be employed to focus on relevant regions or body parts, incorporating spatial context into the tracking process. Further, it enable learning and adaptation in SSKT. By training neural networks on diverse data sets, they can learn to generalize from examples and adapt to individual variations, such as different body types or movement styles. Neural networks can learn the correlations between sensor data and pose parameters, enabling them to accurately estimate poses even in challenging scenarios [25]. Transfer learning techniques can also be applied, where pre-trained neural network models on large-scale datasets are fine-tuned for specific tracking tasks, reducing the need for extensive training data. Overall, neural networks are instrumental in SSKT for feature representation, pose estimation, semantic separation, incorporating contextual information, and learning/adaptation. They empower the system to accurately track body movements, estimate poses, and separate body parts or objects in complex and dynamic environments. The use of neural networks enhances the performance and robustness of SSKT, making it a powerful tool for applications such as motion analysis, rehabilitation, sports performance monitoring, and virtual reality interactions [26].

14.5   CHALLENGES

SSKT with the integration of IoT and AI brings significant advancements in motion tracking. However, this combination also presents several challenges that need to be addressed for the successful implementation and deployment of SSKT systems. Let's explore some of the key challenges in SSKT with IoT and AI [27; 28]:

    i. Data Quality and Variability: SSKT relies on the collection of high-quality sensor data from IoT devices. However, ensuring data quality and dealing with data variability pose significant challenges. IoT devices may suffer from sensor inaccuracies, noise, or signal drift, which can adversely affect tracking accuracy. Variability in sensor characteristics, data acquisition setups, or user-specific factors further adds complexity. Robust pre-processing techniques, calibration methods, and sensor fusion algorithms are needed to mitigate these challenges and ensure consistent and reliable tracking performance.

    ii. Computational Complexity and Efficiency: SSKT algorithms, especially those based on AI techniques, can be computationally intensive. Real-time tracking and analysis of complex body movements require efficient algorithms that can run on resource-constrained IoT devices. Balancing the computational complexity of AI algorithms with the limited processing capabilities of IoT devices is a challenge. Optimization techniques, such as model compression, lightweight network architectures, or edge computing strategies, are necessary to ensure efficient processing and real-time performance in IoT-based SSKT systems.

    iii. Privacy and Security: IoT-enabled SSKT systems involve the collection, transmission, and storage of sensitive user data, raising privacy and security concerns. Personal motion data may contain personally identifiable information or reveal sensitive health conditions. Ensuring data privacy, protecting against unauthorized access or data breaches, and complying with privacy regulations are critical challenges. Encryption, secure communication protocols, and privacy-preserving techniques, such as data anonymization or differential privacy, need to be implemented to address these challenges and build trust in SSKT systems.

    iv. Adaptability and Generalization: SSKT systems should be adaptable and capable of generalizing to diverse users, body types, and movements. Individual variations, such as different anatomical structures, joint ranges, or movement styles, pose challenges in accurately tracking and estimating poses across different individuals. AI algorithms need to be trained on diverse datasets to learn and adapt to individual characteristics. Transfer learning and domain adaptation techniques can help improve generalization capabilities and handle individual differences, ensuring accurate tracking performance across a broad user base.

    v. Robustness to Environmental Factors: Tracking accuracy in SSKT can be affected by various environmental factors, such as lighting conditions, occlusions, or complex backgrounds. IoT devices may operate in different physical environments with varying lighting conditions or dynamic obstacles. Handling these challenges requires robust computer vision algorithms that can handle varying illumination, handle occlusions or partial visibility, and differentiate between the body parts of interest and the background. Advanced sensor fusion techniques that combine data from multiple modalities, such as cameras and wearable sensors, can enhance robustness to environmental factors.

vi. Integration and Interoperability: IoT-based SSKT systems involve the integration of multiple devices, sensors, and platforms. Ensuring seamless interoperability and compatibility among different IoT devices, data formats, and communication protocols is a significant challenge. Integration of data from various sensors and platforms, such as cameras, wearable devices, or cloud-based processing units, requires standardization and well-defined interfaces. Interoperability standards, open APIs, and data exchange formats need to be established to enable easy integration and collaboration among different components of the SSKT system.

vii. Ethical Considerations: The deployment of SSKT systems raises ethical considerations, particularly regarding data ownership, consent, and transparency. Users need to have control over their motion data and understand how it is being collected, stored, and used. Clear consent mechanisms, transparent data handling practices, and ethical guidelines are necessary to address these concerns. Additionally, bias mitigation techniques and fairness considerations should be integrated into AI algorithms to ensure unbiased tracking results and avoid discriminatory outcomes.

Addressing these challenges requires multidisciplinary research and collaboration between experts in computer vision, AI, IoT, data privacy, and ethics. By overcoming these hurdles, SSKT with IoT and AI can unlock the full potential of accurate and context-aware motion tracking, enabling applications in healthcare, rehabilitation, sports analysis, human-computer interaction, and virtual reality, among others.

14.5.1 Future Scope

The future scope of integrating neural networks in SSKT with IoT and AI holds immense potential for advancing motion tracking technologies. Neural networks can be further optimized to enhance the accuracy of pose estimation and motion tracking. Ongoing research aims to develop more sophisticated neural network architectures and training strategies that can better handle complex motion patterns, occlusions, and challenging environmental conditions. By leveraging larger datasets, advanced regularization techniques, and novel network architectures, it is possible to achieve even higher accuracy and robustness in SSKT systems [29]. As the deployment of IoT devices continues to increase, there is a growing need for real-time processing and analysis on edge devices. Future research will focus on developing lightweight neural network models that can run efficiently on resource-constrained IoT devices. Model compression, quantization, and pruning techniques will be explored to reduce the memory and computational requirements while maintaining acceptable tracking performance, enabling real-time tracking capabilities on edge devices. SSKT can benefit from the fusion of data from multiple sensors and modalities. Neural networks can play a vital role in integrating information from diverse sources, such as cameras, depth sensors, wearable devices, or inertial sensors. Future research will explore innovative ways to fuse data from these different modalities using neural network–based architectures, allowing for more comprehensive and accurate tracking of body movements. Neural networks offer the potential for adaptive and personalized tracking systems. By continuously learning from user feedback and adapting to individual characteristics, neural networks can improve tracking performance and adapt to user-specific requirements. Personalization can be achieved by incorporating user-specific training data or employing transfer learning techniques to fine-tune pre-trained models for individual users. Adaptive tracking systems can dynamically adjust tracking parameters based on real-time feedback, ensuring optimal performance in different contexts and activities. With the increasing concern for data privacy, future research will focus on developing privacy-preserving techniques for SSKT [30]. Neural networks can be leveraged to enable on-device processing and analysis, reducing the need to transmit sensitive data to external servers. Techniques such as federated learning, differential privacy, and encrypted computation can be explored to ensure user privacy while still achieving accurate tracking results. These privacy-preserving approaches will enhance user trust and facilitate the widespread adoption of SSKT technologies. The integration of SSKT with AI-based decision support systems holds great potential for various applications. By combining pose estimation and tracking data with AI algorithms, it becomes possible to provide real-time feedback, recommendations, or interventions based on the tracked movements. For example, in rehabilitation settings, AI models can analyze the tracked data to provide personalized exercise plans or detect deviations from correct movements [31]. The integration of SSKT with AI decision support systems can greatly enhance the effectiveness and efficiency of various domains, such as healthcare, sports training, and virtual reality experiences. The future of neural network–based SSKT with IoT and AI is promising. Advancements in neural network architectures, real-time processing on edge devices, multi-modal fusion, adaptive tracking, privacy-preserving techniques, and integration with AI decision support systems will pave the way for more accurate, personalized, and context-aware motion tracking systems [32]. These advancements will have a profound impact on various domains, improving healthcare, sports analysis, rehabilitation, human-computer interaction, and immersive experiences in virtual reality [7].

14.6   CONCLUSION

While much of the program's framework is currently insufficiently optimized for field testing, this project has provided modest results, and has laid the foundation for future implementations by the authors. Future work on the project will be oriented at generating exportable rigging key-frame matrices for third-party applications, and optimization of the framework as a whole. In addition, the author would like to begin field testing with multi-source material once improvements have been made. The integration of SSKT with IoT and AI offers tremendous potential for revolutionizing motion tracking technologies. By combining advanced computer vision techniques, IoT connectivity, and the power of artificial intelligence, SSKT systems can accurately estimate poses, track body movements, and provide valuable insights for a wide range of applications. The utilization of neural networks in SSKT has proven to be instrumental in achieving accurate pose estimation, semantic separation of body parts, incorporating contextual information, and adapting to individual variations. Neural networks excel in learning complex patterns and relationships from data, enabling them to capture the nuances of human motion and improve tracking accuracy. With ongoing research and advancements in neural network architectures, training strategies, and optimization techniques, the future holds even greater potential for improving the accuracy and robustness of SSKT systems. The integration of IoT in SSKT expands the possibilities by allowing the collection of real-time sensor data from connected devices. IoT devices, such as cameras, wearable sensors, or inertial measurement units, provide a rich source of information for tracking body movements. The seamless integration of IoT devices enables a comprehensive and holistic approach to motion tracking, capturing data from multiple modalities and creating a more accurate representation of human motion. This integration also enables real-time processing and analysis on edge devices, reducing the reliance on cloud infrastructure and ensuring timely feedback for users. The incorporation of AI techniques in SSKT enhances the system's capabilities by enabling adaptive tracking, personalized experiences, and decision support systems. AI algorithms can continuously learn and adapt to individual characteristics, improving tracking performance and tailoring the system to the specific needs of users. Additionally, the integration of AI-based decision support systems can provide real-time feedback, recommendations, or interventions based on the tracked movements, opening up new possibilities for applications in healthcare, rehabilitation, sports analysis, and virtual reality. While SSKT with IoT and AI offers numerous benefits, it also presents several challenges that need to be addressed. Data quality, computational complexity, privacy and security concerns, adaptability to individual variations, robustness to environmental factors, and interoperability among different devices and platforms are among the challenges that need careful consideration. Research and development efforts are required to develop robust pre-processing techniques, lightweight neural network models, privacy-preserving methods, and interoperability standards to overcome these challenges and ensure the successful deployment of SSKT systems. In conclusion, the integration of SSKT with IoT and AI holds immense potential for advancing motion tracking technologies. By leveraging the power of neural networks, IoT connectivity, and AI algorithms, SSKT systems can provide accurate and context-aware motion tracking, enabling applications in healthcare, sports analysis, rehabilitation, human-computer interaction, and virtual reality. Continued research and innovation in this field will pave the way for even more sophisticated and impactful SSKT systems, improving the understanding of human motion and unlocking new possibilities for various domains.

FUNDING

There is no funding support in this work.

Compliance with ethical standards.

CONFLICT OF INTEREST

All authors do not have any conflict of interest.

ETHICAL APPROVAL

This chapter does not contain any studies with human participants or animals performed by any of the authors.

REFERENCES

1. Huang, Y., Huang, T. S. and Niemann, H. Segmentation-based object tracking using image warping and Kalman filtering. *Proceedings International Conference on Image Processing* 2002, 3, 601–604. 10.1109/ICIP.2002.1039042.
2. Kumar, A., Albreem, M. A., Gupta, M., Alsharif, M. H. and Kim, S. Future 5G network based smart hospitals: Hybrid detection technique for latency improvement. *IEEE Access* 2020, 8, 153240–153249. 10.1109/ACCESS.2020.3017625.
3. Vesper, C., Schmitz, L. and Knoblich, G. Modulating action duration to establish nonconventional communication. *Journal of Experimental Psychology: General* 2017, 146(12), 1722–1737. 10.1037/xge0000379.supp.
4. Trujillo, J. P., Simanova, I., Bekkering, H. and Özyürek, A. Communicative intent modulates production and comprehension of actions and gestures: A kinect study. Cognition 2018a, 180, 38–51. 10.1016/j.cognition.2018.04.003.
5. Thompson, P. and Galata, A. Hand tracking from monocular RGB with dense semantic labels. 2020 15th IEEE International Conference on Automatic Face and Gesture Recognition (FG 2020), 2020, pp. 394–401. 10.1109/FG47880.2020. 00113.
6. Trujillo, J. P. et al. Toward the markerless and automatic analysis of kinematic features: A toolkit for gesture and movement research. *Behavior Research Methods* 2019, 51, 769–777. 10.3758/s13428-018-1086-8.
7. Chakravarty, S. and Kumar, A. PAPR reduction of GFDM signals using encoder-decoder neural network (autoencoder). *National Academy Science Letters* 2023, 46, 213–217. 10.1007/s40009-023-01230-1.
8. Kumar, A., Sharma, H., Gour, N. and Pareek, R. A hybrid technique for the PAPR reduction of NOMA waveform. *International Journal of Communication Systems* 2023, 36, 10.1002/dac.5412.
9. Kumar, A., Sharma, H., Mathur, S., Sharma, D., Khandelwal, G. and Sharma, G. Computer vision, machine learning based monocular biomechanical and security analysis. *Journal of Discrete Mathematical Sciences & Cryptography* 2023, 26, 685–693. 10.47974/jdmsc-1741.

10. Sharma, M. K. and Kumar, A. NOMA waveform technique using orthogonal supplementary signal for advanced 5G networks security. *Journal of Discrete Mathematical Sciences and Cryptography* 2022, 25, 1125–1136. 10.1080/09720529. 2022.2075088.

11. Jia et al. Caffe: Convolutional architecture for fast feature embedding. Computer vision and pattern recognition. *Computer Science* 2014, 2014, 1–4. arXiv:1408.5093, 2014.

12. Tsung et al. Microsoft COCO: Common objects in context. Computer vision and pattern recognition. *Computer Vision and Pattern Recognition* 2014, 2014, 1–15. arXiv:1405.0312.

13. Alvear, O., Calafate, C. T., Cano, J. C. and Manzoni, P. Crowdsensing in smart cities: Overview, platforms, and environment sensing issues. *Sensors* 2018, 18, 460. [Google Scholar]

14. Viani, F., Robol, F., Polo, A., Rocca, P., Oliveri, G. and Massa, A. Wireless architectures for heterogeneous sensing in smart home applications: Concepts and real implementation. *Proceedings of the IEEE* 2013, 101, 2381–2396.

15. Bisio, I., Lavagetto, F., Marchese, M. and Sciarrone, A. Smartphone-centric ambient assisted living platform for patients suffering from co-morbidities monitoring. *IEEE Communications Magazine* 2015, 53, 34–41.

16. Corno, F. and Razzak, F. Intelligent energy optimization for user intelligible goals in smart home environments. *IEEE Transactions on Smart Grid* 2012, 3, 2128–2135.

17. Chen, L., Nugent, C. and Okeyo, G. An ontology-based hybrid approach to activity modeling for smart homes. *IEEE Transactions on Human-Machine Systems* 2014, 44, 92–105.

18. Kung, H., Chaisit, S. and Phuong, N. T. M. Optimization of an RFID location identification scheme based on the neural network. *International Journal of Communication Systems* 2015, 28, 625–644.

19. Perera, C., Zaslavsky, A., Christen, C. and Georgakopoulos, D. Sensing as a service model for smart cities supported by Internet of Things. *Transactions on Emerging Telecommunications Technologies* 2014, 25, 81–93.

20. Gil, D., Ferrández, A., Moramora, H. and Peral, J. Internet of Things: A review of surveys based on context aware intelligent services. *Sensors* 2016, 16, 1069.

21. He, X., Wang, K., Huang, H. and Liu, B. QoE-driven big data architecture for smart city. *IEEE Communications Magazine* 2018, 56, 88–93.

22. Kumar, A., Venkatesh, J., Gaur, N., Alsharif, M. H., Uthansakul, P. and Uthansakul, M. Cyclostationary and energy detection spectrum sensing beyond 5G. *Electronic Research Archive* 2023a, 31(6), 3400–3416. 10.3934/era.2023172.

23. Rasch, K. An unsupervised recommender system for smart homes. *Journal of Ambient Intelligence and Smart Environments* 2014, 6, 21–37.

24. Joseph, R., Nugent, C. D. and Liu, J. From activity recognition to intention recognition for assisted living within smart homes. *IEEE Transactions on Human-Machine Systems* 2017, 47, 368–379.

25. Kumar, A. et al. Intelligent conventional and proposed hybrid 5G detection techniques. *Alexandria Engineering Journal* 2022, 61(12), 10485–10494.

26. Silver, D., Huang, A. and Maddison, C. J. Mastering the game of Go with deep neural networks and tree search. *Nature* 2016, 529, 484–489.

27. Cosma, G., Brown, D., Archer, M., Khan, M. and Pockley, A. G. A survey on computational intelligence approaches for predictive modeling in prostate cancer. *Expert Systems with Applications* 2016, 70, 1–19.

28. Dawadi, P. N., Cook, D. J. and Schmitter-Edgecombe, M. Automated clinical assessment from smart home based behavior data. *IEEE Journal of Biomedical and Health Informatics* 2017, 20, 1188–1194.

29. Kumar, A. et al. Hybrid detection techniques for 5G and B5G M-MIMO system. *Alexandria Engineering Journal* 2023b, 75, 429–437.
30. Kumar, A. PAPR reduction in beyond 5G waveforms using a novel SLM algorithm. *National Academy Science Letters* 2023. 10.1007/s40009-023-01289-w.
31. Abdulsalam, Y., Singh, S. and Alamri, A. Mining human activity patterns from smart home big data for healthcare applications. *IEEE Access* 2017, 5, 13131–13141.
32. Jens, L., Järpe, E. and Verikas, A. Detecting and exploring deviating behaviour of smart home residents. *Expert Systems with Applications* 2016, 55, 429–440.

15 Interaction in Real-Time Communication
Artificial Intelligence-Based Face Recognition System with Aging Effect and Other Medical Parameters

Md. Asif Iqbal and Atul Kumar Dadhich
Department of Electrical Engineering, Vivekananda Global University, India

Javed Khan Bhutto
Department of Electrical Engineering, King Khalid University, UAE

Hina Shahnawaz
Department of Applied Science, Poornima University, India

15.1 INTRODUCTION

Weta Digital organizes its operations using a proprietary character simulation system that replicates the famous "Gollum" and "Jack Sully" characters from the *Avatar* films [1]. Similarly, Industrial Light & Magic (ILM) employed a muscle simulation system to re-create the character "Hulk" from the *Avengers* films. Although the SE simulation system accurately replicates real-world tissue and muscle functionality, it does not incorporate aging characteristics. Considering that 3D humanoid characters are simulated with bones, muscles, and hair, similar to real people, aging becomes an essential feature to consider. For instance, in a hypothetical sequel to an *Avatar* movie featuring an older "Jack Sully," the muscles would require remodeling since the older character's musculature would differ from the original character's configuration [2].

15.2 MAJOR FACE RECOGNITION DATABASES

FG-NET is a popular aging database that contains images of individuals taken over a period of 5 to 70 years. The data set was used in a study to evaluate the

DOI: 10.1201/9781003403678-15

performance of different face recognition algorithms on aging faces. The results showed that the use of artificial intelligence–based simulation improved the accuracy of face recognition with aging effects [3]. The CAS-PEAL-R1 database contains images of 1,040 individuals taken under controlled lighting and pose conditions. The database was used in a study to evaluate the performance of different face recognition algorithms on aging faces. The results showed that the use of artificial intelligence–based simulation improved the accuracy of face recognition with aging effects [4]. MegaFace is a large-scale face recognition data set that contains over 1 million images of over 690,000 individuals. The data set was used in a study to evaluate the performance of different face recognition algorithms on aging faces. The results showed that the use of artificial intelligence–based simulation improved the accuracy of face recognition with aging effects [5]. The LFWA+ database contains images of 13,233 individuals, each with 73 attributes, including age, gender, and ethnicity. The database was used in a study to evaluate the performance of different face recognition algorithms on aging faces. The results showed that the use of artificial intelligence–based simulation improved the accuracy of face recognition with aging effects.

15.2.1   SCOPE

Notwithstanding referenced highlights, a few programming dialects was utilized for creating required modules and expansions. Application Programming Points of interaction (programming interface) for Maya are carried out utilizing C++ and Python. Notwithstanding the application programming point of interaction, Maya can be prearranged utilizing Python and Maya Inserted Language (MEL) [6]. However totally related programming and prearranging dialects are irrefutably factual and related to Maya, involving one language in improvement projects is a decent programming practice since it helps in both programming uprightness and upkeep. Python was picked in light of the fact that they are helpful to use in both a prearranging and a programming setting [7].

Assumptions for research include following:

- Possible clients for the proposed reenactment framework will have a piece of decent information for character fixing ory and Autodesk's Maya PC illustrations programming for utilizing this character re-creation framework [8].
- Possible clients for the proposed reenactment framework know the process for character arrangement utilizing the module for planned recreation and will have a piece of careful information for utilization for the device's UI.
- Possible clients for the proposed reenactment framework will decide on maturing properties for the character as per needs for their own creation or task that the apparatus is being utilized for.
- Proposed framework is answerable for joint rotational cutoff points and skin distortions in light of maturing and not character development or motion [9].

Artificial intelligence (AI) has made significant progress in recognizing aging effects in face recognition systems in recent years, but there are still limitations and challenges that can cause failures. One reason for AI failure in understanding the actual aging effect in face recognition systems is the lack of diversity in the training data. If the training data set used to train the AI algorithm is not diverse enough, it may not accurately capture the range of facial features and aging effects that occur in the population. This can lead to errors in the system's ability to recognize faces with aging effects. Another challenge is the limited representation of the aging process in the training data set. The aging process is complex and can vary significantly between individuals, making it difficult to capture in a single data set. Additionally, the aging process can be affected by many factors, such as genetics, lifestyle, and environment, which can make it difficult to accurately predict the aging effects in an individual.

15.3 SYSTEM AND METHODOLOGY

Reasons for research work are to respond to essential examination question which are consideration for maturing character controls and computerization for solid gear process for a humanoid character. These segments for workwill characterize how results that were achieved by framework had been tried by utilizing explicit factual strategies. Research types for this theory are quantitative exploration. Research objectives are to create a module for Autodesk Maya PC design programming (since they are financially the most involved item for liveliness both in industry and the scholarly world) that computerizes the fixing and cleaning process involving muscles with help for maturing. Accomplishment for "Senescence" Framework are estimated in two kinds: one are genuine working for item that can be utilized for mimicking characters in different ages and others are discernment for reproduced ages in characters by target group [10].

15.4 TESTING USEFULNESS FOR FRAMEWORK

The "Senescence" Framework works assuming it can mechanize the fixing/cleaning process and apply indicated maturing boundaries like reach for movement values to joints and width boundary to muscle deformer for character and doesn't work in the event that they can't make it happen [11]. Testing "Discernment" for Age in Reproductions second part are trying discernment for age by crowd in character that are being manipulated by utilizing "Senescence" Situation. Productivity for the module in reproducing a character for an age is characterized by exactness for discernment. This will be tried by utilizing a reviewing cycle that will be characterized in later parts of this section. UI for the module has maturing controls for the two skeletons and muscles in which the client can openly set properties for the character's skeleton and muscles utilizing an XML document that goes with it [12]. Boundaries for muscle and skeleton joints were picked in light of the fact that they intently look like form in Figure 15.1 and the properties that change when people age. Additionally, preceding choice joints and muscles for the character will be put and arranged as per real associations among bones and muscles in the human outer muscle framework, which will be examined in the next area.

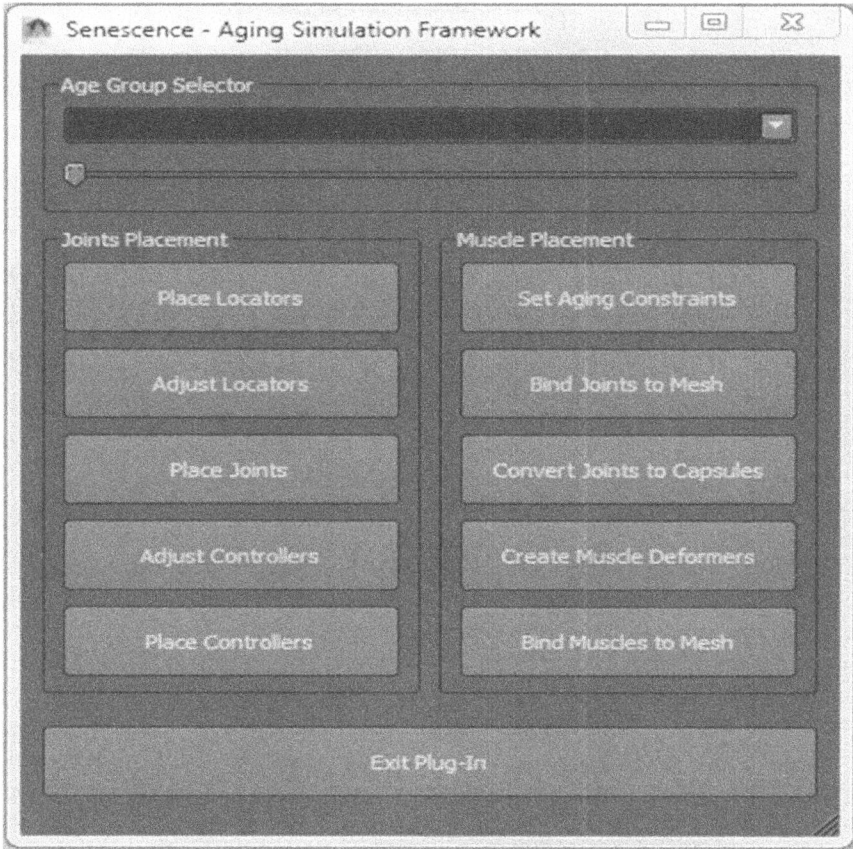

FIGURE 15.1 User interface for "Senescence" plug-in.

A more profound comprehension and information for human outer muscle framework and its workings during development for each joint are required to foster areas of strength for reenactment. Following is a set for pictures for the human outer muscle framework.

15.4.1 PROCESS FLOW

The process of developing an artificial intelligence (AI)-based simulation for a face recognition system with aging effects involves several steps. Here are some of the key steps:

- Data Collection: The first step in developing an AI-based face recognition system with aging effects is to collect data. This typically involves gathering a large data set of facial images that shows people of various ages, ethnicities, and genders [13].

- Data Preprocessing: The collected data needs to be pre-processed to remove any noise or inconsistencies. This step may involve resizing images, applying filters, and adjusting lighting and color.
- Training a Deep Learning Model: Once the data is pre-processed, the next step is to train a deep learning model. This involves feeding the pre-processed images into a neural network, which learns to recognize facial features and patterns.
- Adding Aging Effects: After the deep learning model is trained to recognize faces, the next step is to add aging effects. This can be done by applying filters or other techniques to the images to simulate the effects of aging.
- Testing and Evaluation: The final step is to test and evaluate the AI-based simulation. This involves measuring its accuracy in recognizing faces with aging effects and comparing it to other existing face recognition systems.

15.4.2 METHODOLOGY

Artificial intelligence (AI) can understand aging effects in face recognition systems through the use of deep learning algorithms. Deep learning is a subset of machine learning that uses artificial neural networks to learn from large data sets. To understand aging effects in face recognition systems, AI algorithms are trained on large data sets of facial images that include images of people at different ages. The neural network learns to identify the features that change as people age, such as wrinkles, sagging skin, and changes in facial structure. During the training process, the neural network adjusts the weights and biases of its connections to minimize the difference between the predicted age and the actual age of the person in each image. This process allows the network to learn how aging affects facial features and to recognize these changes in new images [14]. Once the AI algorithm is trained, it can be used to analyze new images and predict the age of the person in the image. The algorithm can also be used to simulate the effects of aging on an individual's face, allowing the system to recognize faces with aging effects more accurately. AI algorithms can understand aging effects in face recognition systems through the use of deep learning techniques, which allow the system to learn how aging affects facial features and to recognize these changes in new images (Figures 15.2 and 15.3).

15.5 LIMITATIONS

Artificial intelligence (AI) algorithms can sometimes fail to accurately understand the actual aging effects in face recognition systems for a few reasons. Here are some examples.

Limited Training Data: One of the main reasons AI algorithms may fail to accurately understand aging effects is due to a lack of diverse training data. If the algorithm is not trained on a sufficiently diverse data set, it may not learn to recognize the subtle variations in aging that occur across different individuals, ethnicities, and genders.

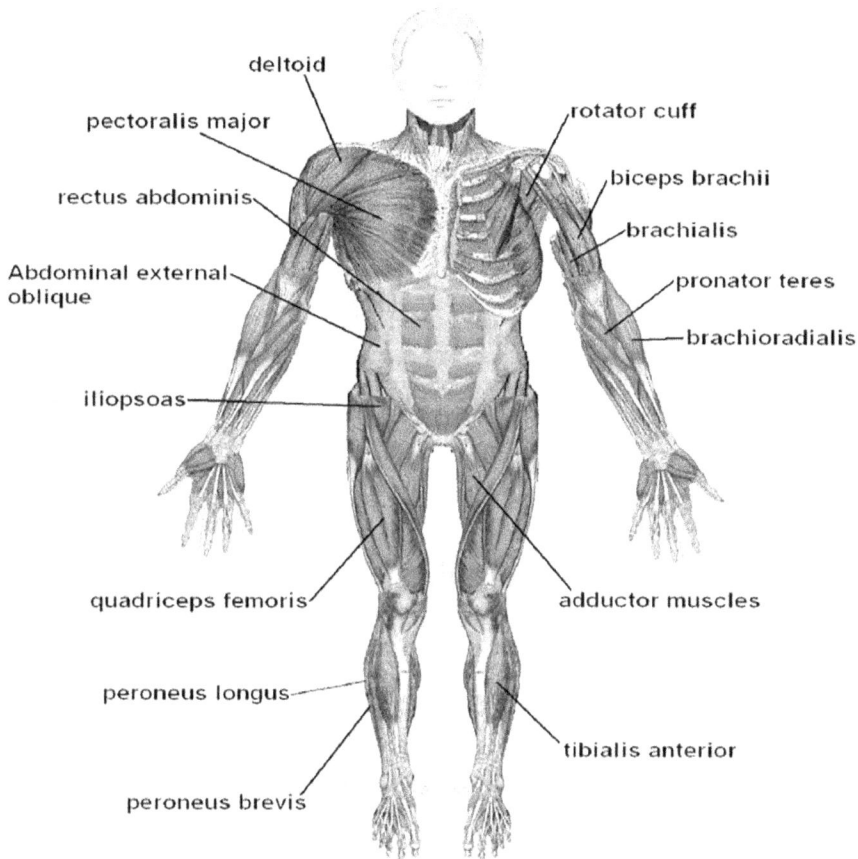

FIGURE 15.2   Muscles for human body: anterior view.

Biased Data: AI algorithms can also be biased if the training data is not representative of the entire population. For example, if the data set used to train the algorithm contains mostly young or middle-aged individuals, it may not learn to accurately recognize the aging effects in older individuals.

Changes in Appearance: As people age, their appearance can change significantly due to factors such as weight gain, illness, or changes in hairstyle. AI algorithms may not be able to accurately recognize these changes, which can lead to errors in face recognition.

Environmental Factors: The accuracy of face recognition systems can also be affected by environmental factors such as lighting, camera angle, and background. AI algorithms may not be able to account for these factors, leading to errors in recognition [11].

Limitations of Technology: Finally, it's important to remember that AI technology is still evolving, and there are limitations to what it can accurately recognize. Some aging effects may be more subtle or difficult to recognize than others, and AI algorithms may struggle to accurately identify them.

Generation Phase

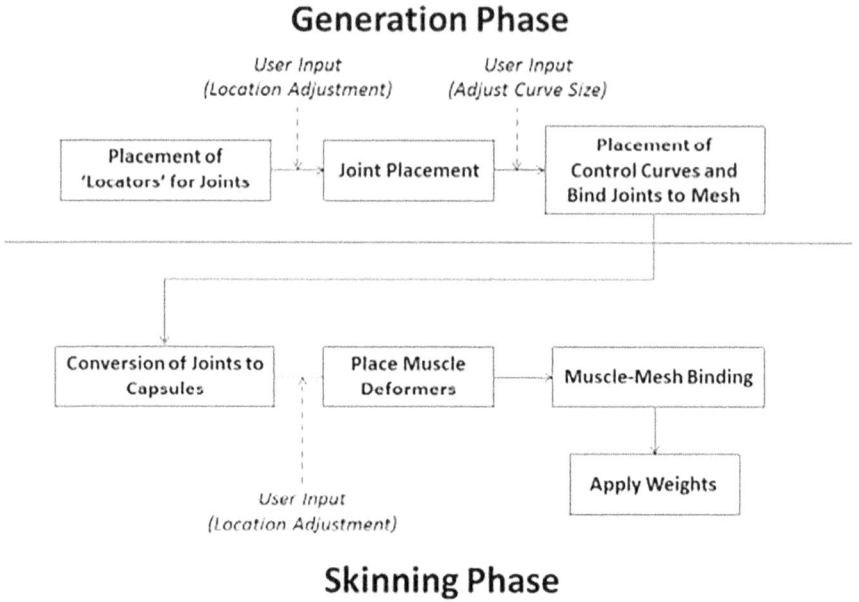

FIGURE 15.3   System pipeline.

Overall, while AI algorithms can be highly accurate in recognizing aging effects in face recognition systems, there are several reasons why they can fail to understand the actual aging effects. Addressing these limitations requires careful attention to training data, bias, appearance changes, environmental factors, and limitations of the technology [15].

15.6   RESULTS

One hundred members in electronic overview circulated utilizing departmental messages. We were effectively able to get 100 members who were over 18 years of age altogether. Among them, 60 were non-illustrators who had a place with a general gathering, and the other 40 members were prepared in liveliness; this can be seen in Figure 15.4. Finally, the performance of AI algorithms in face recognition systems can also be affected by technical limitations such as the quality of the input images, lighting conditions, and variations in poses and expressions.

Among 100 members, 51 distinguished character reenactments were intended to address the age bunch 11 to 20 years. Re-creation, which addressed the 21 to 30 years age class, was distinguished by 60 members, which are most noteworthy and considered as a part of all of the age classifications. Forty-eight members accurately recognized the 31 to 40 age bunch accurately. Reenactment, which addressed 41 to 50 years, was recognized by 55 members. Second most noteworthy reaction recognizable proof rate was for the 51 to 70 years age class (Figure 4.2). In view of the pattern in reactions, we can reason that most members had the option to distinguish the 21 to 30 years age class and 51 to 70 age classification (Figure 15.5).

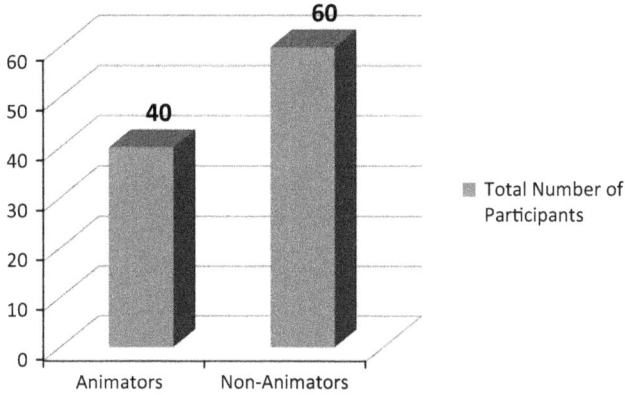

FIGURE 15.4   Survey participants.

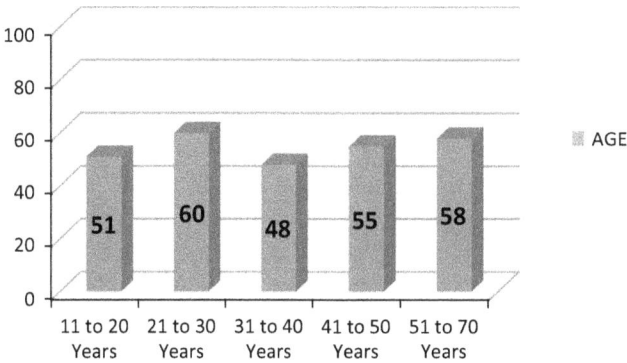

FIGURE 15.5   Successful age perception.

This "Complete Deviation/Distinction" recurrence dissemination was made to comprehend where most client reactions lie; for example, how close a member was close to reply and gauge normal conflict for each subject (Figures 5.1 and 5.2). We have a deviation of 0 to 4 for each question in view of the member's reactions. As a matter of course, we permit a distinction for not exactly or equivalent to 1 for every reaction demonstrated by members for each character re-creation addressing a particular age bunch. Therefore, for progress, a mean contrast or deviation ought to not be exactly or equivalent to 1. As shown by the recurrence histogram and box plot, we have a mean deviation of 3.64 with a standard deviation of 3.428 for every member. This is higher than whatever we had expected for fruitful insight for age, which are less than or equivalent to 1. Therefore, we can't dismiss the invalid hypo sister, H0 (1), which is in contrast to reenacted age bunches for the character isn't seen well by members. Bunch I members have a mean of 3.28 with a standard deviation of 3.948 while

Gathering II members have a mean of 5.25 with a standard deviation of 2.790. We have a planning incentive for 0.013, which are not exactly $\alpha = 0.05$. Here, for this situation, we have sufficient proof to say that Gathering I members (members who were artists) showed improvement over members who were not artists. Before, for this situation, we hold elective hypo sister, Ha (2), which implies that we are a distinction in discernment for mimicked age in character between an illustrator and a non-artist. We can unhesitatingly say that illustrator members were more effective in relating reproduced characters' ages to genuine ages than non-artist members. During the training process, the deep learning algorithm learns to identify the features that change as people age, such as wrinkles, sagging skin, and changes in facial structure. By analyzing a large data set of facial images, the algorithm is able to learn how aging affects facial features and to recognize these changes in new images.

Overall, the algorithm used by AI to understand aging effects in face recognition systems involves a combination of data collection, preprocessing, deep learning, aging simulation, and testing and evaluation. By using these techniques, the system is able to accurately recognize faces with aging effects and improve its accuracy over time.

15.7 CONCLUSION

In this study, we reject one for our null hypotheses and retain one for our alternative hypotheses.

  I. H_0 (1) = difference in simulated age groups for character is not perceived well by participants.
 II. H_a (2) = re are a difference in perception for simulated age in character between an animator and a non-animator.

Accordingly, we can with certainty say that artists had the option to distinguish different maturing reenactments better than other members. Likewise, we can presume that all members noted changes in various age classes; however, not changes connected with a particular age classification. Members saw huge outrageous contrasts (e.g., 21 to 30 years age bunch when contrasted with 51 to 70 years) in age bunches better compared to or mimicked age bunches with unpretentious contrasts. Therefore, for fruitful distinguishing proof for maturing by crowd, contrasts ought to be extremely unmistakable than exceptionally unobtrusive. The process of developing an AI-based simulation for a face recognition system with aging effects requires a combination of data collection, pre-processing, deep learning, and testing and evaluation. Overall, while AI has made significant progress in recognizing aging effects in face recognition systems, there are still limitations and challenges that can cause failures. Addressing these limitations will require more diverse training data sets, advanced algorithms that can better capture the complexities of the aging process, and better image quality and processing techniques.

REFERENCES

1. Kumar, A., Dhanagopal, R., Albreem, M. A., and Le, D. A comprehensive study on the role of advanced technologies in 5G based smart hospital. *Alexandria Engineering Journal*, vol. 60, pp. 5527–5536, 2021.
2. Saito, Y., Kishiyama, Y., Benjebbour, A., Nakamura, T., Li, A., and Higuchi, K. Non-orthogonal multiple access (NOMA) for cellular future radio access. In *2013 IEEE 77th Vehicular Technology Conference (VTC Spring)*, pp. 1–5. IEEE, 2013.
3. Murudkar, C. V., and Gitlin, R. D. Optimal-capacity, shortest path routing in self-organizing 5G networks using machine learning. In *2019 IEEE 20th Wireless and Microwave Technology Conference (WAMICON)*, pp. 1–5. IEEE, 2019.
4. Iqbal, M. A., and Dwivedi, A. D. Modelling & efficiency analysis of InGaP/GaAs single junction PV cells with BSF. *International Journal of Engineering and Advanced Technology*, vol. 8, no. 6, pp. 623–627, 2019.
5. Chimnani, M., et al. Efficiency improvement approach of InGaN based solar cell by investigating different optical and electrical properties. In *Proceedings of International Conference on Sustainable Computing in Science, Technology and Management (SUSCOM), Amity University Rajasthan*, Jaipur-India. 2019.
6. Ramakrishnan, B., Kumar, A., Chakravarty, S., Masud, M., and Baz, M. Analysis of FBMC waveform for 5G network based smart hospitals. *Applied Sciences*, vol. 11, no. 19, p. 8895, 2021. 10.3390/app11198895.
7. Kumar, A., and Gupta, M. A review on activities of fifth generation mobile communication system. *Alexandria Engineering Journal*, vol. 57, no. 2, pp. 1125–1135, 2017.
8. Tong, J., Ping, L., and Ma, X. Superposition coded modulation with peak-power limitation. *IEEE Transactions on Information Theory*, vol. 55, no. 6, pp. 2562–2576, 2009.
9. Miridakis, N. I., and Vergados, D. D. A survey on the successive interference cancellation performance for single-antenna and multiple-antenna OFDM systems. *IEEE Communications Surveys & Tutorials*, vol. 15, no. 1, pp. 312–335, 2012.
10. Lee, J., Kim, Y., Kwak, Y., Zhang, J., Papasakellariou, A., Novlan, T., Sun, C., and Li, Y. LTE-advanced in 3GPP Rel-13/14: An evolution toward 5G. *IEEE Communications Magazine*, vol. 54, no. 3, pp. 36–42, 2016.
11. Kumar, A., Albreem, M. A., Gupta, M., Alsharif, M. H., and Kim, S. Future 5G network based smart hospitals: Hybrid detection technique for latency improvement. *IEEE Access*, vol. 8, pp. 153240–153249, 2020. 10.1109/ACCESS.2020.3017625.
12. Tsai, Y., Zhang, G., and Wang, X. Variable spreading factor orthogonal polyphase codes for constant envelope OFDM-CDMA system. In *IEEE Wireless Communications and Networking Conference, 2006. WCNC 2006*, vol. 3, pp. 1396–1401. IEEE, 2006.
13. Baig, I., ul Hasan, N., Zghaibeh, M., Khan, I. U., and Saand, A. S. A DST precoding based uplink NOMA scheme for PAPR reduction in 5G wireless network. In *2017 7th International Conference on Modeling, Simulation, and Applied Optimization (ICMSAO)*, pp. 1–4. IEEE, 2017.
14. Kumar, A., Venkatesh, J., Gaur, N., Alsharif, M. H., Uthansakul, P., and Uthansakul, M. Cyclostationary and energy detection spectrum sensing beyond 5G. *Electronic Research Archive*, vol. 31, no. 6, pp. 3400–3416, 2023a. 10.3934/era.2023172.
15. Kumar, A. et al. Hybrid detection techniques for 5G and B5G M-MIMO system. *Alexandria Engineering Journal*, vol. 75, pp. 429–437, 2023b.

16 An Intelligent IoT-Based Smart Healthcare Monitoring System Using Machine Learning

R. Krishnamoorthy
Centre for Advanced Wireless Integrated Technology, Chennai Institute of Technology, India

Meenakshi Gupta
School of Engineering and Technology, Sushant University, India

Gundala Swathi
School of Information Technology and Engineering, Vellore Institute of Technology, India

Kazuaki Tanaka
Kyushu Institute of Technology, Japan

Ch. Raja
Department of ECE, Mahatma Gandhi Institute of Technology, India

Janjhyam Venkata Naga Ramesh
Department of Computer Science and Engineering, Koneru Lakshmaiah Education Foundation, India

16.1 INTRODUCTION

The traditional adage that "health is wealth" still holds true today. The poor and ill quality of human existence is a result of modern society's fast pace, its rising pollution, and the emergence of epidemic and pandemic viruses. More than 90% of the population has been exposed to toxic environments, according to recent data. The bulk of people's living conditions have deteriorated as a result of the industrial revolution and population increases. Therefore, it is important to keep an eye on

DOI: 10.1201/9781003403678-16

healthy lifestyles and work to improve them [1]. The genesis and spread of diseases have become an urgent problem in present situation, quickly growing scientific and evolutionary environment. The problems just mentioned can be fixed by implementing a smart health monitoring (SHM) system. Smart, low-cost sensors that can monitor an individual's health in real time have been made possible by the recent revolutions in industry 5.0 and 5G [2]. Previously, it was not possible to perform health monitoring from remote areas quickly, affordably, and reliably; with the SHM, this has become a reality. Patient information is now more secure and private because to blockchain's incorporation, reducing the risk of data exploitation. Using DL and ML to examine health data for numerous goals has aided in achieving both preventative healthcare and fatality management. As a result, chronic diseases can now be identified earlier than ever before. Integrating cloud-computing and cloud storage has been executed to make the services more real time and cost-effective [3].

SHM relies heavily on the IoT, particularly the IoMT. The original notion behind the "Internet of Things" was the networking of smart tools to facilitate information exchange within a particular field of study or industry. The term "Internet of Medical Things" refers to the network of interrelated smart tools specifically designed for use in medical settings, including but not limited to patient observation, conditioning, and viewing systems, disease and anomaly detection systems, and remote and telemedicine care delivery infrastructures [4]. The Internet of Things and the Science of Human Minds are just two examples of how hospitals are expanding their medical systems to better serve their patients. Our technologies have been developed over the past few decades with a focus on lowering inspection costs and protecting people's lives. In Figure 16.1, we see the SHM in action in a variety of contexts [5].

16.1.1   SHM AND IoMT

SHM health tools include a number of useful functions, such as reducing the need for patients to make unneeded trips to the hospital and allowing medical professionals to remotely monitor patients' conditions in real time. The information that is generated by these devices is safe from being hacked. These technologies serve to solve an issue that is a significant progression in the medical sector, and that problem is the high expense of healthcare services in today's world [6]. The job of IoMTs and SHM will have a constant part in the on the whole progression and expansion if people continue to place more demands on the smartness of gadgets and believe that digitalization will bring about this level of intelligence. SHM, an emerging technology in the field of medicine, has the potential to be utilized to vaguely regulate medical amenities, thereby helping to save the lives of critically ill patients suffering from conditions such as heart attacks, asthma attacks, diabetic patients, and so on. For various conclusions to converge, the data that are produced by the SHM system and the IoMT tools need to undergo regressive processing [7]. The analysis and computation of this data helps to achieve numerous aims, including the control of the breakout of specific diseases, the predictive monitoring of patients' health, the prevention of chronic diseases, and the reduction of fatalities

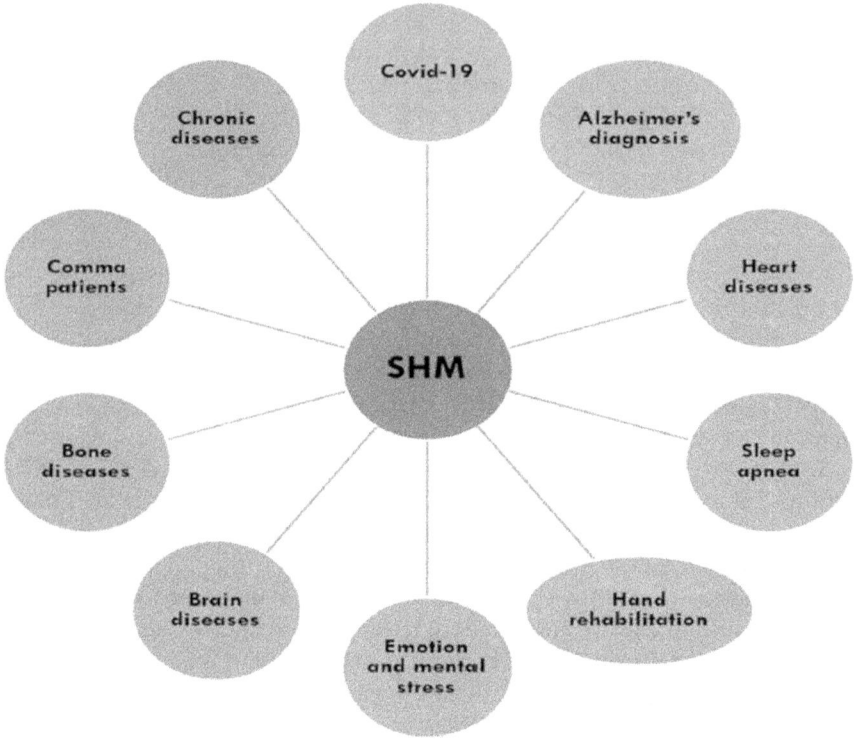

FIGURE 16.1   Applications of SHM.

among patients. The examination of data pertaining to medical treatment requires the application of AI. In the public domain, there are a great number of frameworks and proposed architects that can be used for the scrutiny of healthcare data in SHM networks [8].

16.1.2   ROLE OF DL AND TRANSFER LEARNING IN SHM

DL and transfer learning (TL) are both subfields of ML. In both of these subfields, multiple layers are utilized to accumulate effectual data, which then gradually dig higher level knowledge from historical data. This is pursued by its applications handling hefty amounts of data that have been successfully validated on any platform. DL offers useful information by unearthing previously concealed material with the use of staked blocks of layers within the DL skeleton. This process is known as data mining. DL models are utilized in a wide diversity of fields, including research, SHM, and telemedicine, among others [9]. While transfer learning (TL) is an essential component of the learning machine, which refers to the process by which people apply what they have learned from prior experiences, TL can be problematic for researchers and engineers when it comes to their work. The relationship between DL, ML, and TL may be seen to correlate in Figure 16.2.

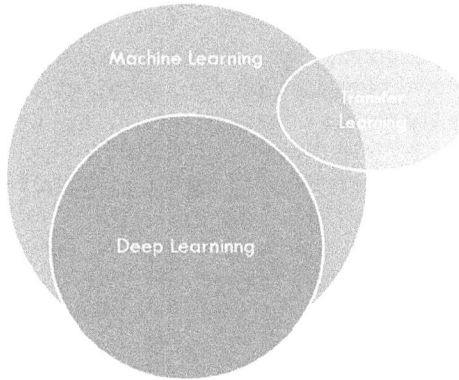

FIGURE 16.2   Relation of DL, ML, and TL.

Utilizing DL in a SHM network comes with a wide variety of benefits. The information that DL models provide is accurate and effective, and they are also beneficial in the process of collecting large amounts of data. Reduce the amount of time that passes before serious cases are reported, and make diagnosis as simple and quick as possible [10]. A computational learning system, a self-healing medical (SHM) device, the Internet of Things (IoT), and knowledgeable medical professionals who are able to sense the real-time state of patients and have the appropriate anticipation of the future and glitches of diabetes, and other conditions are all necessary. By analyzing a patient's genes, which may be done with the assistance of deep learning, it is possible to easily detect general disorders. As a result, medical professionals are able to find future remedies as well as future drugs. ML and DL can both identify normal and aberrant patient data, allowing medical professionals to more accurately diagnose their patients and improve patient outcomes [11].

In today's modern society, monitoring one's health is one of the most important aspects of both treating and diagnosing medical conditions. The electrocardiogram (ECG), electromyography (EMG), and electro-dermal-activity (EDA) are the three diagnostic tools that are utilized in order to evaluate the aberrant situations that are present in a human body. Because of these factors, a conventional analysis carried out by a person and, consequently, the data may be necessary. The prevention of falls is one of the most important concerns for people of advanced age [12]. These days, there are a lot of wearable devices that are popular on the market. Some of these devices may monitor your heart rate or detect your body mass index, and they are often inexpensive and lightweight. With the assistance of a gateway, the information data that has been acquired is both stored and delivered to wherever location is required. However, there is a possibility that the wearable will have downsides and failures in terms of the data collecting and energy monitoring owing to a lack of battery backup, data transfer, faulty network connectivity, and other factors. It is anticipated that there will be approximately 20 billion items in 2020 and 25 billion things in 2025 [13]. The majority of people and businesses are currently utilizing these things because of the low-energy limits, low-memory dispensation, faster-transmission, and increased steadfastness. For regular people, these products are being utilized as smart houses, smart farms, devices for monitoring pets and children, printers, voice assistants, and other similar applications.

The performance of deployment, the adaptability, and the usefulness of fall detection are the primary focuses of the obstacles and restrictions imposed on fall detection. The aged person may become accustomed to the system that has been suggested, and it is imperative to make appropriate use of flexible methods. The key concern here is the flexibility of the suggested system, as well as the privacy concerns that come along with it because of the sensor issues that come into play while monitoring an elderly person's fall detection. In addition, it is unreasonable to anticipate that an elderly person will always use their smartphone in order to navigate the complex surroundings [14]. The identification of the problem that needs to be solved by the proposed system has proven to be a significant challenge in the data set. The conventional method makes use of wired cameras, and one of the problems with this setup is that there is insufficient battery backup. As a result, the suggested system will be able to circumvent this problem by using edge connectivity devices. The proposed section is able to cope with the problems both inside and outside in their respective surroundings [15].

The suggested method has undergone thorough evaluation, during which the health histories of senior people, their use of assistive devices, their levels of gait deficit, and every other concern specific to elderly people were taken into account. Nevertheless, the development of technology has an effect on the adaptability of the proposed model in terms of how far older people can use it. A unified design for decrease detection using AI and IoT is presented in this work. The suggested model creates a comprehensive framework for IoT-based health care solutions, which allows these solutions to transcend the limits that currently exist in terms of data storage, acceleration, and monitoring. Edge gateways are being utilized in conjunction with artificial intelligence to make the detection of a human illness more accurate and to perform a calculation that is more extract [16].

The IoT-ONN model is an innovative and intelligent healthcare monitoring system that is based on contemporary technologies such as the IoT, optimization techniques, and ML. This model is introduced in this chapter. This system is equipped with a medical decision support system that enables it to sense and process data relating to patients. This technology offers a solution at a reduced cost to customers who live in more remote locations. The following is a list of the primary contributions that will be made by the proposed work:

1. The optimal characteristics are selected with the use of an ant-colony-optimization (ACO) method to speed up both the training and testing processes.
2. The IoT-ONN model is an intelligent healthcare monitoring system that makes use of the Internet of Things (IoT), optimization methods, and machine learning to categorize human health using the most appropriate features.
3. To check how well the healthcare IoT-ONN model you built does in several real-time health databases.
4. To evaluate the healthcare IoT-ONN model against other newly established models.

The remaining work is distributed among the many groups that will follow. Previous work in this field is presented in Section 16.2, while the framework being proposed is outlined in Section 16.3. The explanation and the investigational outcomes are included in Section 16.4 of the document. In Section 16.5, the task is brought to a close.

16.2   RELATED WORKS

One of the most significant contributors to poor health among older adults all across the world is falling. A fall can pose a functional danger to elderly people, leading to a reduction in mobility and impairment in their ability to participate in life quality matters. The Internet of Things is being used to detect falls in interior spaces, and low-power sensor nodes are actively participating in the network alongside smart gadgets and cloud-computing. It is proposed that a 3D axis accelerometer be used to establish the utilization of the 6LowPan device in order to enable the data gathering linked to the movements of old people in a real-time environment [17]. Because of the large proportion of senior persons in the population, fall detection has become one of the most pressing issues facing healthcare providers today. It has been noticed that the age group of 65 is represented by 50% of wounded people [18]. It is believed that the fall detection systems are prohibitively expensive and that not all age groups will be able to purchase them. As a result, an adjustable tool has been presented for the old-age homes, and a smart city is intended with medical details beared by the intelligence driven by AI and the Internet of Things [19].

Using the information that is streamed from the accelerometer, it has been suggested that a smart watch, which is part of the Internet of Things, may be used to detect falls. The smart watch is connected to the smartphone in order to carry out the computation; this connection is essential for determining the position of a fall based on a real-time premise without experiencing any delays when interacting with the cloud server [20]. The information that is provided is not sufficient for the protection of the information in this technique. Because fall detection systems as a whole require an increased amount of technology and programming, they are thus more expensive and out of reach for the general population. One of the benefits of using the smart watch to collect the information is that it can help differentiate the fall findings. The SVM and NB are used in conjunction with one another to assist in the process of fall detection. It is possible to show the drop detection model by modifying the frequency with which the spilled information occurs [21]. Through this demonstration, an accurate positive rate of decrease recognition in real-universal conditions has been achieved with a precision of 93.33%. These results hold their own in comparison to those obtained using bespoke and pricey sensors [22].

Elderly folks have a significant opportunity to improve their overall health if they can avoid falling. In the event that the situation is not brought to the attention of the appropriate parties in a timely manner, it will result in the loss of life or impairment among the elderly, which will lower their excellence of life. The exactness of the data set that was produced came out to be 98.75% overall, and individually it was 90.59%. As a result, it was determined that K-NN provides a higher level of accuracy when identifying falls; hence, this method is the one that is used for classification [23]. Through the use of a Python module, a notification will be delivered to a pre-registered phone number in the event that a fall takes place. This notification will provide information regarding the nature of the fall [24]. One further strategy for generating an honest instance acknowledgment has been suggested as a way to cut down on the mischievous consequences that occur following the effect of falling. Because of its close connection to the medical treatment of older persons, fall detection is the most essential and leading topic of study now being conducted [25]. The artificial intelligence for fall detection is consolidated as a result of all the developed researches and methodologies that have been tried. Methods of this kind are evaluated based on the pros and drawbacks that are associated with them. The suggested method focuses on identifying the various fall detection methods and concentrating on the consolidated automated fall detection methods, with vibration measurement serving as a major instrument [26]. This is the primary objective of the method. Additionally, the applicability of the methodologies and the obstacles that are associated with the fall anticipation utilizing the vibration measurement tools are discussed in this section. The purpose of providing an overview of the key methods involved in the decrease anticipation design is to define a diverse strategy depends on united sensors that can be utilized to progress the general performance of the system.

The IoT system has the potential to be exploited for the prediction of the behavior of an individual using machine learning techniques. These approaches would be applied by analyzing the behavior, gestures, health factors, and so on [27]. An IoT and wireless sensor network (WSN)–based cloud system was developed for the identification and dealing of cancer patients [28]. The authors focused on the most significant difficulties, such as safety and effectiveness. Another Internet of Things system was established for the purpose of identifying possible COVID-19 patients. This system was built with the assistance of eight diverse learning strategies, which helped to differentiate the symptoms of a cold from those of COVID-19 [29]. In the study, the usage of an Internet of Things system to monitor patients in smart cities so that ambulances and other forms of assistance can get to patients more quickly is discussed. The authors built a wearable Internet of Things health monitoring system with its own network, which is referred to as a body area network. Within this network, several sensors are continuously measuring and storing the parameters [30]. All of the Internet of Things technology was either implemented in a hospital, a home, or a wearable, which means that in each of these application areas, the system is plagued by some of the same problems. Explain some of the elements that need to be taken into consideration in order to build and execute an automated IoT health monitoring system [31]. Some of these factors include the infrastructure of the IoT layer, intelligent computing, big data analytics, and network traffic. When an IoT-based health monitoring system is built, developers are faced with a number of significant challenges, the most significant of which include the inappropriate use of patient information, instances of cybercrime, data aggregation, etc. [32]. The monitoring of COVID-19 instances is of utmost importance since it enables government officials to monitor patients and, as a result, stop the disease from spreading further. This can be accomplished with the use of an Internet of Things (IOT)–based monitoring system [33].

Real-time monitoring of COVID-19 patients with the assistance of big data on biological signals may have the potential to reduce the number of COVID-19 transmission cases [34]. The suggested design is primarily composed of three levels, which are denoted as the application layer, the data distribution layer, and the data acquisition layer. However, the majority of health systems based on IoT have a few issues, such as a delay in communication, latency, and other similar issues. Utilizing data mining algorithms in conjunction with fog computing can provide a solution to all of these issues [35]. This will allow for the resolution of all of these issues. The safety of the patient data is one of the primary concerns of the IoT-based smart health system; hence, a model that is based on block encryption might be applied to protect data stored in the cloud [36]. This would be in addition to the common disease detection that is accomplished by measuring the vital parameters of the body.

16.2.1 CHALLENGES OF SHM

Big data, often known as health data, refers to the information that is gathered through medical equipment and networks such as SHM networks. The management of this healthcare data necessitates the use of extensive computer resources and a large capacity for data storage. Cloud computing and storage on the cloud are the solutions to the problem of handling medical records [37]. On the other hand, the majority of this information is strictly confidential to the patient. The most significant difficulties in SHM are related to the protection of personal information and data. It is important to prevent specific users, individuals, and organizations from misusing this confidential data for the purpose of gaining personal benefits as much as possible. The protection of the data encompasses not only the storage security but also the authentication, network security, computer security, and physical location security. More and more people are using ciphering and deciphering techniques, as well as cryptography, data encryption, and genetic algorithms. The majority of the frameworks for security and privacy offer third parties in situations [38]. In recent years, blockchain has been recognized for their contributions to the development of secure data exchange technologies in the banking and financial industries and cryptographic means are used to validate new blocks as they are added to the chain. A resilient and highly secure method of data transport, blockchain is characterized by the presence of a time stamp as well as the value of the block hash of the preceding block. In the current context, the blockchain has been successfully deployed in a variety of industries, including manufacturing, management, medical services, and supply chain logistics. There are a few different frameworks that can be found in the public domain, and they have all been proven to be successful in the medical healthcare and SHM systems [34].

There are several restrictions associated with these SHM and medical IoT tools, such as the collection of heterogeneous data by a variety of sensors, which increases the likelihood of errors and makes it more difficult to understand the data or diagnose the patients' conditions. Because wearable sensors, especially those

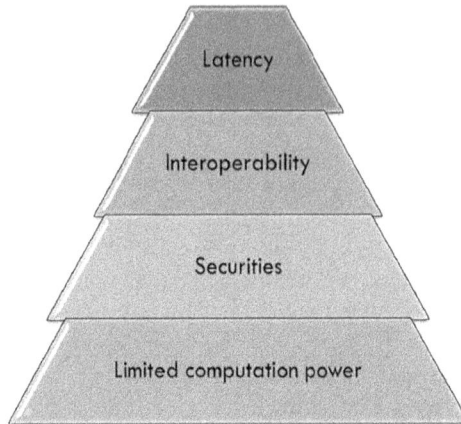

FIGURE 16.3 The different challenges of SHM.

designed for youngsters, can be a source of annoyance, wireless sensors are typically the better option [39]. Because of the sensitive patient information that is at
risk of being compromised, security concerns cannot be ignored. By utilizing an
Internet of Things healthcare system, the topic of fraudulence is also brought up. To
put it simply, chronic patients stand to benefit more from an intelligent medical
system than they would from standard healthcare services. The Internet of Things
and Medical Technologies (IoMT) tools operate on batteries and/or continuous
power, neither of which is accessible in distant places. Figure 16.3 illustrates the
significant difficulties that must be overcome. Real-time monitoring calls for a
network connection that is both quick and dependable can be challenging to establish with devices that have low power output and in distant places [40]. Because
these limits are not directly related to the expansion of innovative technologies, they
can be defeated with enough time and the right tools.

16.3 PROPOSED METHODOLOGY

Figure 16.4 depicts the design of the intelligent IoT for the smart healthcare
monitoring system that makes use of the optimum neural network (IoT-ONN)
model.

16.3.1 DATA COLLECTION

IoT devices such as implanted and external sensors are utilized in the process of
data collection from patients. Implanted sensors that are integrated into patients'
bodies are used to collect data from the internal environment, while the everlasting
sensor is utilized to collect data from the external world. Patients are provided with
conveniently accessible and low-cost IoT sensors to capture medical data, regardless of whether they are at home or in the hospital [41]. These Internet of Things
sensors capture patients' health data and transmit it to an IoT agent for analysis.

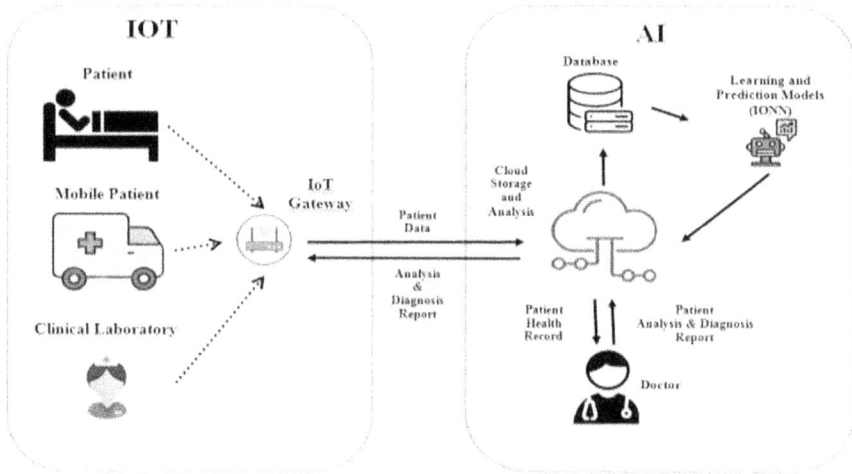

FIGURE 16.4 Concept diagram of the SHM.

In the event that a patient shows up at a clinic or laboratory at a time when there are no doctors accessible, each and every resource is at their disposal. The medical support staff was responsible for collecting the patient's information. IoT sensors are used to collect patient data and communicate it to doctors in real time in order to provide patients who live in inaccessible areas or who are located a significant distance from hospitals with the ability to obtain improved medical treatment. These three sensors are connected to one another by means of an Arduino board in order to collect patient data [42].

16.3.2 LEARNING AND PREDICTION PROCESS

Following the completion of the data collection process, the data are then sent to a fog server within the IoT cloud for additional analysis. The transmission described above will be managed by the devices responsible for communication and networking. Using IoT-ONN techniques, the fog server performs analysis on the data that has been stored. In the process of developing the IoT-ONN model, numerous machine learning methods, such as optimization and classification algorithms, were utilized in order to analyze and categorize the gathered data in order to differentiate between healthy and unhealthy individuals [43]. Figure 16.5 provides an explanation of the suggested workflow for the model.

The research examination has been carried out making use of a three-layer feed forward neural network (NN) that consists of many layers [44]. In the architecture of the neural network that has been proposed, N neurons are used for input, P neurons are used for hiding information, and O neurons are used for output. The features of the training data set are reflected in the number of neurons that are present in the input layer. Because the stated NN is fully incorporated, the neurons in each layer before the one being discussed are connected to each neuron in the layer that comes after it. Following the completion of the study, the data is then

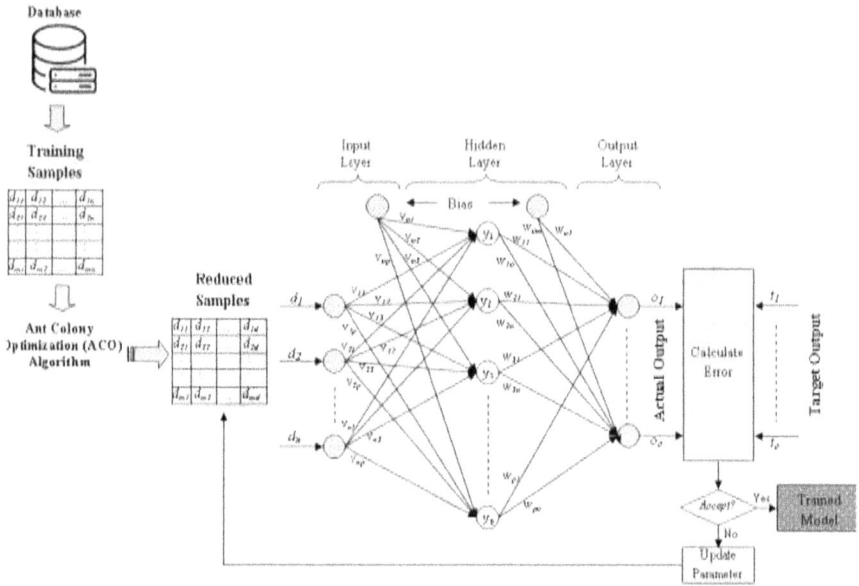

FIGURE 16.5   Flow diagram of the proposed model.

stored on a fog server within the IoT cloud, where it will be accessible to clinicians for the sake of early diagnosis. The physician will conduct an evaluation of the patient's health using the information that has been supplied and will offer recommendations regarding the subsequent measures that should be taken to ensure the very best therapy [45].

16.4 RESULTS AND DISCUSSIONS

In this section, the results of numerous different classification algorithms such as ANN and IONN are discussed and analyzed. The IONN model that has been presented is evaluated with the help of four real-world healthcare data sets that can be found in the UCI Machine Learning Repository [46]. These data sets include breast cancer, liver disorders, SPeCT heart, and thyroid disease. Table 16.1 has an

TABLE 16.1

Data Set Characteristics

Data set	No. of Features	No. of Samples	No. of Classes	Classification Type
SpeCT Heart (SCTH)	34	352	2	Binary
Liver Disorders (LD)	8	468	2	Binary
Breast Cancer Wisconsin (BCW)	41	721	2	Binary
Thyroid Disease (TD)	30	8435	3	Multi

organized list of the information pertaining to each of the data sets. Python is used for the implementation work that is being done on a processor with an Intel Core i5-3210M and a CPU M60 running at 2.50 GHz.

Training time and accuracy are the two performance indicators that are utilized in the process of evaluating the effectiveness of each classifier. The term "training time" refers to the entire amount of time that the classifier uses up during the training process. A classifier's accuracy is measured according to its total performance, which is determined by the formula:

$$\text{Accuracy (Acc)} = \frac{\textit{Total number of correctly classified samples}}{\textit{Total number of samples in testing dataset}} \times 100$$

$$(16.1)$$

Both the existing ANN model and the proposed IONN model, which makes use of every piece of training data to achieve a higher level of accuracy in the training process, are both trained with the tenfold cross-validation technique [47]. In tenfold cross-validation, the outcomes of several learning models for training on different data sets, such as ANN and IONN for the entire fold, are summarized in Table 16.2 and Figure 16.6. When compared to the methods that are already in use, the accuracy of the IOI-ONN model that has been proposed sees a boost of between 4% and 15%. In addition, as compared to ANNs that make use of the BPN algorithm, the overall training time required by the IOI-ONN framework is condensed by anywhere from 15% to 52%. Figure 16.7 depicts the average accuracy of ANN and IOT-ONN models with respect to all data sets.

When compared across all data sets, the IOI-ONN model's training process requires significantly less time than that of the ANN model. The IoT-ONN model

TABLE 16.2
All Data Sets Comparison Outcomes

Data Set	SCTH		LD		BCW		TD	
Folds	ANN	IOT-ONN	ANN	IOT-ONN	ANN	IOT-ONN	ANN	IOT-ONN
1	86.5	98.24	86.5	89.25	76.25	98.54	86.56	99.68
2	69.2	93.41	81	89.34	91.2	95.67	90.24	99.52
3	83.4	89.67	78.23	98.35	81	99.24	84.21	93.64
4	79.3	99.34	86.21	85.36	81.25	99.27	88.28	93.68
5	75.4	86.21	79	85.27	85.23	88.24	86	91.25
6	93.6	84.12	89	95.27	78.24	95.68	91	95.24
7	72.3	98.29	71	98.63	72.68	83.24	85.24	95.12
8	61.2	89.34	83.57	98.57	88.63	93.61	93.61	98.54
9	72.5	98.35	78.29	78.2	78.26	99.32	90.14	98.94
10	92.7	86.24	86.31	98.68	76.24	99.12	86.24	97.37
Avg.	78.61	92.321	81.911	91.692	80.898	95.193	88.152	96.298

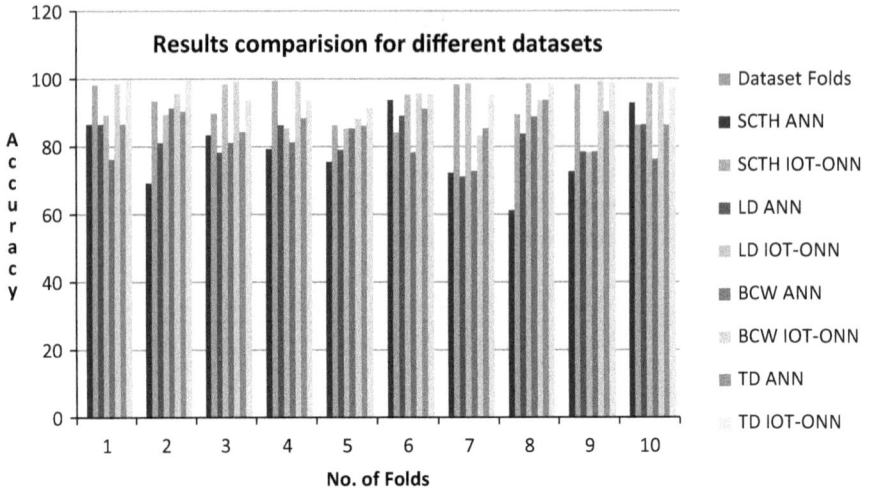

FIGURE 16.6 Data set-based accuracy comparison of ANN and IoT-ONN models.

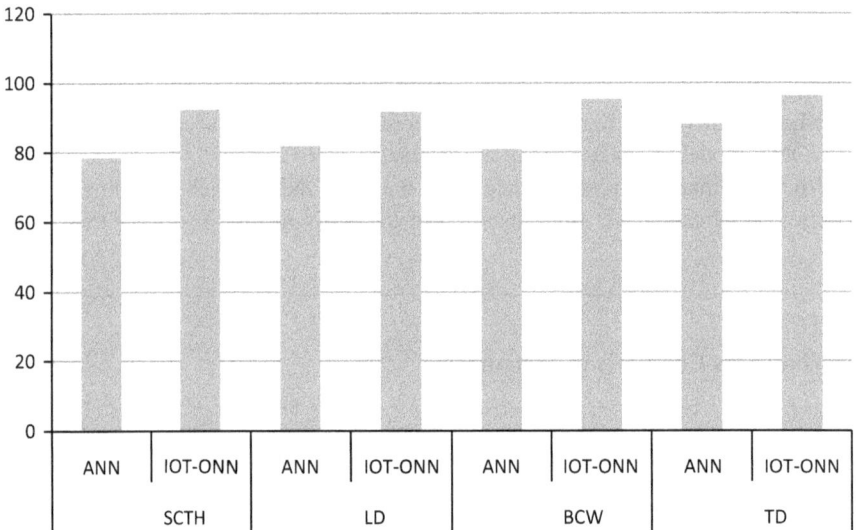

FIGURE 16.7 Avgerage accuracy of the ANN and IoT-ONN models with respective of data sets.

required 15% less time to train in order to perform the evaluation of the SPeCT heart data sets when compared to the ANN model. When it came to evaluating the data sets associated with liver disorders, the IONN model required 19% less time to train than the ANN model did. When it came to the evaluation of the breast cancer Wisconsin (diagnostic) data sets, the IoT-ONN model required 52% less time to train compared to the ANN model. When it came to reviewing data sets related to thyroid disease, the IoT-ONN model required 31% less time to train than its ANN counterpart did. Figure 16.6 demonstrates that while training on the data set presented in Table 16.1, the IONN model achieves a higher percentage of correct predictions than the ANN model does for any and all data sets. When comparing their performance on the SPeCT heart data sets, the IoT-ONN model was 14% more effective than the ANN model. When it came to examining data sets related to liver disorders, the IoT-ONN model performed 10% better than the ANN model. In the evaluation of breast cancer data sets from Wisconsin with a diagnostic focus, the IoT-ONN model performed 15% better than the ANN model. In the evaluation of data sets relating to thyroid disease, the IoT-ONN model performed 4% better than the ANN model.

Table 16.3 and Figure 16.8 present the results of a comparison between the precision of the IoT-ONN model and the accuracy of other existing machine learning models. The IOI-ONN model's accuracy for the SCTH is 12%, 9%, 6%, 2%, and 3% greater than that of the ANN model, the K-NN model, the SVM model, and the DT model, respectively. When compared to ANN, NB, K-NN, SVM, and DT, respectively, the accuracy of the IOI-ONN model for the LD is 11%, 23%, 15%, 13%, and 22% higher than other models. When applied to the BCW data set, the accuracy of the IoT-ONN is 14%, 6%, 3%, –2%, and 2% higher, respectively, than that of the ANN, NB, K-NN, SVM, and DT. When compared to ANN, NB,

TABLE 16.3
Accuracy Comparison of Diverse Classifiers with Various Data Sets

Data Set	ANN	NB	K-NN	SVM	DT	IOT-ONN
SCTH	78.61	85.3	88.11	92.37	90.24	92.32
LD	81.91	72.22	75.24	77.27	71.28	91.69
BCW	80.89	91.23	96.24	97.27	94.25	95.19
TD	88.15	81.68	83.67	84.27	82.64	96.29

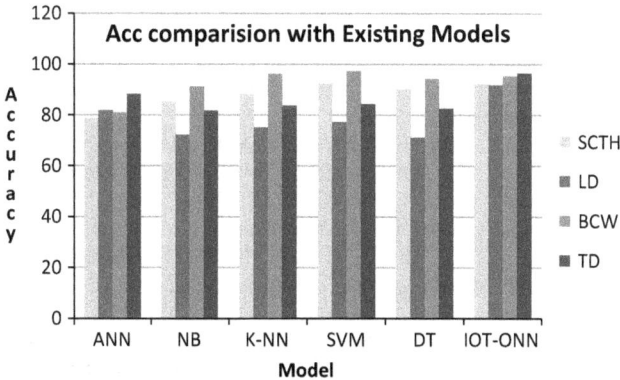

FIGURE 16.8　Accuracy comparison of IoT-ONN with existing models.

K-NN, SVM, and DT, respectively, the accuracy of the IOI-ONN model for the TD data set is 3%, 13%, 15%, 13%, and 14% higher than those other models.

When using a variety of healthcare data sets for training, these results show that the proposed IONN model performs well in terms of the amount of time it takes to train and the accuracy it achieves. The limitation that was found during the course of this research was that the parameters that are utilized by optimization and machine learning algorithms need to be fine-tuned in order to increase the performance of the IoT-ONN model.

16.5 CONCLUSION AND FUTURE WORKS

The Internet of Things (IoT), optimization strategies, and ML are only some of the cutting-edge technologies that are utilized in the IONN model, which is presented in this research. This model represents an innovative and intelligent healthcare system. The performance of the newly built healthcare monitoring system was evaluated utilizing performance metrics as accuracy, and it was compared to a number of different classification algorithms including ANN, NB, K-NN, SVM, and DT. When using a variety of healthcare data sets for training, the findings show that the suggested IONN framework performs quite well in terms of the amount of time it takes to train and the accuracy it achieves. The training algorithm that was presented is capable of solving any kind of categorization challenge that may arise in the actual world. The limitation that was found during the course of this research was that the parameters that are utilized by optimization and machine learning algorithms need to be fine-tuned in order to increase the performance of the IoT-ONN model. The aforementioned limitation can be circumvented through the application of a wide variety of tuning procedures for the parameters. An even more in-depth examination of these factors is recommended for use in subsequent study as it has the potential to yield even more fruitful findings.

REFERENCES

1. Li, W., Chai, Y., Khan, F., Jan, S. R. U., Verma, S., Menon, V. G., & Li, X. (2021). A comprehensive survey on machine learning-based big data analytics for IoT-enabled smart healthcare system. *Mobile Networks and Applications*, 26, pp.234–252.
2. Kumar, A., Dhana, G. R., Albreem, M., & Le, D. (2021). A comprehensive study on the role of advanced technologies in 5G based smart hospital. *Alexandria Engineering Journal*, 2021(60), pp.5527–5536.
3. Ahmed, I., Jeon, G., & Piccialli, F. (2021). A deep-learning-based smart healthcare system for patient's discomfort detection at the edge of Internet of Things. *IEEE Internet of Things Journal*, 8(13), pp.10318–10326.
4. Reddy, P. C. S., Suryanarayana, G., & Yadala, S. (2022). Data analytics in farming: Rice price prediction in Andhra Pradesh. In *2022 5th International Conference on Multimedia, Signal Processing and Communication Technologies (IMPACT)* (pp.1–5). IEEE.
5. Muhammad, K., Khan, S., Del Ser, J., & De Albuquerque, V. H. C. (2020). Deep learning for multigrade brain tumor classification in smart healthcare systems: A prospective survey. *IEEE Transactions on Neural Networks and Learning Systems*, 32(2), pp.507–522.

6. Ramakrishnan, B., Kumar, A., Chakravarty, S., Masud, M., & Baz, M. (2021). Analysis of FBMC waveform for 5G network based smart hospitals. *Applied Sciences.* 11(19), p.8895. 10.3390/app11198895.
7. Liu, L., Shafiq, M., Sonawane, V. R., Murthy, M. Y. B., Reddy, P. C. S., & Kumar Reddy, K. C. (2022). Spectrum trading and sharing in unmanned aerial vehicles based on distributed blockchain consortium system. *Computers and Electrical Engineering*, 103, p.108255.
8. Kumar, A., & Gupta, M. (2017). A review on activities of fifth generation mobile communication system. *Alexandria Engineering Journal*, 57(2), pp.1125–1135.
9. Stone, D., Michalkova, L., & Machova, V. (2022). Machine and deep learning techniques, body sensor networks, and Internet of Things-based smart healthcare systems in COVID-19 remote patient monitoring. *American Journal of Medical Research*, 9(1), pp.97–112.
10. Hemalatha, V., & Sundar, C. (2020). Automatic liver cancer detection in abdominal liver images using soft optimization techniques. *Journal of Ambient Intelligence and Humanized Computing*, 12, 4765–4774. 10.1007/s12652-020-01885-4.
11. Haque, N. I., Rahman, M. A., Shahriar, M. H., Khalil, A. A., & Uluagac, S. (2021). A novel framework for threat analysis of machine learning-based smart healthcare systems. *Cryptography and Security*, 2021, pp.1–15.
12. Pandey, H., & Prabha, S. (2020). Smart health monitoring system using IOT and machine learning techniques. In *2020 Sixth International Conference on Bio Signals, Images, and Instrumentation (ICBSII)* (pp.1–4). IEEE.
13. Singh, B., Somasekhar, K., Anand, K., Gopikrishnan, M., & Krishnamoorthy, R. (2022). Machine learning based predictive modeling of plasma treatment in biomedical surfaces. *Second International Conference on Artificial Intelligence and Smart Energy (ICAIS), 2022*, pp.1043–1046. 10.1109/ICAIS53314.2022.9743031.
14. Kumar, A., Albreem, M. A., Gupta, M., Alsharif, M. H., & Kim, S. (2020). Future 5G network based smart hospitals: Hybrid detection technique for latency improvement. *In IEEE Access*, 8, pp.153240–153249. 10.1109/ACCESS.2020.3017625.
15. Al-Marridi, A. Z., Mohamed, A., & Erbad, A. (2021). Reinforcement learning approaches for efficient and secure blockchain-powered smart health systems. *Computer Networks*, 197, p.108279.
16. Maurya, A. K., Lokesh, K., Kumar, S. R., & Krishnamoorthy, R. (2022). Deep neuro-fuzzy logic technique for brain meningiomasa prediction. 7th International Conference on Communication and Electronics Systems (ICCES), 2022, pp.1244–1248. 10.1109/ICCES54183.2022.9836008.
17. Ahmed, I., Jeon, G., & Chehri, A. (2022). An IoT-enabled smart health care system for screening of COVID-19 with multi layers features fusion and selection. *Computing*, 105, pp.1–18.
18. Lv, Z., Yu, Z., Xie, S., & Alamri, A. (2022). Deep learning-based smart predictive evaluation for interactive multimedia-enabled smart healthcare. *ACM Transactions on Multimedia Computing, Communications, and Applications (TOMM)*, 18(1s), pp.1–20.
19. Guo, B., Ma, Y., Yang, J., & Wang, Z. (2021). Smart healthcare system based on cloud-Internet of Things and deep learning. *Journal of Healthcare Engineering*, 2021, pp.1–10.
20. Kumar, A., Venkatesh, J., Gaur, N., Alsharif, M. H., Uthansakul, P., & Uthansakul, M. (2023a). Cyclostationary and energy detection spectrum sensing beyond 5G. *Electronic Research Archive,* 31(6), pp.3400–3416. 10.3934/era.2023172.
21. Rajan Jeyaraj, P., & Nadar, E. R. S. (2022). Smart-monitor: Patient monitoring system for IoT-based healthcare system using deep learning. *IETE Journal of Research*, 68(2), pp.1435–1442.

22. Krishnamoorthy, R., Liya, B. S., Padmapriya, S., Gunasundari, B., & Thiagarajan, R. (2021). Categorizing the heart syndrome condition by predictive analysis using machine learning approach. *Third International Conference on Advances in Computing, Communication Control and Networking (ICAC3N), 2021*, pp.104–108. 10.1109/ICAC3N53548.2021.9725725.

23. Rajan Jeyaraj, P., & Nadar, E. R. S. (2020). Atrial fibrillation classification using deep learning algorithm in Internet of Things-based smart healthcare system. *Health Informatics Journal*, 26(3), pp.1827–1840.

24. Kumar, A. et al. (2023b). Hybrid detection techniques for 5G and B5G M-MIMO system. *Alexandria Engineering Journal*, 75, pp.429–437.

25. Muthappa, K. A., Nisha, A. S. A., Shastri, R., Avasthi, V., & Reddy, P. C. S. (2023). Design of high-speed, low-power non-volatile master slave flip flop (NVMSFF) for memory registers designs. *Applied Nanoscience*, 13, pp.5369–5378.

26. Subasi, A., Khateeb, K., Brahimi, T., & Sarirete, A. (2020). Human activity recognition using machine learning methods in a smart healthcare environment. In *Innovation in health informatics* (pp.123–144). Academic Press.

27. Basharat, A., Mohamad, M. M. B., & Khan, A. (2022, July). Machine learning techniques for intrusion detection in smart healthcare systems: A comparative analysis. In *2022 4th International Conference on Smart Sensors and Application (ICSSA)* (pp.29–33). IEEE.

28. Balakrishnan, S., Suresh Kumar, K., Ramanathan, L., & Muthusundar, S. K. (2022). IoT for health monitoring system based on machine learning algorithm. *Wireless Personal Communications*, 124, pp.189–205.

29. Chillakuru, P., Madiajagan, M., Prashanth, K. V., Ambala, S., Shaker Reddy, P. C., & Pavan, J. (2023). Enhancing wind power monitoring through motion deblurring with modified GoogleNet algorithm. *Soft Computing*, pp.1–11.

30. Nancy, A. A., Ravindran, D., Raj Vincent, P. D., Srinivasan, K., & Gutierrez Reina, D. (2022). Iot-cloud-based smart healthcare monitoring system for heart disease prediction via deep learning. *Electronics*, 11(15), p.2292.

31. Kute, S., Tyagi, A. K., Sahoo, R., & Malik, S. (2022). Building a smart healthcare system using Internet of Things and machine learning. In *Big Data Management in Sensing* (pp.159–177). River Publishers.

32. Vivekananda, G. N., Ali, A. R. H., Mishra, P., Sengar, R., & Krishnamoorthy, R. (2022). Cloud based effective health care management system with artificial intelligence. *2022 IEEE 7th International conference for Convergence in Technology (I2CT)*, pp.1–6. 10.1109/I2CT54291.2022.9825457.

33. Chatzinikolaou, T., Vogiatzi, E., Kousis, A., & Tjortjis, C. (2022). Smart healthcare support using data mining and machine learning. In *IoT and WSN Based Smart Cities: A Machine Learning Perspective* (pp.27–48). Cham: Springer International Publishing.

34. Tiwari, A., Dhiman, V., Iesa, M. A., Alsarhan, H., Mehbodniya, A., & Shabaz, M. (2021). Patient behavioral analysis with smart healthcare and IoT. *Behavioural Neurology*, 2021, pp.1–9.

35. Alazzam, M. B., Alassery, F., & Almulihi, A. (2021). A novel smart healthcare monitoring system using machine learning and the Internet of Things. *Wireless Communications and Mobile Computing*, 2021, pp.1–7.

36. Khan, M. F., Ghazal, T. M., Said, R. A., Fatima, A., Abbas, S., Khan, M. A., Issa, G. F., Ahmad, M., & Khan, M. A. (2021). An IoMT-enabled smart healthcare model to monitor elderly people using machine learning technique. *Computational Intelligence and Neuroscience*, 2021, pp.1–10.

37. Ismail, A., Abdlerazek, S., & El-Henawy, I. M. (2020). Development of smart healthcare system based on speech recognition using support vector machine and dynamic time warping. *Sustainability*, 12(6), p.2403.

38. Sucharitha, Y., & Shaker Reddy, P. C. (2022). An autonomous adaptive enhancement method based on learning to optimize heterogeneous network selection. *International Journal of Sensors Wireless Communications and Control*, 12(7), pp.495–509.

39. Minopoulos, G. M., Memos, V. A., Stergiou, C. L., Stergiou, K. D., Plageras, A. P., Koidou, M. P., & Psannis, K. E. (2022). Exploitation of emerging technologies and advanced networks for a smart healthcare system. *Applied Sciences*, 12(12), p.5859.

40. Yempally, S., Singh, S. K., & Velliangiri, S. (2022). Analytical review on deep learning and IoT for smart healthcare monitoring system. *International Journal of Intelligent Unmanned Systems* (ahead-of-print). 10.1108/IJIUS-02-2022-0019

41. Riley, A., & Nica, E. (2021). Internet of Things-based smart healthcare systems and wireless biomedical sensing devices in monitoring, detection, and prevention of COVID-19. *American Journal of Medical Research*, 8(2), pp.51–64.

42. Shanmugaraja, P., Bhardwaj, M., Mehbodniya, A., Vali, S., & Reddy, P. C. S. (2023). An efficient clustered M-path sinkhole attack detection (MSAD) algorithm for wireless sensor networks. *Adhoc & Sensor Wireless Networks*, 55, pp.1–21.

43. Sharma, M. K., & Kumar, A. (2022). NOMA waveform technique using orthogonal supplementary signal for advanced 5G networks security. *Journal of Discrete Mathematical Sciences and Cryptography*, 25, pp.1125–1136. 10.1080/09720529. 2022.2075088.

44. Kumar, A. et al. (2022). Intelligent conventional and proposed hybrid 5G detection techniques. *Alexandria Engineering Journal*, 61(12), pp.10485–10494.

45. Sharma, N., & Shambharkar, P. G. (2022, January). Applicability of ML-IoT in smart healthcare systems: Challenges, solutions & future direction. In *2022 International Conference on Computer Communication and Informatics (ICCCI)* (pp.1–7). IEEE.

46. Karunarathne, S. M., Saxena, N., & Khan, M. K. (2021). Security and privacy in IoT smart healthcare. *IEEE Internet Computing*, 25(4), pp.37–48.

47. Talaat, F. M. (2022). Effective prediction and resource allocation method (EPRAM) in fog computing environment for smart healthcare system. *Multimedia Tools and Applications*, 81(6), pp.8235–8258.

Index

For Product Safety Concerns and Information please contact our EU
representative GPSR@taylorandfrancis.com
Taylor & Francis Verlag GmbH, Kaufingerstraße 24, 80331 München, Germany

www.ingramcontent.com/pod-product-compliance
Lightning Source LLC
Chambersburg PA
CBHW060352220326
41598CB00023B/2897

* 9 7 8 1 0 3 2 5 1 7 2 7 8 *